AF758009

CANCER ETIOLOGY, DIAGNOSIS AND TREATMENTS

HYBRID NANOSTRUCTURES IN CANCER THERAPY

Cancer Etiology, Diagnosis and Treatments

Additional books in this series can be found on Nova's website under the Series tab.

Additional e-books in this series can be found on Nova's website under the e-book tab.

Nanotechnology Science and Technology

Additional books in this series can be found on Nova's website under the Series tab.

Additional e-books in this series can be found on Nova's website under the e-book tab.

CANCER ETIOLOGY, DIAGNOSIS AND TREATMENTS

HYBRID NANOSTRUCTURES IN CANCER THERAPY

MOHSEN ADELI
EDITOR

Nova Science Publishers, Inc.
New York

Copyright © 2012 by Nova Science Publishers, Inc.

All rights reserved. No part of this book may be reproduced, stored in a retrieval system or transmitted in any form or by any means: electronic, electrostatic, magnetic, tape, mechanical photocopying, recording or otherwise without the written permission of the Publisher.

For permission to use material from this book please contact us:
Telephone 631-231-7269; Fax 631-231-8175
Web Site: http://www.novapublishers.com

NOTICE TO THE READER

The Publisher has taken reasonable care in the preparation of this book, but makes no expressed or implied warranty of any kind and assumes no responsibility for any errors or omissions. No liability is assumed for incidental or consequential damages in connection with or arising out of information contained in this book. The Publisher shall not be liable for any special, consequential, or exemplary damages resulting, in whole or in part, from the readers' use of, or reliance upon, this material. Any parts of this book based on government reports are so indicated and copyright is claimed for those parts to the extent applicable to compilations of such works.

Independent verification should be sought for any data, advice or recommendations contained in this book. In addition, no responsibility is assumed by the publisher for any injury and/or damage to persons or property arising from any methods, products, instructions, ideas or otherwise contained in this publication.

This publication is designed to provide accurate and authoritative information with regard to the subject matter covered herein. It is sold with the clear understanding that the Publisher is not engaged in rendering legal or any other professional services. If legal or any other expert assistance is required, the services of a competent person should be sought. FROM A DECLARATION OF PARTICIPANTS JOINTLY ADOPTED BY A COMMITTEE OF THE AMERICAN BAR ASSOCIATION AND A COMMITTEE OF PUBLISHERS.
Additional color graphics may be available in the e-book version of this book.

Library of Congress Cataloging-in-Publication Data

Hybrid nanostructures in cancer therapy / editor, Mohsen Adeli.
p. ; cm.
Includes bibliographical references and index.
ISBN 978-1-62100-517-9 (hardcover)
I. Adeli, Mohsen.
[DNLM: 1. Neoplasms--drug therapy. 2. Drug Delivery Systems--methods. 3. Nanostructures--therapeutic use. QZ 267]
LC classification not assigned
616.99'4061--dc23

2011035485

Published by Nova Science Publishers, Inc. † New York

Contents

Preface

Based on the World Cancer Report from the World Health Organization, one of the top three killers in the modern societies has been cancer in 2008, so that 7.6 million deaths from the disease has been estimated in this year. This organization estimates 12 million cancer deaths worldwide in 2030.

Tissues having abnormal cellular and subcellular systems, tumors, are known with active angiogenesis and higher vascular density than normal organs. Due to these characterizes, blood circulates inside them for a longer time in comparison with that for normal tissues which leads to deliver supply more efficiently.

Defective vascular architecture for tumors in combination with poor lymphatic drainage causes a property for tumors which is known as the enhanced permeation and retention (EPR) effect. On the other hand in the subcellular case, the development of tumor genes is different with the normal tissues and often shows genovariation. Therefore the inherent complexity of tumor in the both cellular and subcelluar scales and the existence of biomacromolecules such as P-glycoprotein (Pgp), usually act as barriers to traditional chemotherapy by preventing drug from reaching the target sites, tumor mass. In a successful chemotherapy, therapeutic agents should pass variety of biological barriers including hepatic and renal clearance, enzymolysis and hydrolysis, as well as cell membrane and endosomal/lysosomal degradation. In addition, in the case of anticancer drugs their efficiency could be also limited because of their undesirable properties, such as poor solubility, low chemical and physical stability and their high toxicity for normal tissues and cells.

Nanotechnology has emerged as a key technology which has opened new opportunities to revolutionalize the field of drug delivery, medical diagnostics, biosensors and tissue engineering in the near future. Using nanomaterials as cargos, it has been possible to improve the biodistribution and prolonged blood circulation times of therapeutics, which have significantly improved their pharmaceutical efficacy and dosing of clinically approved ones. They are particularly promising candidates for early diagnosis of cancer cells. Several classes of nanomaterials, including dendritic and supramolecular polymers, carbon nanotubes, graphene and metal nanoparticles, have shown tremendous ability to recognize and destroy cancer cells *in vivo*. In this book, some of these novel systems and their potential applications in cancer therapy are reviewed.

Introduction

In spite of the flourishing developments in a wide variety of life-associated technologies in the recent years, efforts for treatment of cancers have not been effective to manage the patient's diseases optimally with the current therapies. While the new technologies provide the new opportunities and more comfortable life for human, they or their products always introduce into the biological systems and affect their normal cycles in different manners. Unfortunately in some cases these effects are not predictable and lead to developed diseases or apparent new ones. This is why in the modern societies diversity and number of people who are buckled with cancers are more than others. Nanotechnology has emerged a key technology which has opened new vistas to find effective therapies for cancer. In nanotechnology particularly nanomaterials are promising candidates for early diagnosis for cancer cells. Several classes of nanomaterials including dendritic and supramolecular polymers, carbon nanotubes, graphene and metal nanoparticles have shown tremendous ability to recognize and destroyed cancer cells *in vivo*. However hybrid nanomaterials in which several types of these nanomaterials are associated together through different interactions are new systems with a wide collection of useful properties that could be useful for early cancer diagnosis or therapy. They are multivalent nanomaterials with a high ability to perform several useful functions in the same time. In this book some of these novel systems and their potential applications in cancer therapy are reviewed.

The first chapter of this book deals with the short introduction for some of hybrid nanomaterials, their properties and potential applications in nanomedicine. In this chapter advantages of nanomaterials and their hybrid structures over the bulk materials for particular applications in nanomedicine complied.

Since structure, conformation and functions of bioactive moieties such as proteins, antibodies and DNA are regulated by non-covalent interactions; supramolecular polymers in which these types of interactions dominate their physicochemical properties can be used for biomedical applications ranging from tissue engineering to drug delivery systems. Therefore the second chapter of this book explains supramolecular polymers including cyclodextrins building blocks in which polymers are attached to cyclodextrin rings by either covalent links or noncovalent interactions. The biomedical applications of these types of supramolecules are also discussed.

Dendrimers are forth generation of polymers that characterized by their extensively branched three dimensional structures which provide a high degree of surface functionality and versatility. The unique properties associated with dendrimers such as well-known structure, monodispersed size and molecular weight, high functionality, water solubility, multivalency and available internal cavities makes them attractive to use in nanomedicine. Structural properties of dendrimers and their behaviors in the biological systems are reviewed in the third chapter. Different biomedical applications of these macromolecules, their ability to target drugs to tumors by encapsulation or conjugation methods, their potential application in imaging and also their toxicity is discussed in this chapter.

Chapters four and five are focused on the biomedical applications of carbon nanotubes. In these chapters through efforts has been made to discuss the modification of carbon nanotubes by polymers to solublize them in aqueous media has been fully discussed. Based on interactions between polymers and carbon nanotubes this topic is further divided into two parts. In the first part which is also the title of the chapter four, modification of carbon nanotubes by polymers through covalent linkages and potential applications of the resulted hybrid nanometerials as anticancer drug delivery systems are reviewed. In subsequently second part which is more focused on the surface modification of carbon nanotubes. This part deals with non-covalent inateractions of carbon nanotubes –hybrid nanomaterials. Toxicity and uptake of these types of hybrid nanomaterials is also reported briefly. Reading these two chapters it can be found that modified carbon nanotubes are promising candidates to use as novel tolls in nanomedicine and probably come to clinical phases in future.

Due to their size-dependent electrical and optical properties, high stability in biological mediums, easy surface modification and functionalization and their small sizes metal nanoparticles have received considerable attention during the past decade to use in nanomedicine. Therefore three last chapters of this book are devoted to quantum dots, gold and titanium dioxide nanoparticles and their biomedical applications. The synthesis and properties of quantum dot- and gold nanoparticle-polymer hybrid nanomaterials are discussed in chapters 6 and 7 respectively. Promises and challenges for biomedical applications of quantum dots-polymer hybrid nanomaterials and also their toxicity are reviewed in chapter 6. Different biomedical applications of gold nanoparticle-polymer hybrid nanomaterials as promising and highly biocompatible systems including drug delivery, gene delivery, photothermal therapy, photodynamic therapy and molecular imaging are discussed in chapter 7. Lately in the eight chapter application of titanium dioxide nanoparticles for the photocatalytic destruction of biological species and also their potential applications in cancer therapy has been evaluated. In further the mechanism of destruction of biological active species and cancer cells by these nanoparticles is reviewed. Conjugation of biomolecules onto the surface of TiO_2 nanoparticles to improve their biological properties is also comprehensively explained.

Mohsen Adeli
Tehran, 2011

In: Hybrid Nanostructures in Cancer Therapy
Editor: Mohsen Adeli
ISBN: 978-1-62100-517-9
© 2012 Nova Science Publishers, Inc.

Chapter I

Hybrid Nanostructures; Promising Drug Delivery Systems

Mohsen Adeli[1,2]
[1]Department of chemistry, Faculty of Science, Lorestan University, Khoramabad, Iran
[2]Department of chemistry, Sharif University of Technology, Tehran, Iran

1. Introduction

There have been innumerable promises brought in with the emergence of nanomaterials in recent years. This is illustrated in Figure 1, which is based on a search carried out on the "ACS" and "ScienceDirect" bibliographic portal. Over the period from 2000 to 2010, the number of research papers, published by above publishers, dedicated to application of nanomaterials in medicine increased from about 54 per year to almost 800 with a marked acceleration since the year 2005.

Use of nanomaterials and nanostructures for biomedical purposes constitutes a new field called "nanomedicine". Nanomedicine involves a multi-step process from the design, synthesis, in vitro experiments and initial administration to cross the tissue endothelium barrier and introduction into the interstitial space of tissues, through the cell membrane into organelles of cells and even through the perinuclear membrane into the nucleus of cells (Figure 2).

Nanomaterials should be biocompatible and be able to pass different barriers after administration before reaching their target or being eliminated from the blood stream. Each one of the steps described in Figure 2 can have a key role in the *in vivo* fate of any nanosystem administered as a carrier agent. Novel nanomaterials used in nanomedicine have to be biocompatible and go through these barriers in the in vivo and preclinical stages. In the designing and synthesis steps of any system based on nanomaterials, all barriers mentioned in Figure 2 should be taken into account. In the other words, designing and synthesis steps are the basis for nanomedicine and they have a critical role in this case and any system that ignore any *in vivo* barrier in the design and synthesis steps will find it difficult to succeed in application.

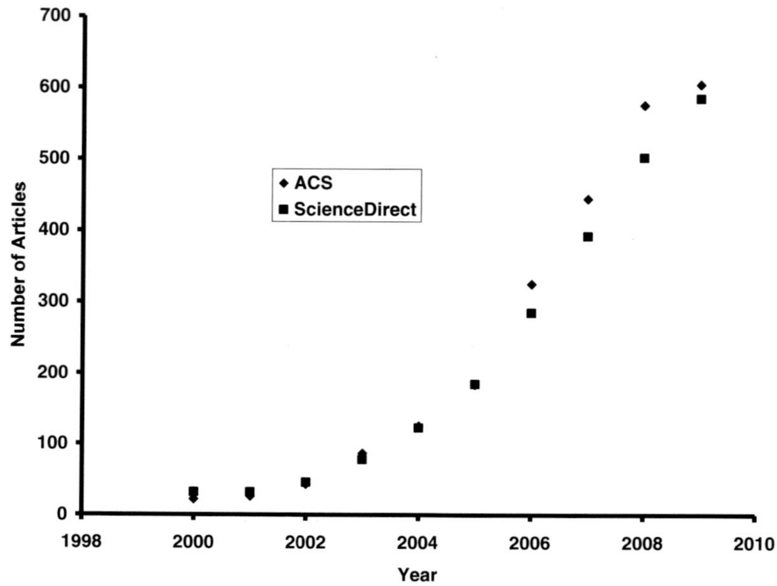

Figure 1. The number of research papers dedicated to "nanomedicine" by searching the "ACS" and "ScienceDirect" publishers.

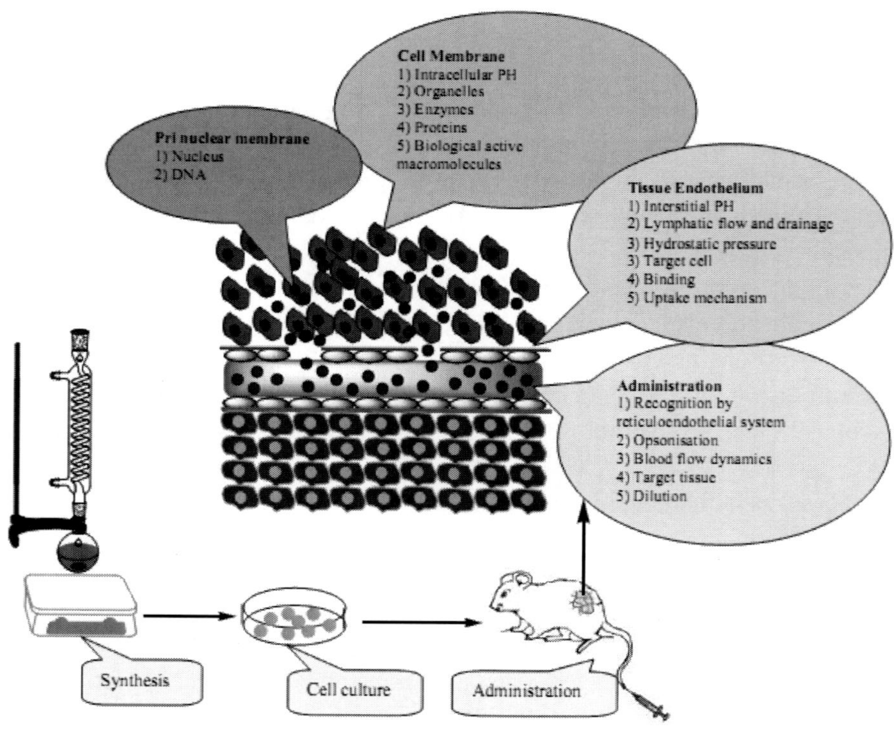

Figure 2. Nanomedicine from synthesis to *in vivo* barriers.

Development of nanostructures in which all above steps are taken into account and are containing a biocompatible backbone, marker, antibody and therapeutic agent for molecular imaging and targeted therapy is an area of high current interest [1–6].

The basic rationale is that nanostructures have functional and structural properties that are not available from either molecule or in bulk scales. For example due to their small size, nanostructures can cross different barriers in body. When conjugated with functional bioactive ligands, such as antibodies, they can be used to target malignant tumors with high specificity [7–10].

2. Cancer

The word "cancer come from the Latin word for crab. An ancient physician from Greece recognized the resemblance of the swollen mass of blood vessels around a malignant tumor to the shape of a crab and so named the disease. Cancer is one of the top three ''killers'' in modern society, which include cardiovascular diseases.

In human it is consist of more than two hundred different disease in which cells divide at an exponential growth rate in an uncontrolled process [11]. This abnormal growth rate of cells leads to the formation of a swollen mass, called malignant tumor.

The tumor tissue grows and invades the adjacent tissues, obstructing normal physiological functions. In some cases, the cancerous cells can separate from its origin place and migrate through circulation to other parts of the body, forming a new tumor site. This is known as cancer metastasis.

Over a period of time, malignant tumors cause not working of various tissues, which turns fatal. According to American Cancer Society's annual report [12], more than 570,000 people are estimated to die of various cancers in the year 2005 in the USA.

Cancer can develop in any living organ or tissue in the body. The most cancer developing sites include the skin, lungs, female breasts, prostate, colon and rectum and corpus uteri. Unfortunately the current treatment options are not effective, in most cases, and cancer patients are not satisfied with them.

3. Nanomedicine in Oncology

In the case of cancer therapy, the goal of nanomedicine is to develop safer and more effective delivery systems for therapeutic and diagnostic agents using nanomaterials and nanostructures.

Oncology benefits nanomedicine in two fashions. i) Early diagnosis of cancer cells, ii) Targeting of anticancer therapeutics to the cancer cells.

The most important attribute to delivery systems based on nanomaterials and nanostructures is their potential to enhance the targeting anticancer drugs to tumors and their accumulation in tumor cells than in healthy tissues by "passive" or "active" delivery or targeting (Figure 3) [13 and 14].

"Passive" or "Active" Delivery or Targeting

Although an effective cancer therapy is still not achieved in the recent years, delivery systems bases on novel nanomaterials have developed rapidly with some exciting results [1-3]. Most of these achievements are due to the abnormal pathophysiology of tumor vasculature because in contrast to normal tissue, tumors are containing a high density of abnormal blood vessels that are dilated and poorly differentiated, with a chaotic architecture and aberrant branching [4, 5]. This especial pathophysiology of tumor vasculature in one hand and lake of functional lymphatic vessels in tumor in the other hand has caused an enhanced permeability and retention effect in tumor tissue which results in an increased accumulation of macromolecules in tumors (Figure 3) [6-8]. This is the first and one of the most important reasons to use nanomaterials in tumor or cancer therapy, because they passively accumulate in solid tumors after their intravenous administration.

However the accumulation of anticancer agents in tumor cells based on pathophysiology of the tumor vasculature which is called "passive drug delivery or targeting" is not an effective way to destroy tumor cells and cancer therapy and it is containing a lot of non-specific interactions between anticancer agents and biological active molecules. Several approaches to overcome the disadvantages of passive targeting have been purposed.

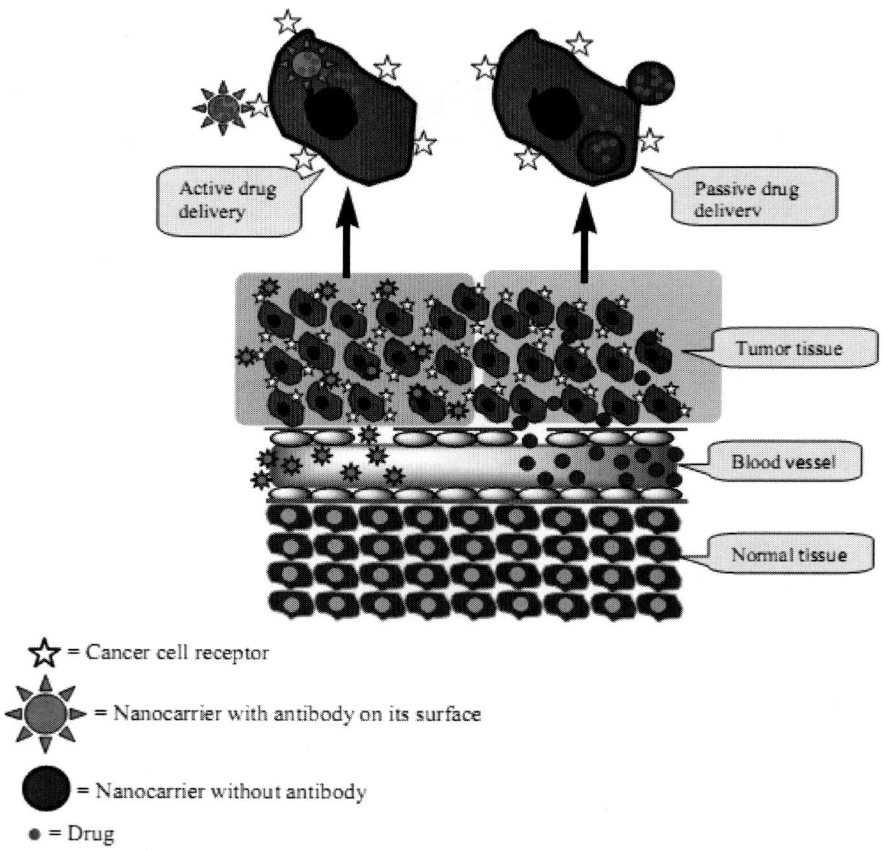

Figure 3. Schematic diagram showing the passive and active drug delivery systems for tumor therapy.

The most commonly used method is antibody- or ligand-mediated targeting of anticancer therapeutics which is called "active targeting". The basic principle that underlies active targeting is that the selective delivery of anticancer drugs to cancer cells can be enhanced by specific interactions between anticancer drugs and cancer cells through conjugating the drugs with molecules that bind to receptors that are either uniquely expressed or overexpressed on cancer cells compared with normal cells (Figure 3) [9-10 and 12-15].

4. Nanoparticles and Nanostructures in Oncology

To be an effective and perfect delivery system, nanostructures should have several characteristics.

I. High functionality to conjugate multiple diagnostic and therapeutic agents on their surface and to have effective interaction with target cells.
II. Biocompatibility and water solubility
III. Inertness against biological active molecules
IV. No *immunogenicity effect*
V. Stability in biological systems
VI. Ability to cross different barriers, especially cell and perinuclear membrane, in body
VII. Release diagnostic and therapeutic agents in destination organelles
VIII. Break down to biocompatible materials in destination organelle and …

There are several classes of nanomaterials which promise to be particularly capable agents in the detection, diagnosis, and treatment of cancer (Figure 4).

i) Dendritic polymers, ii) Carbon nanotubes, iii) Quantum dots and iv) Supramolecules

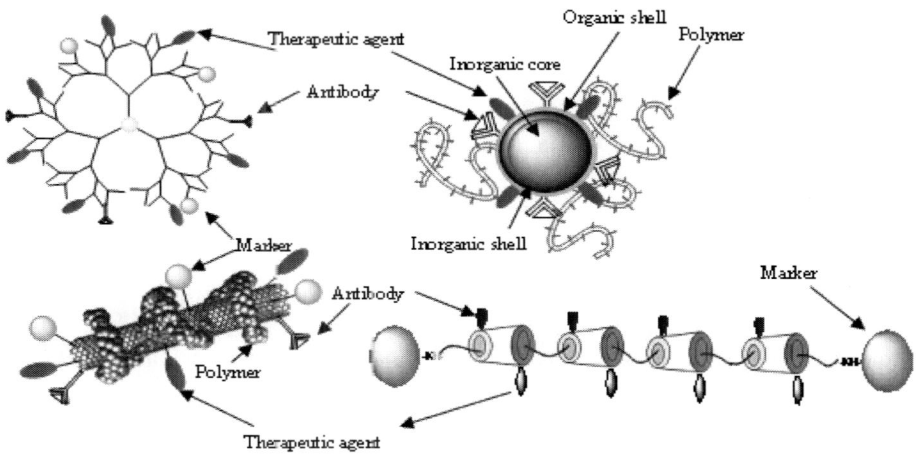

Figure 4. Schematic representations of a) dendrimer b) carbon nanotube c) nanoparticle or quantum dot and d) supramolecules based delivery systems.

Most promising and well studied therapeutic agents that has been transported by dendrimers, carbon nanotubes, quantum dots and supramolecules based delivery systems are methotrexate, adriamycin (doxorubicin), paclitaxel, cisplatin and 5-fluorouracil (Figure 5). Variety of these nanosystems ranging from primary stages to the different clinical trials is reported in past decade [16].

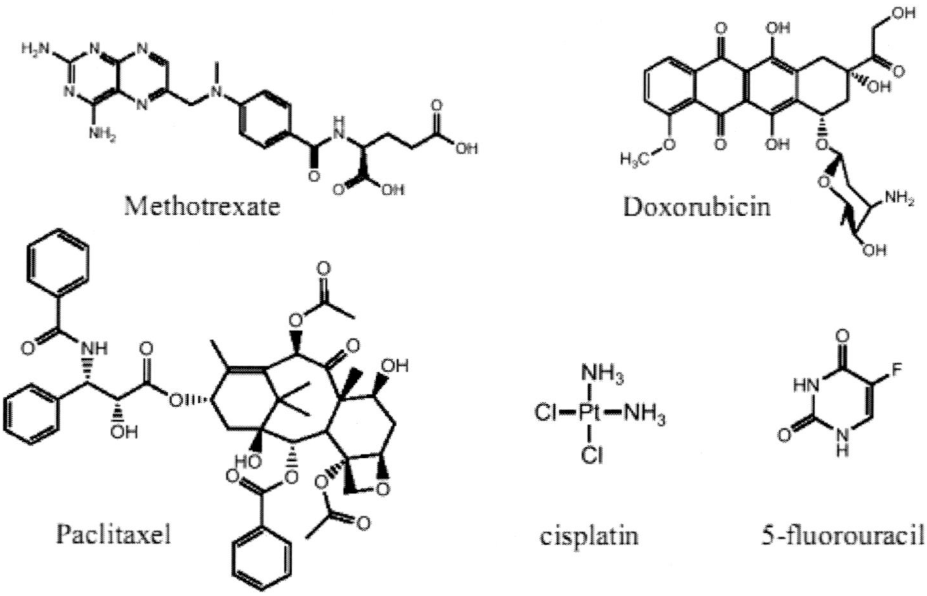

Figure 5. Most studied therapeutic agents transported by dendrimers, carbon nanotubes, quantum dots and supramolecules based delivery systems.

4.1. Dendritic Polymers

Dendritic polymers are nano-size and high functional macromolecules consisting of tree-like arms or branches. They are highly branched and monodisperse three-dimensional macro-molecules with definite molecular weights and encapsulation properties [17]. Dendrimers are synthesized from polyfunctional monomers in a step-wise manner containing protecting-deprotecting reactions or some similar reactions. This strategy causes a possibility to precisely control the properties of dendrimers such as size, functionality, shape, dimension, density, polarity, flexibility, and solubility in the molecular level by choosing different building/branching units and surface functional groups [18]. In general, dendrimers often possess empty internal cavities with defined dimensions and can encapsulate hydrophobic drug molecules that can math their cavities [19]. In addition, they have a large number of surface functional groups in compare to conventional macromolecules that causes an ability to conjugate a large number of drugs to their surface functional groups and enhancing the solubility, biocompatibility and affectivity of the conjugated drugs [20-23]. In addition to drugs, variety of other small molecules such as antibody and markers can be conjugated to the surface functional groups of dendrimer's outer shell to obtain multifunctional drug delivery systems [24, 25]. However, basic scientific advances and perfect synthetic routes for prep aration of varieties of dendrimers with desirable properties, coupled with a high knowledge to conjugate a wide range of biological active molecules to their surface or encapsulate them as guest molecules within their cavities, provide a highly versatile and potentially extremely powerful strategy for drug delivery based on dendritic polymers [26-31]. Recent advances in dendrimer chemistry show that they can be covalently linked with defined numbers of targeting ligands, imaging dyes, and drugs, thus providing a platform for the specific targeting, imaging, and treatment of cancer [32-41]. Different types of dendrimers are commercially available now that among them different generations of polyamidoamine (PAMAM), polypropyleneimine (PPI), biomolecules derived dendrimers such as amino acid dendrimers, carbohydrate-modified dendrimers, nucleic acids-nucleobases dendrimers, and polyester dendrimers are the most extensively studied for biological applications and especially in cancer therapy (Figure 6) [42-44]. They have a three-dimensional architecture with primary amine groups on their surface which are available for the conjugation of different types of biological active molecules, drugs or markers [45]. Their behavior in aqueous solutions and also their biocompatibility as cargo for drugs, ligands and markers has been well studied [46-49]. Some of the issues associated with immunoconjugates, such as decreased solubility and reduced binding efficiency, can be addressed using dendritic polymers as transporter molecules attached to antibodies. Different research groups have studied the conjugation of antibodies to dendrimers for targeting the drugs and biologically active molecules [50-53].

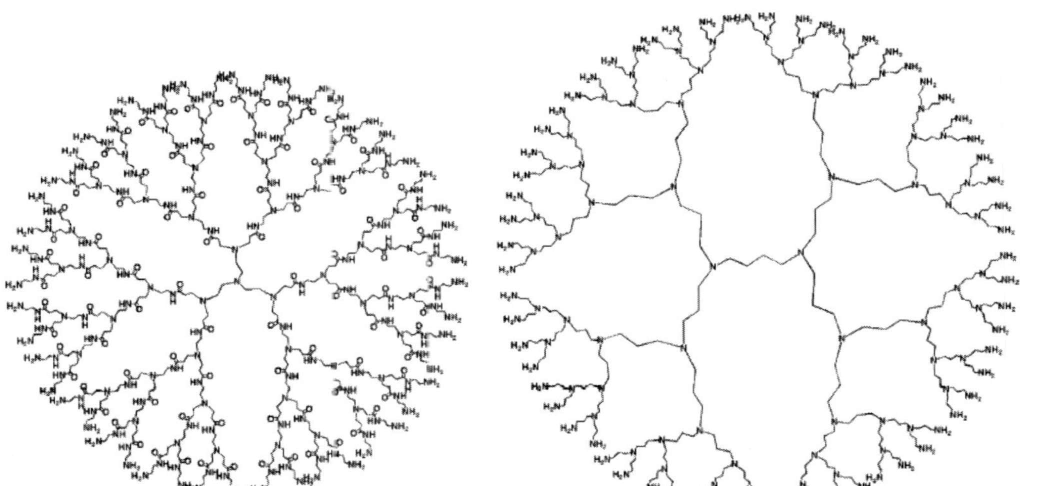

Figure 6. Structure of Commercially available G5 PAMAM (1)and G4 PPI (2)dendrimers.

In some cases anticancer drugs or biologically active molecules are conjugated to the functional groups of dendrimers by linkages sensitive to the external factors through which drugs or biological active molecules released in the tumor sites [54].

It is important to develop a method to specifically deliver an apoptosis-sensing device simultaneously into the desired cells along with a cytotoxic drug to monitor the real-time apoptotic effects of the drug. High functionality of dendrimers give a possibility to synthesize bifunctional dendrimer nanodevice in which targeting agent and apoptosis-detecting reagent are conjugated to dendrimers to monitor the in vitro apoptosis of the cell [55].

Table 1. list of some of drug delivery systems synthesized through conjugation of drugs to dendrimers used in cancer therapy

Dendrimer	Drug	Antibody	Marker	Reference
PAMAM	Doxorubicin	-	-	56 and 54
PAMAM	Cis-platin (CDDP)			57 and 58
PAMAM	-	Folic acid (FA)	Fluorescein isothiocyanate (FITC)	60 and 61
PAMAM	Paclitaxel	FA	FITC	44
PAMAM	Methotrexate	FA	FITC	33
PAMAM	phthalocyanine (DPc)	-	-	59
dendritic polymers having cyclic cores of 1,4,7,10-tetraazacyclododecane	5-Flurouracil	-	-	62
PAMAM	-	Biotin	FITC	38
PAMAM	-	J591 anti-PSMA (prostate specific membrane antigen)	FITC	53b
PAMAM	glycosides	-	-	62c
Glycopeptide dendrimer	colchicine	β-galactoside	fluorescein conjugates	62d

Table 2. list of some of drug delivery systems prepared through noncovalent interactions between drugs and dendrimers used in cancer therapy

Dendrimer	Drug	Antibody	Marker	Reference
hydroxy-terminated dendrimers	Doxorubicin	-	-	62f
PAMAM	5-fluorouracil (5-FU)	micro-RNA 21 (as-miR-21)	-	61b
Typical	Guanosine monophosphate	-	-	61c
Polyester dendrimer	Camptothecins	-	-	61d
PAMAM	Doxorubicin	-	-	61e

4.2. Linear-Dendritic Copolymers

In recent years, combining the advantages of polymers and dendrimers, several groups have prepared hybrid linear– dendritic copolymers. Linear–dendritic copolymers are hybrid structures that combine two types (linear and dendritic) of macromolecular architectures. In a linear–dendritic copolymer, each moiety can have a deep effect on the properties of the other, and they form a macromolecule with modified and advanced properties. For example, the presence of a dendritic portion in a hybrid linear– dendritic copolymer reduces its viscosity, whereas the presence of a linear polymer in a hybrid linear–dendritic copolymer increases its flexibility. In the past several years, a significant number of reports on the preparation of such hybrid copolymers have appeared in the literature [63 and 64].

In general, four types of amphiphilic linear-dendritic copolymers containing PEG have been reported in the literature:

AB linear-dendritic diblock copolymers containing B as the dendritic block and A as the linear block [63b], ABA triblock linear-dendritic copolymers containing B as the linear block and A as the dendritic blocks [65], linear-dendritic star copolymers in which the dendritic blocks are connected to the end of arms of a star polymer [66], and multiarm linear-dendritic block copolymers with a dendrimer core and linear PEG arms [67]. Linear-dendritic copolymers are able to transport drugs either by conjugation methods or non-covalent interactions [68a, b]. Linear-dendritic block copolymers comprising diblock copoly (oxyalkylene) chains to the surfaces of full generation PAMAM dendrimers have been synthesized and their solubilization capacities for poorly water soluble drugs has been investigated [68c]. Molecular self-assemblies and thermoresponsive systems of linear-dendritic copolymers are also used to deliver and controlled release of drugs [68d, e].

4.3. Carbon Nanotubes

Although the molecular and cellular mechanisms for the cytotoxicity of carbon nanotubes (CNTs) are not yet fully understand and their biocompatibility still remain under question [69], in recent years carbon nanotubes (CNTs) have also been used as multipurpose innovative carriers for delivery of drugs and bioactive molecules into the cells because of their unique property: the ability to cross cell membranes [70].

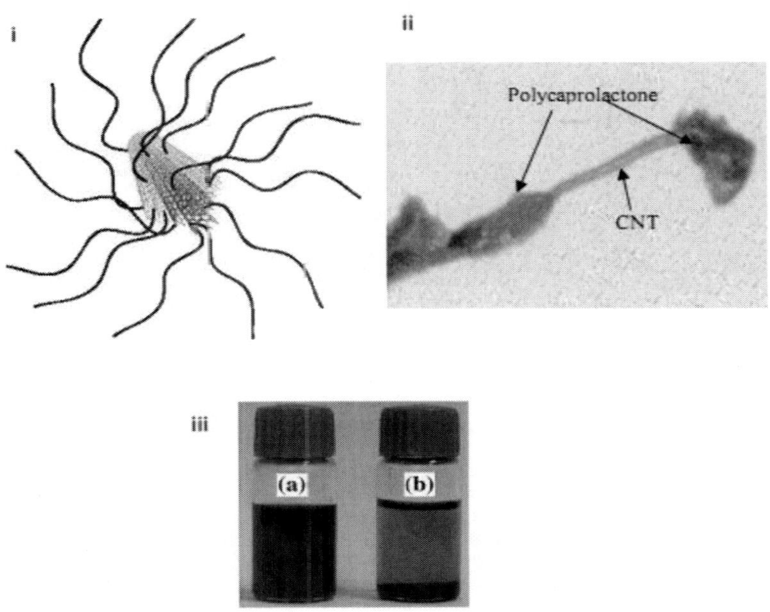

Figure 7. (i) CNT-*graft*-polymers, (ii) TEM image of a MWCNT containing polycaprolactone conjugated to its surface, (iii) Chloroform solution of (a) CNT-graft-PLA-block-PCL and (b) pristine CNT.

However a disadvantage that limits application of CNTs in nanomedicine is their low solubility and processability. Chemical modification and functionalization of carbon nanotubes is a widely used strategy in order to increase their dispersion and solubilization which have evolved into a rather broad research field [71]. Depend on the polymer; modified CNTs can be soluble in aqueous or organic solvents. For example conjugation of polylactide or polycaprolactone onto the surface of carbon nanotubes leads to modified CNTs solublize in organic solvents such as chloroform [71] (Figure 7).

Polymers or bioactive molecules can be fixed on CNTs through covalent or non-covalent methods. Due to their high surface area, in both methods, all requierd objects for an effective cancer therapy including polymers, drugs, antibodies and markers can be transported by CNTs simultaneously. For Example high loading capacity for π-stacking of anticancer drugs and fluorescence molecules with an aromatic structure on water soluble CNTs functionalized by poly(ethylene glycol) (PEG) via non-covalent and covalent methods has been achieved (Figure 8) [72].

Variety of drugs, biological species, proteins, plasmid DNA and markers are trasported by carbon nanotubes in order to internalize to the special cells with no obvious toxicities *in vivo* [73-75]. The release of drugs from drug delivery systems based on CNTs can be controlled by changing the pH. A polysaccharide [sodium alginate (ALG) and chitosan (CHI)] modified SWCNTs for controlled release of DOX, also including folic acid (FA) as a targeting (DOX-FA-CHI/ALG-SWCNTs) group has been rported recently [75a]. These drug delivery systems were found, using transmission electronic microscopy and fluorescence microscopy, to enter cells through the intearction of folic acid with its receptors on the surface of cells, and following internalization the DOX was selectively released into the acidic environment of the lysosomes.

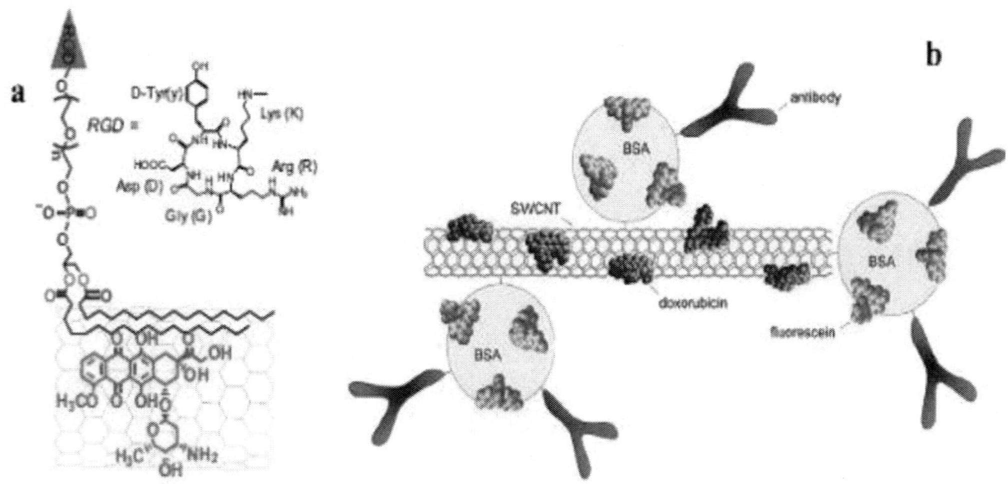

Figure 8. (a) Schematic structure of SWNTs functionalized with cyclic arginine-glycine-aspartic acid at the termini of PEG and loaded with doxorubicin on the sidewall by π-stacking. (b) Schematic illustration of the doxorubicin–fluorescein–BSA–antibody-SWCNT complexes (red = doxorubicin, green = fluorescein, light blue = BSA, dark blue = antibodies). Reprinted with the permission of Ref [72].

The drug delivery system containing SWNTs, sodium alginate, chitosan and DOX together with and without folic acid (DOX-FA-CHI/ALG-SWCNTs and DOX-CHI/ALG-SWCNTs) and also free DOX (used as a control) were incubated with human cervical carcinoma HeLa cells and evaluated using fluorescence microscopy allowing the DOX to be located as it emits red fluorescence under irradiation with green light. Higher intensity for cells incubated with DOX-FA-CHI/ALG-SWCNTs systems compared with other samples proved that the internalization of this system into the HeLa cells is mediated by folic acid. Evaluation the fluorescence microscopy images of these systems indicated that the fluorescence is concentrated in the cytoplasm and suggesting that the nanotubes cannot cross intracellular membranes which is in agree with the reported results [21,22].

Blood circulation half-lives of the order of hours and efficient renal clearance make modified carbon nanotubes suitable as nanovectors for drug delivery purposes [76].

CNTs are able to absorb near-infrared (NIR) radiation (700–1100 nm) and convert it into heat. This property of CNTs opens a new way to make new nanostructures useful for cancer photo-therapy [77] because NIR light can easily and safely penetrate normal tissue or tumors and kill any cell containing them. This property of nanostructures such as gold nanoparticles, gold nanorods and CNTs for thermally killing the cancer cells is being explored and investigates during few years ago [78]. On the other hand this optic-thermal property of CNTs can enhance the permeability of tumor vasculature compared to normal vasculature; therefore it can be used to target the drugs to the cancer cells [79].

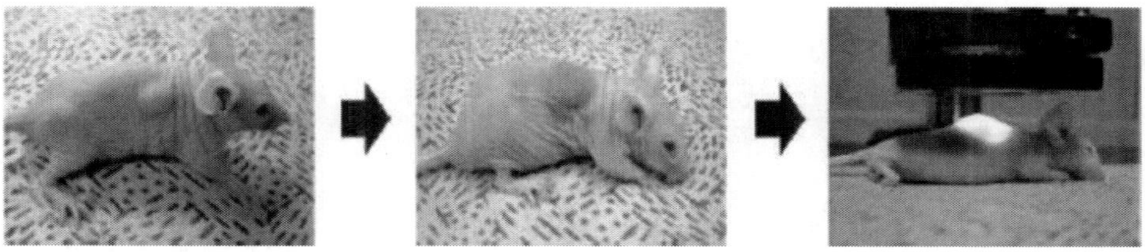

Figure 9. Photothermal treatments for *in vivo* tumor ablation using PEG-SWNTs: (a) photograph of a mouse bearing KB tumor cells (~70mm^3); (b) photograph of a mouse after intratumoral injection of PEG-SWNTs solution (~120 mg/L, 100 μL); (c) photograph of near-infrared irradiation (808 nm, 76 W/cm^3) for 3 min to tumor region. Reprinted with the permission of Ref [77].

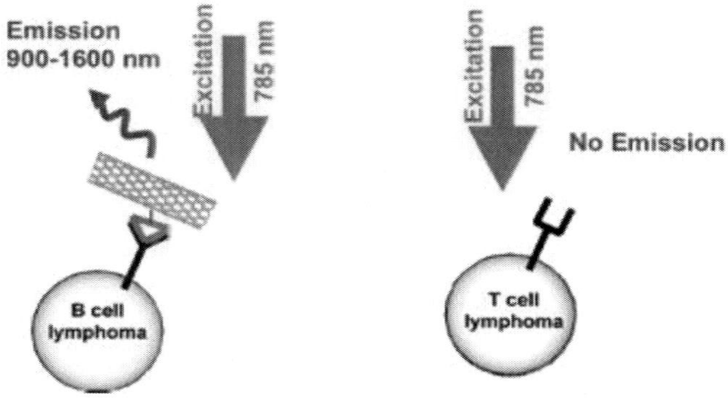

Figure 10. Schematic of NIR photoluminescence (PL) detection of SWNT-Rituxan conjugate selectively bound to CD20 cell surface receptors on B-cell lymphoma (left). The conjugate is not recognized by T-cell lymphoma (right). Reprinted with the permission of ref [80].

A promising application of CNTs is to use them as the near-infrared (NIR, wavelength ~0.8-2 μm) fluorescent tags for selective probing of cell surface receptors and cell imaging, where the fluorescent molecules are relatively rare and have been vigorously required for biological applications because cells and tissues exhibit little auto-fluorescence in this region [80]. A semiconducting SWNTs modified with polyethyleneglycol is conjugated to antibodies such as Rituxan to selectively recognize CD20 cell surface receptor on B-cells to recognize HER2/neu positive breast cancer cells through the intrinsic NIR photoluminescence of nanotubes (Figure 10).

Gene delivery and transfection is an important research filed that continue to draw strong interest because of their potential application for gene therapy and disease prevention [81]. Due to their ability to cross the cell membrane and their strong interactions with DNA and RNA, CNTs can be used as possible transfection vectors [82]. Recently the interaction between CNTs and DNA and the structure of CNT-DNA hybrids has been investigated and determined with a high acuracy. STM provided the direct observation of DNA wrapping around a single CNT with a coiling period of 3.3 nm. The molecular dynamics (MD) simulations confirmed the exprimental results and were in agree with the STM observations so that they result in a DNA coiling geometry, and yield a period of 3.2 nm for (6,5) CNT [83].

As it can be found the combination of CNT's high loading and transport capacity and thermal and optical properties along with chemical functionalization with polymers and DNA promises a broad range of applications in medicine, drug delivery and cancer therapy [84, 85].

4.4. Quantum Dots

Another class of nanomaterials which has been greatly interested for biomedical applications is quantum dots (QDs). Optical and physical properties of QDs extremely depend on their structures and have attracted immense interest in developing them to use in nanomedicine [86, 87]. The general structure of QDs used for imaging tumors or targeting the drugs to cancer cells is combined from an inorganic core, an inorganic shell and an organic shell to which biomolecules, modifier macromolecules, antibodies and therapeutic agents are conjugated (Figure 1c).

One of the most important profits of QDs in nanomedicine over current techniques is their ability to track cells in vivo easily and without needs to sacrificing animals [88]. Recently variety of QDs have been used to early imaging of the cancer cells, study the internalization of therapeutic agents into cancer cells and even compartments of the cancer cells [89].

A promising application for functionalized QDs is multiplexed molecular profiling of biomarkers of different cancer cells, because diagnostic and prognostic classifications of human tumors are currently based on immunohistochemistry (IHC), a technique that has been used in clinical medicine for a long time, which is a single-color technique and is unable to perform multiplexed molecular profiling. For example expression of biomarkers and receptors on different cancer cells by antibody-conjugated quantum dots with different colors has been studied (Figure 11) [90].

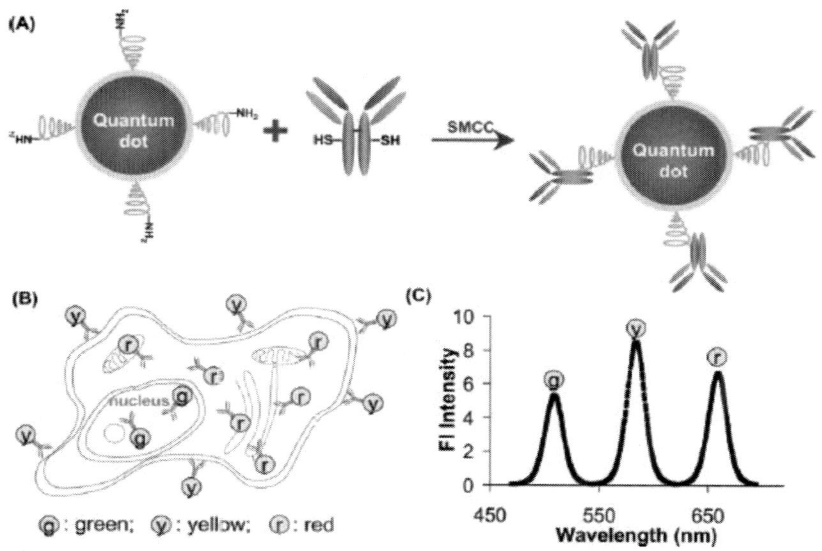

Figure 11. Schematic illustration of bioconjugated QDs for multiplexed in situ molecular profiling. (A) Multicolor QD bioconjugates prepared with functionalized QDs and chemically reduced antibodies. (B) Cell staining using multicolor QD-bioconjugates. (C) Quantification of tumor biomarker expression using wavelength-resolved spectroscopy. Reprinted with the permission of Ref [90].

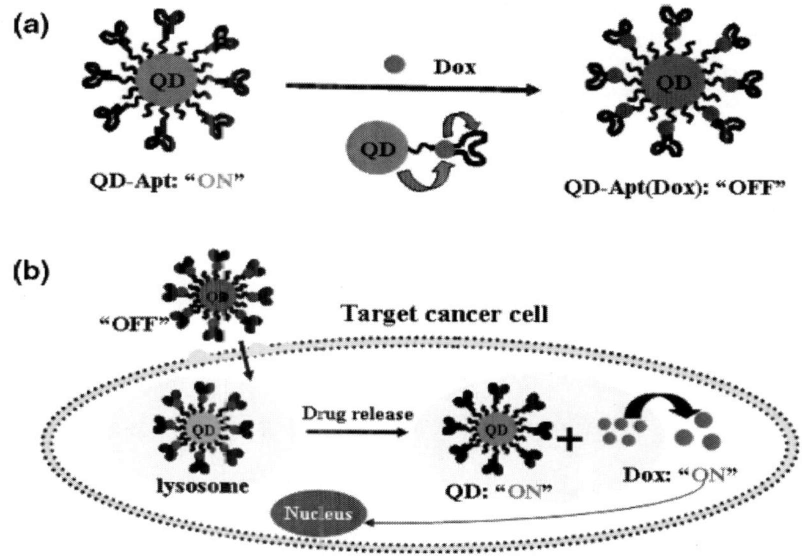

Figure 12. (a) Schematic illustration of QD-Apt(Dox) Bi-FRET system. In the first step, the CdSe/ZnS core-shell QD are surface functionalized with the A10 PSMA aptamer. The intercalation of Dox within the A10 PSMA aptamer on the surface of QDs results in the formation of the QD-Apt(Dox) and quenching of both QD and Dox fluorescence through a Bi-FRET mechanism: the fluorescence of the QD is quenched by Dox while simultaneously the fluorescence of Dox is quenched by intercalation within the A10 PSMA aptamer resulting in the "OFF" state. (b) Schematic illustration of specific uptake of QD-Apt(Dox) conjugates into target cancer cell through PSMA mediate endocytosis. The release of Dox from the QD-Apt(Dox) conjugates induces the recovery of fluorescence from both QD and Dox ("ON" state), thereby sensing the intracellular delivery of Dox and enabling the synchronous fluorescent localization and killing of cancer cells. Reprinted with the permission of Ref [92].

However in order to improve the biocompatibility, solubility and functionality of QDs they should be modified by macromolecules such as polymers. Recently the expression of epidermal growth factor receptor (EGFR) and E-cadherin (E-cad) in different cancer cells has been quantified by using polymer modified antibody-conjugated QDs with different emission wavelengths [91].

QDs have also been used to study the release of drugs inside cells through a donor-acceptor model fluorescence resonance energy transfer (FRET) between them and Dox and a donor-quencher model FRET between Dox and aptamer (Figure 12) [92].

In spite of all above and many other profits of QDs in nanomedicine, toxicity of QDs [93], photobleaching problems [94], their specific and nonspecific interactions with the bioactive molecules in plasma and blood [93] remains a major problem that should be solved before they can be used in clinical setting.

5. Why Hybrid Nanostructures?

As above mentioned nanomaterials with intrinsic properties are unique candidates for cancer therapy, thus forming a hard foundation for further study and improvement but no one have all desirable properties and therefore could not considered as a perfect drug delivery or diagnostic system individually. For example carbon nanotubes are able to cross the cell membrane but they are not soluble in aqueous solutions and blood. Hybridization of these nanomaterials is a new way to make nanostructures with a hybrid of all wanted properties.

6. Hybrid Nanostructures

A very young and promising strategy to overcome disadvantages of above delivery systems and produce perfect targeted drug delivery or diagnostic systems is to make hybrid systems containing all or at least two classes of above nanomaterials. This strategy leads to new nano-scale materials called "hybrid nanostructures" [95].

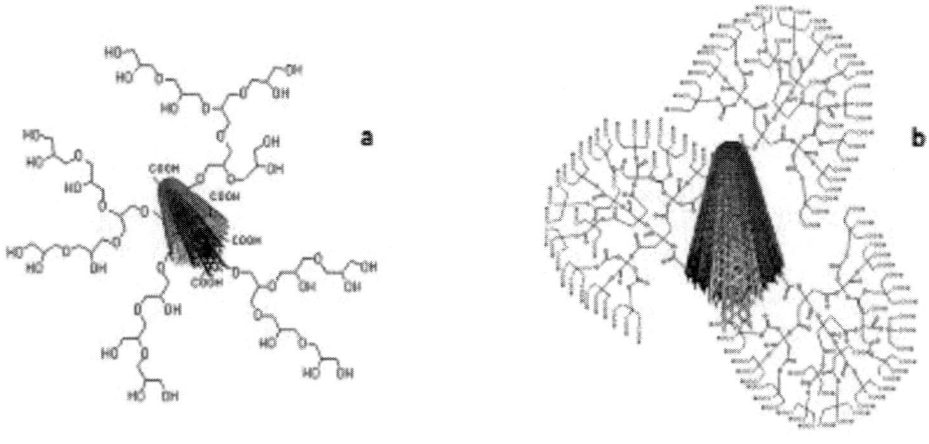

Figure 13. Schematic representation of a) CNT-*graft*-polyglycerol and b) CNT-*graft*-polycitric acid.

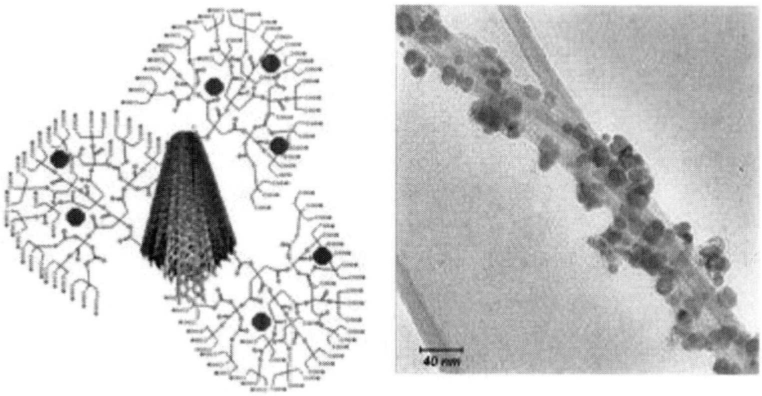

Figure 14. (a) A hybrid nanostructure comprising CNT, dendritic polymers and metal nanoparticles. (b) TEM image of this hybrid nanostructure.

For example conjugation of biocompatible and water soluble dendritic polymers such as polyglycerol (PG) or polycitric acid (PCA) onto the surface of CNTs can raise the water solubility of pristine CNTs, reduce their hydrophobicity, decrease the aggregation and size polydispersity and consequently lessen the toxicity of the CNTs in biological and physiological systems. On the other hand due to the presence of highly hydrophobic CNTs, dendritic polymers are able to cross the cell membrane much better than those without CNTs (Figure 13) [95].

Dendritic polymers grafted onto the surface of carbon nanotubes are able to encapsulate metal nanoparticles and therefore leading to hybrid nanostructure containing three classes of nanomaterials (Figure 14) [96].

Although carbon nanotubes are known to have near-infrared emissions, the luminescence intensities are usually too weak for whole-body *in vivo* imaging. Conjugation of QDs onto the surface of CNTs through chemical linkages raises their luminescence intensities and provides a possibility to track them inside the body [97].

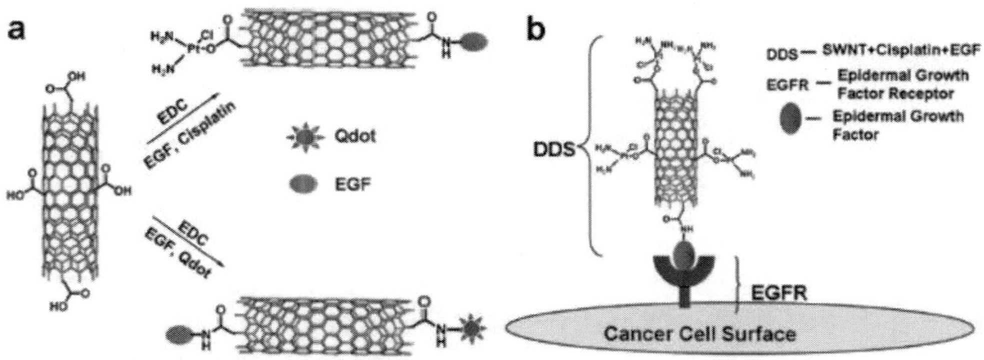

Reprinted with the permission of Ref [97].

Figure 15. (a) Synthesis of hybrid nanomaterials-based delivery system. (b) Schematic presentation SWNT bundles bioconjugated with EGF and cisplatin targeting the cell surface receptor EGFR on a single head and neck squamous carcinoma cells cell.

Targeted, *in vivo* killing of cancer cells using drug-CNT bioconjugate hybrid materials has been reported recently. Cisplatin and epidermal growth factor (EGF) has been attached to the functional groups of hybrid nanomaterials consisting CNTs and QDs to specifically target squamous cancer (Figure 15).

QDs conjugated onto the surface of CNTs provide a possibility to track hybrid nanostructures incubated with cancer cells while CNTs causes fast transferring through the cell membrane (Figure 16) [98].

Conjugation of DNA aptamer to dendrimer-modified quantum dot leads to hybrid nanostructures that can recognize the extracellular matrix protein tenascin-C on the surface of human glioblastoma cells and can specifically target U251 human glioblastoma cells [99]. Folate-decorated nanoparticles of biodegradable polymers containing QDs for targeted and sustained imaging for cancer diagnosis at its early stage have been reported recently [100]. Several types of multifunctional hybrid nanostructures based on dendritic polymers, CNTs, QDs and polyrotaxanes as intracellular anticancer drug carriers, providing new tools in cancer therapy, has been synthesized by our groups [101]. Those consist of linear-dendritic copolymers, CNTs, Fe_3O_4 nanoparticles, antibody and anticancer drugs with several key features such as (a) their ability to cross cell membranes and also high surface area per unit weight for high drug loading assigned to CNTs, (b) high functionality, water solubility and biocompatibility assigned to linear-dendritic copolymers and (c) targeting to tumors using a magnetic field assigned to Fe_3O_4 nanoparticles were used for killing the cancer cells and targeting drugs to tumor cells, then it was proved that they are promising systems for future cancer therapy (Figure 17) [102].

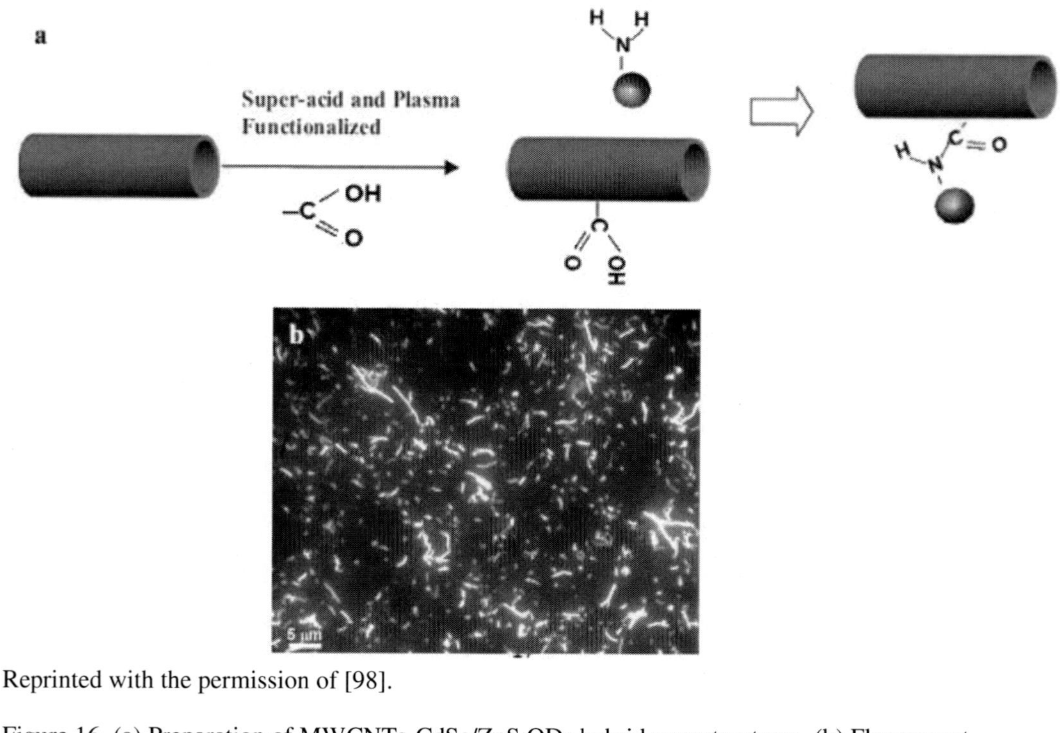

Reprinted with the permission of [98].

Figure 16. (a) Preparation of MWCNTs-CdSe/ZnS QDs hybrid nanostructures. (b) Fluorescent microscopy image of MWCNTs-CdSe/ZnS QDs hybrid nanostructures.

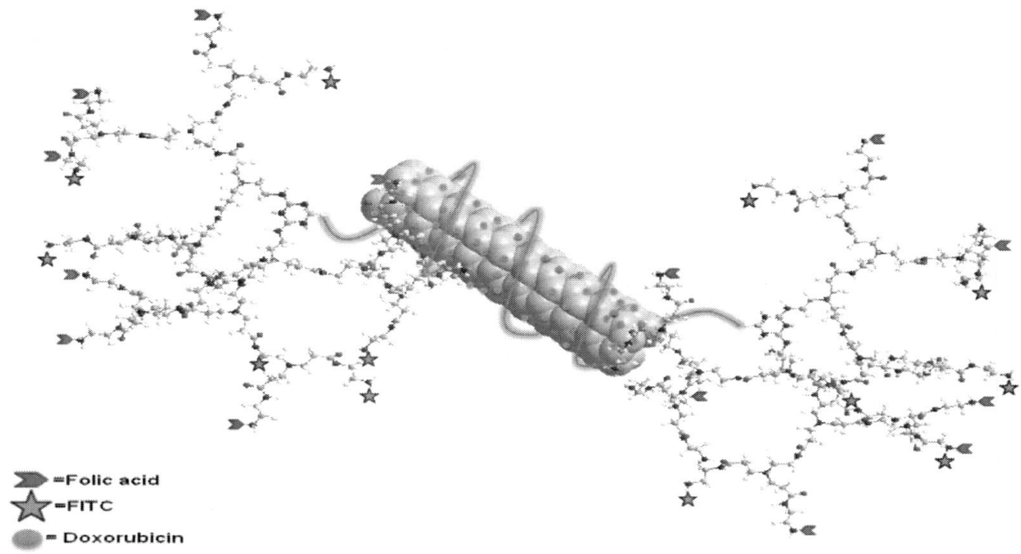

Figure 17. Structure of a hybrid nanostructure consists of linear-dendritic copolymers, CNT, Fe_3O_4 nanoparticles, FITC and doxorubicin used for cancer therapy.

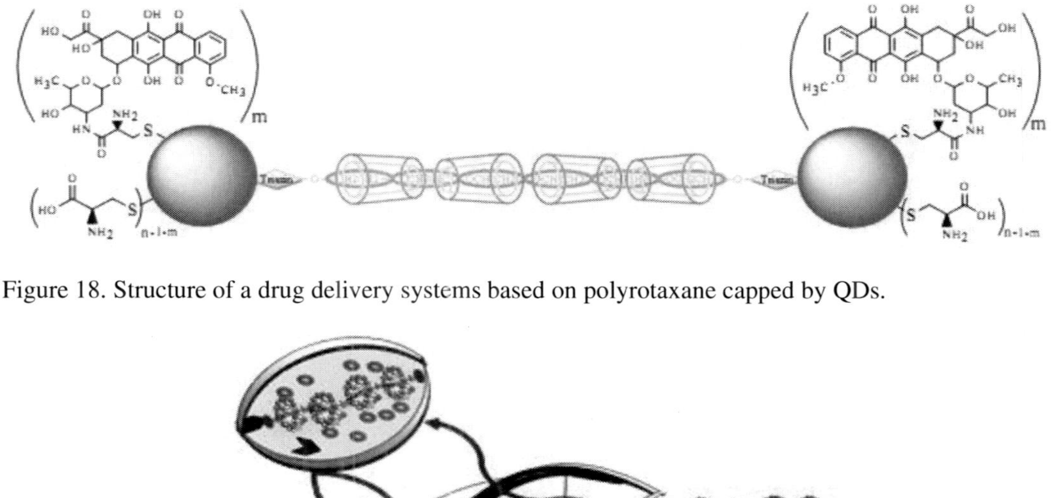

Figure 18. Structure of a drug delivery systems based on polyrotaxane capped by QDs.

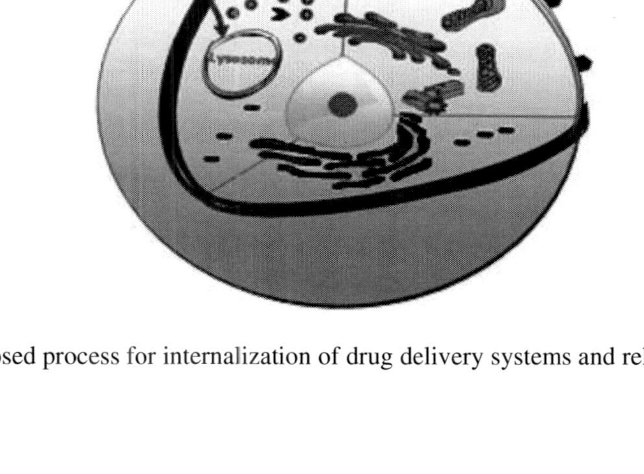

Figure 19. The purposed process for internalization of drug delivery systems and release the drug.

Polyrotaxanes consist of cyclodextrin rings, polyethylene glycol axes and quantum dot stoppers were also synthesized and to prove the efficacy of their molecular self-assemblies as drug delivery systems, doxorubicin was conjugated to their functional groups and they were subjected to the endocytosis and release the drug inside the cancer cells, mouse tissue connective fibroblast adhesive cell line (L929), then it was found that the molecular self-assemblies transfer through the cell membrane quickly and release drug into the intracellular environment slowly (Figure 18) [103].

Based on microscopy observations and cytotoxicity tests it seems the drug delivery systems are enough stable to escape the cytoplasm and insert the cell metabolism and drugs release after disassociation of self-assemblies and break down to their individual molecules by the cells (Figure 19).

Hybrid nanomaterials and nanostructures open a new and promising way to use all desirable properties of nanomaterials simultaneously in order to targeting anticancer drugs to tumors and early diagnosis of cancer cells. In the next chapters some of these systems will be discussed.

Conclusion

Successfulness of nanomaterials in cancer therapy and diagnosis depends on their ability to cross the biological barriers, to receive the targeted sites, and also their cytotoxicity directly. A well-known and promising strategy to improve this ability and decrease their toxicity is hybridization with other nanomaterials. Based on this fact hybrid nanomaterials and nanostructures are the best candidates to be use in nanomedicine thus forming a rigid foundation for further study and improvement.

References

[1] (a) de Villiers, M.M.; Aramwit, P.; Kwon, G.S. *Nanotechnology in Drug Delivery* (Biotechnology: Pharmaceutical Aspects), Springer, 2008. (b) Amiji, M.M. *Nanotechnology for Cancer Therapy*. CRC Press, 2006. (c) Grobmyer, S. R.; Moudgil, B.M. *Cancer Nanotechnology: Methods and Protocols* (Methods in Molecular Biology), Humana Press, 2010.

[2] Challa, S.; Kumar, S. R. *Nanotechnologies for the life sciences*, Wiley, 2007.

[3] Agrawal, A.; Deo, R.; Wang, G. D.; Wang, M. D.; Nie, S. *PNAS* 2008, 105, 3298-3303.

[4] VanHandel, M.; Alizadeh, D.; Zhang, L.; Kateb, B.; Bronikowski, M.; Manohara, H.; Badie, B. *Journal of Neuroimmunology* 2009, 208, 3-9.

[5] Choi, J. H.; Chen, K. H.; Han, J-H.; Chaffee, A. M.; Strano, M. S. *Small* 2009, 5, 672-675.

[6] Byrne, J. D.; Betancourt, T.; Brannon-Peppas, L. *Advanced Drug Delivery Reviews* 2008, 60, 1615-1626.

[7] Yang, L.; Mao, H.; Wang, Y.A.; Cao, Z.; Peng, X.; Wang, X.; Duan, H.; Ni, C.; Yuan, Q.; Adams, G.; Smith, M.Q.; Wood, W.C.; Gao, X.; Nie, S. *Small* 2009, 5, 235-243.

[8] Liu, Z.; Cai, W.B.; He, L.N.; Nakayama, N.; Chen, K.; Sun, X.M.; Chen, X.Y.; Dai, H.J. *Nat. Nanotech.* 2007, 2, 47–52.
[9] Weissleder, R.; Kelly, K.; Sun, E.Y.; Shtatland, T.; Josephson, L. *Nat. Biotechnol.* 2005, 23, 1418-1423.
[10] Ross, R.W.; Zietman, A.L.; Xie, W.; Coen, J.J.; Dahl, D.M.; Shipley, W.U.; Kaufman, D.S.; Islam, T.; Guimaraes, A.R.; Weissleder, R.; Harisinghani, M. *Clinical Imaging* 2009, 33, 301-305.
[11] Tannock, I.F.; Hill, R.P. (Eds.), *The Basic Science of Oncology*, 3rd edn., McGraw-Hill, Health Professions Division, New York, 1998.
[12] Cancer Facts and Figures 2005, American Cancer Society, Atlanta, 2005, p. 1.
[13] Sunderland, C.J.; Steiert, M.; Talmadge, J.E.; Derfus, A.M.; Barry, S.E. *Drug. Dev. Res.* 2006, 67, 70–93.
[14] Orive, G.; Gascon, A.R.; Hernandez, R.M.; Dominguez-Gil, A.; Pedraz, J.L. *Trends Pharm. Sci.* 2004, 25, 382–387.
[15] a) Küchler, S.; Radowski, M.R.; Blaschke, T.; Dathe, M.; Plendl, J.; Haag, R.; Schäfer-Korting, M.; Kramer, K.D. *Eur. J. Pharm. and Biopharm.* 2009, 71, 243-250.
[16] D'Emanuele, A.; Attwood, D. *Advanced Drug Delivery Reviews* 2005, 57, 2147-2162.
[17] Esfand, R. Tomalia, D.A. *Drug Discov. Today* 2001, 6, 427-436.
[18] Tomalia, D.A. *Prog. Polym. Sci.* 2005, 30, 294-324.
[19] Jansen, J.F.G.A.; Debrabandervandenberg, E.M.M.; Meijer, E.W. *Science* 1994, 266, 1226-1229.
[20] Bhadra, D.; Bhadra, S.; Jain, S.K ; Jain, N.K. *Int. J. Pharm.* 2003, 257, 111-124.
[21] Najlah, M.; Freeman, S.; Attwood, D.; D'Emanuele, A. *Int. J. Pharm.* 2006, 308, 175-182.
[22] Najlah, M.; Freeman, S.; Attwood, D.; D'Emanuele, A. *Int. J. Pharm.* 2007, 336, 183-190.
[23] D'Emanuele, A.; Jevprasesphant, R.; Penny, J.; Attwood, D. *J. Control. Release* 2004, 95, 447-453.
[24] a) Majoros, I.J.; Myc, A.; Thomas, T.P.; Mehta, C.B.; Baker Jr., J.R. *Biomacromolecules* 2006, 7, 572-579. b) Johansson, E. M. V.; Dubois, J.; Darbre, T.; Reymond, J-L. *Bioorganic and Medicinal Chemistry* 2010, 18, 6589–6597.
[25] Thomas, T.P.; Majoros, I.J.; Kotlyar, A.; Kukowska-Latallo, J.F.; Bielinska, A.; Myc, A.; Baker Jr., J.R. *J. Med. Chem.* 2005, 48, 3729-3735.
[26] Svenson, S.; Tomalia, D.A. *Adv. Drug Deliv. Rev.* 2005, 57, 2106-2129.
[27] Boas, U.; Heegaard, P.M.H. *Chem. Soc. Rev.* 2004, 33, 43-63.
[28] Cheng, Y.Y.; Wang, J.R.; Rao, T.L.; He, X.X.; Xu, T.W. *Front. Biosci.* 2008, 13, 1447-1471.
[29] Cheng, Y.Y.; Gao, Y.; Rao, T.L.; Li, Y.W.; Xu, T.W. *Comb. Chem. High Throughput Screen* 2007, 10, 336-349.
[30] D'Emanuele, A.; Attwood, D. *Adv. Drug Deliv. Rev.* 2005, 57, 2147e2162.
[31] a) Majoros, I.J.; Williams, C.R.; Baker Jr. J.R. *Current Topics in Medicinal Chemistry* 2008, 8, 1165-1179.
[32] Gurdag, S.; Khandare, J.; Stapels, S.; Matherly, L.H.; Kannan, R.M. *Bioconjugate Chem.* 2006, 17, 271-283.
[33] Majoros, I.J.; Thomas, T.P.; Mehta, C.B.; Baker, Jr., J.R. *J. Med. Chem.* 2005, 48, 5892.

[34] Thomas, T.P.; Majoros, I.J.; Kotlyar, A.; Kukowska-Latallo, J.F.; Bielinska, A.; Myc, A.; Baker, Jr., J.R. *J. Med. Chem.* 2005, 48, 3729.
[35] Lutz, J-F.; Börner, H.G. *Prog. Polym. Sci.* 2008, 33, 1-39.
[36] Wiener, E.C.; Konda, S.; Shadron, A.; Brechbiel, M.; Gansow, O. *Invest. Radiol.* 1997, 32, 748.
[37] Duncan, R.; Izzo, L. *Adv. Drug Deliv. Rev.* 2005, 57, 2215-2237.
[38] Yang, W.; Cheng, Y.; Xu, T.; Wang, X.; Wen, L. *European Journal of Medicinal Chemistry* 2009, 44, 862-868.
[39] Svenson, S.; Tomalia, D.A. *Advanced Drug Delivery Reviews* 2005, 57, 2106-2129.
[40] Quadir, M.A.; Treiber, C.; Multhaup, G.; Körner, M.; Haag, R. *J. Controlled Release* 2008, 132, 32-33.
[41] (a) Kukowska-Latallo, J. F.; Candido, K. A.; Cao, Z.; Nigavekar, S. S.; Majoros, I. J.; Thomas, T. P.; Balogh, L. P.; Khan, M. K.; Baker, J.R., Jr. *Cancer Res.* 2005, 65, 5317-5324. (b) Thomas, T. P.; Shukla, R.; Kotlyar, A.; Kukowska-Latallo, J.; Baker Jr, J. R. *Bioorganic and Medicinal Chemistry Letters* 2010, 20, 700–703.
[42] Patri, A. K.; Majoros, I.; Baker, J. R., Jr. *Curr. Opin. Chem. Biol.* 2002, 6, 466-471.
[43] Cloninger, M. J. *Curr. Opin. Chem. Biol.* 2002, 6, 742-748.
[44] (a) Mullen, D. G.; Fang, M.; Desai, A.; Baker, J. R.Jr., Orr, B. G.; Holl, M. M. B. *ACS Nano*, 2010, *4*, 657-670. (b) Farrell, D.; Alper, J.; Ptak, K.; Panaro, N. J.; Grodzinski, P.; Barker, A. D. *ACS Nano*, 2010, 4 , 589-594.
[45] Singh, P. *Bioconjugate Chem.* 1998, 9, 54-63.
[46] Wu, C.; Brechbiel, M. W.; Kozak, R. W.; Gansow, O. A. *Bioorg. Med. Chem. Lett.* 1994, 4, 449-454.
[47] Kojima, C.; Kono, K.; Maruyama, K.; Takagishi, T. *Bioconjugate Chem.* 2000, 11, 910-917.
[48] Agrawal, A.; Min, D-H.; Singh, N.; Zhu, H.; Birjiniuk, A.; von Maltzahn, G.; Harris, T. J.; Xing, D.; Woolfenden, S. D.; Sharp, P. A.; Charest, A.; Bhatia, S. *ACS Nano*, 2009, *3* , 2495–2504.
[49] Baker, J. R.; Quintana, A.; Piehler, L. T.; Banazak-Holl, M.; Tomalia, D. A. Raczka, E. *Biomed. Microdevices* 2001, 3, 61-69.
[50] Ong, K. K.; Jenkins, A. L.; Cheng, R.; Tomalia, D. A.; Durst, H. D.; Jensen, J. L.; Emanuel, P. A.; Swim, C. R.; Yin, R. *Anal. Chim. Acta* 2001, 444, 143-148.
[51] Kobayashi, H.; Sato, N.; Saga, T.; Nakamoto, Y.; Ishimori, T.; Toyama, S.; Togashi, K.; Konishi, J.; Brechbiel, M. W. *Eur. J. Nucl. Med.* 2000, 27, 1334-1339.
[52] (a) Barth, R. F.; Adams, D. M.; Soloway, A. H.; Alam, F.; Darby, M. V. *Bioconjugate Chem.* 1994, 5, 58-66. (b) Navarro, G.; de ILarduya. C. T. *Nanomedicine: Nanotechnology, Biology, and Medicine* 2009, 5, 287-297.
[53] (a) Wu, G.; Barth, R. F.; Yang, W.; Chatterjee, M.; Tjarks, W.; Ciesielski, M. J.; Fenstermaker, R. A. Bioconjugate Chem. 2004, 15, 185-194. (b) Patri, A. K.; Myc, A.; Beals, J.; Thomas, T. P.; Bander, N. H.; Baker, J. R. Jr. *Bioconjugate Chem.* 2004, 15, 1174□-1181.
[54] Lai, P-S.; Lou, P-J.; Peng, C-L.; Pai, C-L.; Yen, W-N.; Huang, M-Y.; Young, T-H.; Shieh, M-J. *Journal of Controlled Release* 2007, 122, 39-46.
[55] Myc, A.; Majoros, I.J.; Thomas, T.P.; Baker, J. R. Jr. *Biomacromolecules* 2007, 8, 13-18.

[56] Wang, D.; Kopeckova, J. P.; Minko, T.; Nanayakkara, V.; Kopecek, J. *Biomacromolecules* 2000, 1, 313.

[57] Malik, N.; Evagoro, E. G.; Duncan, R. *Anticancer Drugs* 1999, 10, 767.

[58] Duncan, R.; Malik, N. *Proc. Int. Symp. Control. Release Bioact. Mater.* 1996, 23, 105.

[59] Nishiyama, N.; Nakagishi, Y.; Morimoto, Y.; Lai, P-S.; Miyazaki, K.; Urano, K.; Horie, S.; Kumagai, M.; Fukushima, S.; Cheng, Y.; Jang, W-D.; Kikuchi, M.; Kataoka, K. *Journal of Controlled Release* 2009, 133, 245-251.

[60] Shi, X.; Wang, S.H.; Shen, M.; Antwerp, M.E.; Chen, X.; Li, C.; Petersen, E. J.; Huang, Q.; Weber, W. J.; Baker, J.R. Jr. *Biomacromolecules* 2009, 10, 1744-1750.

[61] (a) Wang, S.H.; Shi, X.; Van Antwerp, M.; Cao, Z.; Swanson, S. D.; Bi, X.; Baker, J. R. Jr. *Adv. Funct. Mater.* 2007, 17, 3043-3050. (b) Mei, M.; Ren, Y.; Zhou, X.; Yuan, X-B.; Li, F.; Jiang, L-H.; Kang, C-S.; Yao, Z. *Journal of Applied Polymer Science* 2009, 114, 3760-3766. (c) Hu, J.; Fang, M.; Cheng, Y.; Zhang, J.; Wu, Q.; Xu, T. J. Phys. Chem. B 2010, 114, 7143-7157. (d) Morgan, M. T.; Nakanishi, Y.; Kroll, D. J.; Griset, A. P.; Carnahan, M. A.; Wathier, M.; Oberlies, N. H.; Manikumar, G.; Wani, M. C.; Grinstaff, M. W. *Cancer Res* 2006, 66, 11913-11921. (e) Ke, W.; Zhao, Y.; Huang, R.; Jiang, C.; Pei, Y. *Journal of Pharmaceutical Sciences* 2008, 97, 2208-2216.

[62] (a) Zhuo, R. X.; Du, B.; Lu, Z. R. J. *Control. Release* 1999, 57, 249-257. (b) Bhadra, D.; Bhadra, S.; Jain, S.; Jain, N. K. *Int. J. Pharm.* 2003, 257, 111-124. (c) Winnicka, K.; Bielawski, K.; Bielawska, A. *Pharmacological Reports* 2010, 62, 414-423. (d) Johansson, E. M. V.; Dubois, J.; Darbre, T.; Reymond, J-L. *Bioorganic and Medicinal Chemistry* 2010, 18, 6589-6597. (e) Yao, H.; Veine, D. M.; Zeng, Z-Z.; Fay, K.S.; Staszewski, E. D.; Livant, D. L. *Clin Exp Metastasis* 2010, 27, 173-184. (f) Gardikis, K.; Hatziantoniou, S.; Bucos, M.; Fessas, D.; Signorelli, M.; Felekis, T.; Zervou, M.; Screttas, C. G.; Steelee, B. R.; Ionov, M.; Micha-Screttas, M.; Klajnert, B.; Bryszewska, M.; Demetzos, C. *Journal of Pharmaceutical Sciences* 2010, 99, 3561-3571.

[63] (a) Gitsov, I. In Advances in Dendritic Macromolecules; Newkome, G. R., Ed.; Elsevier: Amsterdam, 2002; Vol. 5, p 45; (b) Gitsov, I.; Fréchet, J. M. *J. Macromolecules* 1993, 26, 6536. (c) Pesak, D. J.; Moore, J. S. *Macromolecules* 1997, 30, 6467. (d) Gitsov, I.; Wooley, K. L.; Hawker, C. J.; Ivanova, P. T.; Fréchet, J. M. J. *Macromolecules* 1993, 26, 5621; (e) Santini, C. M. B.; Johnson, M. A.; Boedicker, J. Q.; Hatton, T. A.; Hammond, P. T. *J. Polym. Sci. Part A: Polym. Chem.* 2004, 42, 2784. (f) Al-Muallem, A. H.; Knauss, D. M. *J. Polym. Sci. Part A: Polym. Chem.* 2001, 39, 152. (g) Zhu, L.; Tong, X.; Li, M.; Wang, E. *J Polym Sci Part A: Polym Chem* 2000, 38, 4282.

[64] (a) Fréchet, J. M. J.; Gitsov, I. *Macromol. Symp.* 1995, 98, 441. (b) Johnson, M. A.; Iyer, J.; Hammond, P. T. *Macromolecules* 2004, 37, 2490. (c) Gitsov, I.; Zhu, C. J. *Am. Chem. Soc.* 2003, 125, 11228. (d) Glauser, T.; Stancik, C. M.; Moller, M.; Voytek, S.; Gast, A. P.; Hedrick, J. L. *Macromolecules* 2002, 35, 5774. (e) Carnahan, M. A.; Middleton, C.; Kim, J.; Kim, T.; Grinstaff, M. W. *J. Am. Chem. Soc.* 2002, 124, 5291. (f) Johnson, M. A.; Santini, C. M. B.; Iyer, J.; Satija, S.; Ivkov, R.; Hammond, P. T. *Macromolecules* 2002, 35, 231. (g) Wursch, A.; Moller, M.; Glauser, T.; Lim, L. S.; Voytek, S. B.; Hedrick, J. L.; Frank, C. W.; Hilborn, J. G. *Macromolecules* 2001, 34, 6601.

[65] (a) Namazi.H.; Adeli. M. *Journal of Polymer Science: Part A: Polymer Chemistry* 2005, 43, 28-41. (b) Adeli, M.; Zarnegar, Z.; Dadkhah, A.; Hossieni, R.; Salimi, F.; Kanani, A. *Journal of Applied Polymer Science* 2007, 104, 267. (c) Namazi, H.; Adeli, M. *J. Polym. Sci. A: Polym. Chem.* 2005, 43, 28. (d) Namazi, H.; Adeli, M. Polymer 2005, 45, 10788. (e) Namazi, H.; Adeli, M. *European Polymer Journal* 2003, 39, 1491.

[66] Gitsov, I.; Fréchet, J. M. J. *J. Am. Chem. Soc.* 1996, 118, 3785.

[67] (a) Adeli, M.; Haag, R. *Journal of Polymer Science Part A: Polymer Chemistry* 2006, 44, 5740. (b) Adeli. M.; Zarnegar. Z.; Kabiri. R.; Salimi. F.; Dadkhah. A. *International Journal of Nanoscience and Nanotechnology* 2007, 2, 53. (c) Adeli, M.; Haag, R.; Zarnegar, Z. *Journal of Nanoparticle Research* 2007, 9, 1057.

[68] (a) Adeli, M.; Namazi, H.; Jafari, S.; Dadkhah, A.; Shukla, A.; Zarnegar, Z. *Colloid and Polymer Science* 2007, 285, 1527. (b) Namazi, H.; Adeli, M. *Biomaterials* 2005, 26, 1175. (c) Zhou, Z.; D'Emanuele, A.; Lennon, K.; Attwood, D. *Macromolecules* 2009, 42, 7936-7944. (d) Wood, K. C.; Little, S. R.; Langer, R. L.; Hammond, P. T. *Angew. Chem. Int. Ed.* 2005, 44, 6704-6708. (e) Stovera, T. C.; Kimb, Y. S.; Loweb, T. L.; Kester, M. *Biomaterials* 2008, 29, 359–369.

[69] (a) Haniu, H.; Matsuda, Y.; Takeuchi, K.; Kim, Y. A.; Hayashi, T.; Endo, M. *Toxicology and Applied Pharmacology* 2010, 242, 256-262. (b) Firme, C. P.; Bandaru, P. R. *Nanomedicine: Nanotechnology, Biology, and Medicine* 2010, 6, 245-256. (c) Ding, L.; Stilwell, J.; Zhang, T.; Elboudwarej, O.; Jiang, H.; Selegue, J. P.; Cooke, P. A.; Gray, J. W.; Chen, F. F. *Nano Lett.,* 2005, 5, 2448-2464. (d) Chou, C-C.; Hsiao, H-Y.; Hong, Q-S.; Chen, C-H.; Peng, Y-W.; Chen, H-W.; Yang, P-C. *Nano Lett.,* 2008, 8, 437-445.

[70] (a) Kang, B.; Yu, D.; Dai, Y.; Chang, S.; Chen, D.; Ding, Y. *Small* 2009, 5, 1292-1301. (b) Bhirde, A. A.; Patel, V.; Gavard, J.; Zhang, G.; Sousa, A. A.; Masedunskas, A.; Leapman, R. D.; Weigert, R.; Gutkind, J. S.; Rusling, J. F. *ACS Nano* 2009, *3*, 307-316. (c) Kam, N.W.S.; Liu, Z.; Dai, H. *Angew. Chem. Int. Ed.* 2006, 45, 577-581: Angewandte Chemie 2006, 118, 591-595. (d) Heister, E.; Neves, V.; Tîlmaciu, C.; Lipert, K.; Beltrán, V. S.; Coley, H. M.; Silva, S. R. P.; McFadden, *J. Carbon* 2009, 47, 2152-2160.

[71] (a) Adeli, M.; Sepahvand, R.; Astinchap, B. *International Journal of Nanoscience.* 2009, 8, 533. (b) Adeli. M.; Bahari. A.; Hekmatara. H. *Nano Brief Reports and Reviews* 2008, 3, 1.

[72] Liu, Z.; Sun, X.; Nakayama-Ratchford, N.; Dai, H. *ACS Nano* 2007, 1, 50.

[73] (a) Adeli, M.; Sepahvand, R.; Astinchap, B. *Journal of Nanoparticle Re*search 2008, 10, 1309. (b) Ali-Boucetta, H.; Al-Jamal, K. T.; McCarthy, D.; Prato, M.; Bianco, A.; Kostarelos, K. *Chem. Commun.* 2008, 459. (c) Liu, Z.; Sun, X.; Nakayama-Ratchford, N.; Hai, D. *ACS Nano* 2007, 1, 50.

[74] (a) Kam, N. W.; Liu, Z.; Dai, H. *Angew. Chem. Int.* Edn 2006, 45 577. (b) Singh, R.; Pantarotto, D.; McCarthy, D.; Chaloin, O.; Hoebeke, J.; Partidos, C. D.; Briand, J. P.; Prato, M.; Bianco, A.; Kostarelos, K. *J. Am. Chem. Soc.* 2005, 127, 4388. (b) Burke, A.; Ding, X.; Singh, R.; Kraft, R. A.; Levi-Polyachenko, N.; Rylander, M. N.; Szot, C.; Buchanan, C.; Whitney, J.; Fisher, J.; Hatcher, H. C.; D'Agostino, R.; Kock, N. D.; Ajayan, P.M.; Carroll, D. L.; Akman, S.; Torti, F. M.; Torti, S. V. *PNAS* 2009, 106, 12897–12902.

[75] (a) Liu, Z.; Cai, W.; He, L.; Nakayama, N.; Chen, K.; Sun, X.; Chen, X.; Dai, H. *Nat. Nanotechnol.* 2007, 2, 47. (b) Schipper, M. L.; Nakayama-Ratchford, N.; Davis, C. R.; Sh Kam, N. W.; Chu, F.; Liu, Z.; Sun, X.; Dai, H.; Gambhir, S. S. *Nat. Nanotechnol.* 2008, 3, 216. (c) Zhang, X.; Meng, L.; Lu, Q.; Fei, Z.; Dyson, P.J. *Biomaterials* 2009, 30, 6041-6047.

[76] Liu, Z.; Davis, C.; Cai, W.; He, L.; Chen, X.; Dai, H. *Proc. Natl. Acad. Sci. USA* 2008, 105 1410.

[77] (a)Weissleder, R. A. *Nat. Biotechnol.* 2001, 19, 316-17. (b) Kam, N.W.S.; O'Connell, M.; Wisdom, J. A.; Dai, H. *Proc. Natl. Acad. Sci. USA* 2005, 102,11600. (c) Liu, Z.; Cai, W.; He, L.; Nakayama, N.; Chen, K.; Sun, X.; Chen, X.; Dai, H. *Nat. Nanotechnol.* 2007, 2, 47-52. (d) Marches, R.; Chakravarty, P.; Musselman, I. H.; Bajaj, P.; Azad, R. N.; Pantano, P.; Draper, R. K.; Vitetta, E. S. *Int. J. Cancer* 2009, 125, 2970–2977.

[78] (a) Gobin, A. M.; Lee, M. H.; Halas, N. J.; James, W.D.; Drezek, R. A.; West, J. L. *Nano Lett.,* 2007, 7, 1929-1934. (b) Loo, C.; Lowery, A.; Halas, N.; West, J.; Drezek, R. *Nano Lett.*, 2005, 5,709-11. (c) Huang, X.; El-Sayed, I. H.; Qian, W.; El-Sayed, M. A. *J. Am. Chem. Soc.* 2006, 128, 2115–20. (d) Hirsch, L. R.; Stafford, R. J.; Bankson, J. A.; Sershen, S. R.; Rivera, B.; Price, R. E.; Hazle, J. D.; Halas, N. J.; West, J. L. *Proc. Natl. Acad. Sci. USA* 2003, 100,13549-54. (e) Moon, H. K.; Lee, S. H.; Choi, H. C. *ACS Nano* 2009, 3, 3707.

[79] (a) Shao, N.; Lu, S.; Wickstrom, E.; Panchapakesan, B. *Nanotechnology* 2007, 18, 315101–9. (b) Falk, M. H.; Issels, R. D. *Int. J. Hyperthermia* 2001, 17, 1–18. (c) Wust, P.; Hildebrandt, B.; Sreenivasa, G.; Rau, B.; Gellermann, J.; Riess, H.; Felix, R.; Schlag, P. M. *Lancet Oncol.* 2002, 3, 487–97.

[80] Welsher, K.; Liu, Z.; Daranciang, D.; Dai, H. *Nano Lett.*, 2008, 8, 586-590.

[81] Dubruel, P.; Christiaens, B.; Rosseneu, M.; Vandekerckhove, J.; Grooten, J.; Goossens, V.; Schacht, E. *Biomacromolecules* 2004, 5, 379.

[82] Lu, Q.; Moore, J. M.; Huang, G.; Mount, A. S.; Rao, A. M.; Larcom, L. L.; Ke, P. C. *Nano Lett.,* 2004, 4, 2473-2477.

[83] Yarotski, D. A.; Kilina, S. V.; Talin, A. A.; Tretiak, S.; Prezhdo, O. V.; Balatsky, A. V.; Taylor, A. *J. Nano Lett.*, 2009, 9, 12-17.

[84] Kam, N. W. S.; O'Connell, M.; Wisdom, J. A.; Dai, H. J. *Proc. Natl. Acad. Sci. U.S.A.* 2005, 102, 11600.

[85] Bi, S.; Zhou, H.; Zhang, S. *Biosensors and Bioelectronics* 2009, 24, 2961-2966.

[86] (a) Chan, W. C. W.; Nie, S. *Science* 1998, 281, 2016-2018. (b) Phan, J. H.; Moffitt, R. A.; Stokes, T. H.; Liu, J.; Young, A. N.; Nie, S.; Wang, M. D. *Trends in Biotechnology* 2009, 27, 350-358. (c) Jamieson, T.; Bakhshi, R.; Petrova, D.; Pococka, R.; Imani, M.; Seifalian, A. M. *Biomaterials* 2007, 28, 4717-4732. (d) Bhang, S. H.; Won, N.; Lee, T-J.; Jin, H.; Nam, J.; Park, J.; Chung, H.; Park, H-S.; Sung, Y-E.; Hahn, S. K.; Kim, B-S.; Kim, S. *ACS Nano* 2009, *3*, 1389–1398. (e) Chen, C.; Peng, J.; Xia, H-S.; Yang, G-F.; Wu, Q-S.; Chen, L-D.; Zeng, L-B.; Zhang, Z-L.; Pang, D-W.; Li, Y. *Biomaterials* 2009, 30, 2912-2918.

[87] (a) Pan, J.; Feng, S-S. *Biomaterials* 2009, 30, 1176-1183. (b) Smith, B. R.; Cheng, Z.; De, A.; Koh, A. L.; Sinclair, R.; Gambhir, S. S. *Nano Lett.*, 2008, *8*, 2599-2606. (c) Weng, K. C.; Noble, C. O.; Papahadjopoulos-Sternberg, B.; Chen, F. F.; Drummond, D. C.; Kirpotin, D. B.; Wang, D.; Hom, Y. K.; Hann, B.; Park, J. W. *Nano Lett.*, 2008, 8, 2851-2857.

[88] Gao, X.; Cui, Y.; Levenson, R. M.; Chung, L. W. K.; Nie, S. *Nat. Biotechnol.* 2004, 22, 969-74.

[89] (a) Orndorff, R. L.; Rosenthal, S. J. *Nano Lett.*, 2009, 9, 2589-2599. (b) Yong, K-T.; Ding, H.; Roy, I.; Law, W-C.; Bergey, E. J.; Maitra, A.; Prasad, P. N. *ACS Nano* 2009, 3, 502-510. (c) Manzoor, K.; Johny, S.; Thomas, D.; Setua, S.; Menon, D.; Nair, S. *Nanotechnology* 2009, 20, 065102 (13pp). (d) Zhang, J.; Jia, X.; Lv, X-J.; Deng, Y-L.; Xie, H-Y. *Talanta* 2010, 81, 505-509.

[90] (a) Zhang, H.; Sachdev, D.; Wang, C.; Hubel, A.; Gaillard-Kelly, M.; Yee, D. *Breast Cancer Res. Treat.* 2009, 114, 277-285. (b) Yezhelyev, M. V.; Al-Hajj, A.; Morris, C.; Marcus, A. L.; Liu, T.; Lewis, M.; Cohen, C.; Zrazhevskiy, P.; Simons, J. W.; Rogatko, A.; Nie, S.; Gao, X.; O'Regan, R. M. *Adv. Mater.* 2007, 19, 3146-3151. (c) Hu, M.; Yan, J.; He, Y.; Lu, H.; Weng, L.; Song, S.; Fan, C.; Wang, L. *ACS Nano* 2009, *4*, 488-494. (d) Ghazani, A. A.; Lee, J. A.; Klostranec, J.; Xiang, Q.; Dacosta, R. S.; Wilson, B. C.; Tsao, M. S.; Chan, W. C. W. *Nano Lett.*, 2006, 6, 2881-2886.

[91] (a) Huang, D-h.; Su, L.; Peng, X-h.; Zhang, H.; Khuri, F. R.; Shin, D. M.; Chen, Z. *Nanotechnology* 2009, 20, 225102 (9pp). (b) Zaman, M. B.; Baral, T. N.; Zhang, J.; Whitfield, D.; Yu, K. *J. Phys. Chem.* C, 2009, 113, 496-499.

[92] Bagalkot, V.; Zhang, L.; Levy-Nissenbaum, E.; Jon, S.; Kantoff, P. W.; Langer, R.; Farokhzad, O. C. *Nano Lett.*, 2007, 7, 3065-3070.

[93] (a) Dobrovolskaia, M. A.; Mcneil, S. E. *Nat. Nanotech.* 2007, 2, 469-478. (b) Soltesz, E. ; Kim, S.; Laurence, R.; DeGrand, A.; Parungo, C.; Dor, D.; Cohn, L.; Bawendi, M.; Frangioni, J.; Mihaljevic, T. *Ann. Thorac. Surg.* 2005, 79, 269-277. (c) Ballou, B.; Lagerholm, B. C.; Ernst, L. A.; Bruchez, M. P.; Waggoner, A. S. *Bioconjug. Chem.* 2004, 15, 79-86. (d) Fischer, H. C.; Liu, L. C.; Pang, K. S.; Chan, W. C. W. *Adv. Funct. Mater.* 2006, 16, 1299-1305.

[94] Weissleder, R. *Nat. Biotechnol.* 2001, 19, 316-317.

[95] (a) Adeli, M.; Mirab, *N. Polymer* 2009, 50, 3528. (b) Adeli, M.; Mirab, N. *Nanotechnology* 2009, 20, 485603 (10pp). (c) Herrero, M. A.; Guerra, J.; Myers, V. S.; Gomez, V.; Crooks, R. M.; Prato, M. *ACS Nano*, 2010, 4 , 905–912.

[96] (a) Adeli, M.; Mehdipour, E.; Bavadi, M. *Journal of Applied Polymer Science* 2010, 116, 2188-2196. (b) Bahari, A.; Adeli, M.; Hekmetara, H. *Nano Brief Reports and Reviews* 2009, 4, 217-223.

[97] Bhirde, A. A.; Patel, V.; Gavard, J.; Zhang, G.; Sousa, A. A.; Masedunskas, A.; Leapman, R. D.; Weigert, R.; Gutkind, J. S.; Rusling, J. F. *ACS Nano* 2009, 3, 307.

[98] Shi, D.; Guo, Y.; Dong, Z.; Lian, J.; Wang, W.; Liu, G.; Wang, L.; Ewing, R. C. *Adv. Mater.* 2007, 19, 4033-4037.

[99] Li, Z.; Huang, P.; He, R.; Lin, J.; Yang, S.; Zhang, X.; Ren, Q.; Cui, D. *Materials Letters* 2010, 64, 375-378.

[100] Pan, J.; Feng, S-S. *Biomaterials* 2009, 30, 1176-1183.

[101] (a) Tavakoli, A.; Adeli, M.; Vosoughi, M. *Nanomedicine: Nanotechnology, Biology, and Medicine* 2010, 6, 556-562.

[102] Mehdipoor, E.; Adeli, M.; Bavadi, M.; Sasanpour, P.; Ashiri, M.; Rashidian, B. *Journal of Materials Chemistry* 2011, Submitted.

[103] Adeli, M.; Kalantari, M.; Sadeghi, E.; Mahmoudi, M. *Nanomedicine: Nanotechnology, Biology, and Medicine* 2011, In press.

In: Hybrid Nanostructures in Cancer Therapy
Editor: Mohsen Adeli

ISBN: 978-1-62100-517-9
© 2012 Nova Science Publishers, Inc.

Chapter II

Biomedical Applications of Cyclodextrin-Polymers

Mohsen Adeli[1,2] ***and Mahdieh Kalantari***[1]
[1]Department of chemistry, Faculty of Science, Lorestan University, Khoramabad, Iran
[2]Department of chemistry, Sharif University of Technology, Tehran, Iran

Abstract

This chapter explains biomedical applications of cyclodextrin-polymers. Cyclodextrins (CDs) are a class of natural cyclic oligosaccharides with 6, 7, or 8 D-(+)-glucose units linked by α-1, 4-linkages. The geometry of CDs gives a hydrophobic internal cavity that various organic, inorganic and biological molecules can be fitted in it. Many hydroxyl groups are situated on the outer parts of the rings, which make some of CDs water-soluble. These unique physicochemical properties of CDs make them promising materials to design polymeric systems. In the present chapter, first, the effect of CDs on solubility, stability and bioavailability of drugs is described. Second, polymeric systems based on CDs, such as polyrotaxanes, micelles, physical hydrogels and chemical hydrogels are discussed. Finally, based on a summary of the recent papers potential applications of these systems in drug and gene delivery are discussed.

1. Introduction

Cyclodextrins (CDs) are a class of natural cyclic oligosaccharides with D-(+)-glucose units linked by α-1, 4-linkages [1-4]. CDs can be produced by glucosyl transferase enzyme (CGTase) [5, 6]. CGTase itself is produced by the microorganisms such as Bacillus macerans, Klebsiella oxytoca and Bacillus [6]. Among CDs, the rings consist of six, seven and eight glucopyranose units are the most important for biomedical applications and are commonly named α-, β- and γ-CD, respectively. It is assumed that CDs are hollow cone [7] with the primary hydroxyl groups at the narrow edge and secondary hydroxyl groups at the wide edge.

As a result of the orientation of hydroxyl groups to the outside of cone, CDs have hydrophilic exterior and a lipophilic cavity [8]. Hydrophobic cavity of CDs is capable of forming inclusion complexes with many organic, inorganic and biological molecules with suitable polarity and size [9]. Pharmaceutical properties of the drugs such as solubility and stability can be improved by forming complex with CDs. In addition, hydroxyl functional groups of CDs can be converted to other useful functional groups that can be used for attachment of the cyclodextrin to various compounds. CDs with this unique molecular structure are widely used in biomedical applications particularly in drug and gene delivery. But, due to their some undesirable properties such as hemolytic activity and low aqueous solubility of β-CD, many modified CDs, particularly polymeric systems based on CDs, with better properties than natural cyclodextrins have been synthesized. Some of the polymeric systems based on CDs and their biomedical applications will be described in this chapter.

2. The Effect of CDs on the Pharmaceutical Properties of Drugs

2.1. Solubility

High-throughput screening approaches to generate drugs have led to an increasing number of lipophilic drugs that their clinical applications are restricted, due to their poor water-solubility [10].

CDs and their derivatives have been used to improve the aqueous solubility of poorly water-soluble drugs. CDs have many hydroxyl functional groups at the outer surfaces of their rings, which make them hydrophilic and water-soluble [11]. In addition, they can form inclusion complexes with various drugs by taking up the drug molecule or some aromatic moiety of the molecule in to their hydrophobic cavities without changing molecular structure of guest [12]. For example, CDs and cyclodextrin systems have been tested for transporting anticancer drugs with suitable aromatic groups such as phenyl groups [13].

The main driving forces for the inclusion complex formation are hydrophobic interactions, van der Waals interactions, and hydrogen bonds [14]. Therefore no covalent linkages are formed between host and guest during the formation of inclusion complex. Various methods are used to form drug/cyclodextrin complexes such as co-precipitation, slurry complexation, past complexation, damp mixing, heating method, extrusion and dry mixing [15]. UV-vis absorbance, NMR-spectra, X-ray diffraction patterns, and DSC thermograms are applied to investigate changes in the characteristic analytical features of a drug molecule upon complexation as an indication that a complex has been formed [16]. Phase solubility profiles, described by Higuchi and Connors [17], show the effect of solubilizer, i.e. cyclodextrin or ligand, on the substrate solubility, such as drug solubility. These profiles are classified in two main categories, A- and B-types. A-type curves can be obtained when forming soluble inclusion complexes. In contrast to A-type profiles, B-type profiles show the formation of poorly soluble inclusion complexes. Studies show that the water-soluble modified CDs give A-type curves while natural cyclodextrins with less solubility, particularly β-CD, give B-type curves [18]. The use of parent CDs in most pharmaceutical formulations is limited for a variety of reasons including their inherent low solubility, high molecular weight, possible parenteral toxicity and relatively high cost [19].

Thus, it is necessary to find methods to improve the properties of CDs such as their complexation and solubilization efficiency.

Improvement of the solubilization efficiency of CDs can be obtained by their modification and synthesis of their water-soluble derivatives. The addition of small amount of water-soluble and biocompatible polymers such as polyvinylpyrrolidone (PVP), polyethylene glycol (PEG) and chitosan to the complexation medium can also result in considerable enhancement of the drug/cyclodextrin complexation, drug solubilization capacity of the CDs and drug permeability from aqueous CD solutions through biological membranes [19, 20].

2.2. Stability

A very important factor for the drug formulations is their stability against degradation processes such as hydrolysis that can occur in an aqueous environment. The most common consequence for the drug degradation is the loss of potency. However, sometimes harmful degradation products may also be formed. Allergy, for example, is in many cases due to drug degradation products rather than to the drug itself [21]. Therefore, there is a need to prepare new drug formulations with sufficient stability. CDs are able to increase the drug resistance to hydrolysis, oxidation, racemization and photodegradation by the formation of complex with drug molecules. In fact, the encapsulation protects the drugs molecules against attack of various reactive molecules and thus reduces the rate of various degradation processes [22]. They may also sterically hinder the guest molecule from undergoing the structural changes that result in degradation processes [23]. In addition, CDs improved the solid state stability and shelf life of drugs [24]. 20(*S*)-Camptothecin (CPT) as an antineoplastic agent show a wide spectrum of antitumor activity for various cancers such as prostate, human lung and breast via inhibition of topoisomerase I [25], enzyme that catalyze the reaction of DNA relaxation [26]. However, the clinical use of CPT has been limited due to the reversible and pH-dependent conversion of its lactone ring to the water-soluble carboxylate form while only the lactone form can poison topoisomerase I [27]. To overcome the destability of CPT a group of researchers [28] showed that randomly substituted dimethyl-β-cyclodextrin, RDM-*β*-CD, is effective complexing agent and can be used to improve the stability of CPT. There was approximately a 10-fold increase in the stability of CPT in the presence of a 25% w/v concentration of RDM-*β*-CD, corresponding to an increase in the half-life of CPT from 58.7 min in 0.02 M HCl to 587.3 min.

Under specific condition, CD can have a destabilizing effect on drugs depending on the CD concentration, the stability constant of the complex and degradation rate constant for the drug degradation within the CD cavity [10].

For example, at relatively high concentrations of CDs, tranilast antiallergic drug forms a 2:1 (guest: host) complex with *γ*-CD and 5500-fold enhancement in the rate of degradation process (dimerization) are created. While with increasing CD concentrations, 1:1 and 1:2 inclusion complexes are obtained and the rate of dimerization decrease [29].

Complex stability constant has important role in determining the extent of protection [24, 30-32]. 2-Hydroxypropyl-*β*-cyclodextrin, HP-*β*-CD, with very low concentrations (1% or lower) do not protect taxol anticancer drug as effectively as higher CD concentrations because of the formation of a more physically unstable complex in low CD concentrations [33].

2.3. Bioavailability

Bioavailability as one of the main pharmacokinetic properties of drugs explains the rate and extent to which the active drug component is absorbed from a drug product and becomes available at the site of drug action [34]. Destability, low solubility and low permeability of drugs will often result in their poor bioavailability. Therefore, novel drug delivery systems should be designed to increase the bioavailability of drugs for various administration routes. Pharmaceutical literatures show that CDs can have a positive, negative or no effect on drug bioavailability. There are many parameters that determine the negative or positive effect of CDs on bioavailability of drugs. However, in many cases the importance of drug solubility, dissolution, stability and permeability is emphasized.

One of the main administration routes is via the oral, often referred to as the oral drug delivery, mainly due to patient convenience and compliance [35]. A first need for the oral bioavailability of a drug is that the drug must be dissolved before it reaches the site of action [36]. In the Biopharmaceutical Classification System (BCS), drugs are classified into the following groups based on their solubility and permeability properties [37, 38]:

- Class I: highly soluble and highly permeable
- Class II: poorly soluble and highly permeable
- Class III: highly soluble and poorly permeable
- Class IV: poorly soluble and poorly permeable

An increase in dissolution rate and apparent solubility of class II drugs with low solubility and high permeability, which can increase via the formation of complex between drug and CD by a factor of 10^1 to 10^3 [39], will cause an increased drug permeating through the gut wall, leading to higher oral bioavailability [36].

CDs are not irritant, thus bioavailability enhancement can be obtained by the improvement of the drug contact time at the absorption site [10, 18].

3. Modification of Cyclodextrins

Although, CDs have been extensively used in the field of pharmaceutical, they are not always ideal due to their some undesirable properties and effects such as low aqueous solubility of *β*-CD or created toxicity by the formation of crystalline precipitates of CDs and their complexes with cholesterol in the kidneys after parenteral administration of CDs at high doses [40].

To improve or modify the properties of CDs many modified CDs, particularly cyclodextrin-polymers, with desired properties and biomedical applications have been designed [41, 42].

Depends on the interactions between CDs and polymers there is two ways to combine CDs with polymers:

In the first way noncovalent, physical, interactions causes an affinity between CDs and polymers.

In the second way polymers are attached to CDs through chemical bonding [43].

Some of the CD-containing polymeric systems that are useful for biomedical application are discussed briefly below.

3.1. Hydrogels

Hydrogels as three-dimensional hydrophilic polymer networks are able to absorb large quantities of water or biological fluids while maintaining their structure. Hydrogels are widely used as drug delivery systems, particularly delicate protein and peptide drug delivery, tissue engineering and medical devices because of their good biocompatibility and other desirable properties [44, 45]. The ability of hydrogels to absorb water is assigned to the presence of hydrophilic groups such as OH, –CONH–, $-CONH_2-$, and $-SO_3H$ in polymeric networks of hydrogels [46]. The amount of water in the polymeric network is at least 20% and can reach values of 99% by weight. Hydrogels contain of more than 95% water possess excellent biocompatibility because of their large degree of water retention and their physiochemical similarity with the native extracellular matrix both compositionally and mechanically [47].

Although hedrogels are suitable for drug delivery, their highly hydrophilic property may make the loading of hydrophobic drugs difficult and restricts their ability to control the release of hydrophilic molecules. The attachment of CDs to the polymers forming hydrogel structures has recently been used as a promising method to overcome these disadvantages [48].

CDs with torus-shaped structure possess ability to include peptides and proteins such as cyclosporin, insulin, human growth hormone and other drug molecules [49] and this leads to change the interactions between drug and polymer in polymeric drug delivery systems. Mechanisms of drug loading and release may therefore be modified by using CDs [50].

On the other hand, the binding of CDs to a polymeric matrix prevents the fast decomplexation of the drug that usually occurs when CD–drug solutions are diluted in physiological fluids [51]. Thus, CD-based hydrogels can combine both the favorable properties of CDs and hydrogels. Hydrogels can be classified into two groups based on type of their crosslink: physical hydrogels or chemical hydrogels. Chemical hydrogels can be obtained by covalent interactions between hemopolymers or copolymers with suitable cross-linking agents. Chemical gels have excellent mechanical stability due to their strong covalent crosslinks. Chemical crosslinking methods contain radical polymerization, chemical reaction of complementary groups, high energy irradiation and enzyme usage [47]. In chemical CD-hydrogels, CD moieties are coupled to a polymeric backbone via various strategies. In many cases, they are prepared by copolymerization of CD monomeric derivatives with acrylic or vinyl monomers [48]. Chemical CD-hydrogels can also be synthesized by the reaction between CDs and polymers with reactive end functional groups such as poly(ethylene glycol) (PEG) with isocyanate [52] or amino [53] end groups.

The unique characteristics of hydrogels, as mentioned above, have led to more and more attention to them as drug loading carriers. For example, Xu et al. reported pHEMA/β-CD hydrogel contact lenses prepared by photopolymerization of 2-hydroxyethyl methacrylate (HEMA), mono-methacrylated β-CD (mono-MA-β-CD) and trimethylolpropane trimethacrylate [54]. Drug loading and the *in vitro* and *in vivo* sustained release behavior of the resulting hydrogel contact lenses were investigated using puerarin as a model drug. Puerarin which is capable of forming inclusion complex with β-CD has been used for cataracta glauca and ocular hypertension in China due to its ability to lower intraocular pressure, and improve ocular blood flow. However, as a result of its poor solubility and permeability across biomembrane, it has low bioavailability and therefore its clinical applications have been limited [55]. pHEMA/β-CD hydrogel contact lenses showed high puerarin loading because of the formation of inclusion complexes between puerarin and β-CD. They could effectively deliver puerarin through the cornea and had higher drug bioavailability and longer precorneal retention time than the commercially available puerarin eye drops.

In another study, Zawko et al. functionalized hyaluronic acid (HA) hydrogels with a methacryloyl-β-cyclodextrin, a photocrosslinkable monomer [56]. HA is a type of polysaccharides found ubiquitously in the connective tissues of vertebrates [57]. Hydrogels based on hyaluronic acid are promising materials for biomedical applications because of their biocompatible, porous and biodegradable structure. However, low solubility of drug within aqueous hyaluronic acid hydrogel environment can be limited incorporation of bioactive drugs. The presence of β-CD in HA hydrogels improved drug–hydrogel interactions by the mechanism of inclusion complexation and enhanced the uptake of hydrocortisone as less soluble drug in water [56].

One of the main hydrogels is smart hydrogel [58-66]. This type of polymers is able to change its volume or other physical properties in response to environmental stimuli [67]. There are physical and chemical stimuli. Temperature [68-70], electricity, light, pressure, sound, and magnetic field are examples of the physical stimuli whereas pH [71, 72], solvent composition and ions are chemical stimuli. Temperature-sensitive hydrogels and pH-responsive hydrogels have obtained more attention because of their ability for repeated swelling–deswelling conversion in response to the environmental temperature and pH changes, respectively [73].

If a hydrogel contains a segment with the property of inclusion complex formation and a sensitivity segment, the copolymer obtained may not only possess the ability to include organic compounds, but also may respond to different external stimuli. This strategy can be effectively used to develop new biomedical and pharmaceutical products [74-77].

For example, Liu et al. prepared a smart hydrogel via copolymerization of maleic anhydride-modified β-CD (MAH-βCD) with N-isopropylacrylamide (NIPA) [74]. The resulting gel revealed good combination of pH and temperature sensitivities with a molecular inclusion ability.

Although covalent crosslinking reactions produce gel with excellent mechanical chemical stability, they may conjugate the drug to the hydrogel or impair the integrity of drugs. Moreover, chemical hydrogels are often used as implantables, and the incorporation of drugs by solution sorption may restrict the loading level and be time consuming [78]. To overcome these limitations, physical hydrogels can be useful. Physical hydrogels are formed by non-covalent interactions such as hydrophobic interaction, ionic interaction, hydrogen bonds, crystallization, specific biomimetic interactions and host-guest interactions, and thus can avoid the use of such chemical cross-linking agents and the related reactions [79, 80]. Host-guest interaction between CD and appropriate guest is a promising method to prepare physical hydrogels [81-86].

3.2. Polyrotaxanes

Interlocked molecules such as (pseudo)rotaxanes, catenanes, molecular knots, and molecular necklaces have received much attention due to their potential application in molecularscale functional devices and machines [87-89]. Pseudorotaxanes are mechanically interlocked molecules consisting one or more cyclic components as rings and one or more axes. Pseudorotaxanes are stable sufficiently. It is therefore necessary to locate bulky groups, so-called stoppers, at both ends of the axis to hinder the dissociation of ring from axis. In this term supramolecular system is called rotaxane. Although there is no chemical bonding between rings and axis, rotaxanes are stable compounds, due to a high free activation energy needed to withdraw a ring from the axis of a rotaxane. Rotaxanes can be covalently linked together to obtain polyrotaxanes [90]. Many types of cyclic components, such as calix[*n*]arenes, crown ethers, cyclodextrins, cucurbituril and cyclophanes have been used as ring for synthesizing of rotaxanes [91]. However, CDs have received more interest than other alternatives.

Both polymers and copolymers have been extensively used as axes to construct (pseudo)rotaxane. The first inclusion complex between CD and polymer was reported by Harada et al. in 1990 [92]. CD-based polyrotaxanes can be used as multivalent carrier for drug and biological active molecules due to their high functionality. High functionality of CD-based polyrotaxanes is attributed to the several cyclodextrin rings in their backbone. Each CD has several hydroxyl or other functional groups and a polyrotaxane containing 10 α-CD rings, for example, have 180 hydroxyl functional groups in its backbone [93]. To be biomaterials, polyrotaxanes must preferably be biodegradable.

Biodegradable polyrotaxane is a macromolecule consisting of CDs and a polymer capped with cleavable chain stoppers. Cleavable chain stoppers can be obtained through a biodegradable linkage such as peptide or disulfide linkages. These types of linkages are susceptible to photodegradation, enzymatic degradation, thermo-oxidative degradation or degradation under pH conditions. For example hydrazone bonds, Boc-Trp ester bonds and vinyl ether bonds undergo degradation under acidic conditions, basic conditions and acidic conditions, respectively.

Therefore, pH can be used as stimuli because the environment in different parts of the body shows different pH ranging from 1 to 8 [94]. When the biodegradable linkages are degraded by various stimuli, the polyrotaxane degrades to CDs, polymer and stoppers. In 1995, the first example of biodegradable polyrotaxanes as novel drug delivery system was prepared. This polyrotaxane was composed of threaded α-CDs onto PEO chain end-capped with L-phenylalanine (L-Phe) via biodegradable peptide linkages [95]. The supramolecular structure of this polyrotaxane could be dissociated by enzymatic degradation of peptide linkages. Some of the nanomedical applications of CD-based polyrotaxanes will be discussed later.

3.3. Polymeric Micelles

Due to the prolonged blood circulation time, high stability, the enhanced permeability and retention effect, polymeric micelles have been widely studied as drug/gene delivery systems compared to small molecular surfactant micelles [96]. Polymeric micelles consist of a hydrophobic core and hydrophilic corona. Core acts as a carrier part which accommodates poorly water-soluble drugs, such as doxorubicin [97-100] and paclitaxel [101-109], and hydrophilic corona stabilizes the nanoparticles in aqueous solution [110, 111] and allows the drug molecules to remain in blood circulation for longer [112].

Upon encapsulation of drug within the micelles, they are protected from possible degradation processes by biological surrounding and thus undesirable side effects of cytotoxic drugs are decreased [113]. The size of copolymer micelles is often in the range of 20-100 nm. This range of size is suitable to prevent rapid renal exclusion. On the other hand, it is small enough to avoid undesirable uptake by the reticuloendothelial system [114]. Polymer micelles are able to penetrate inside the certain biological sites, such as tumors, and accumulate at these tissues [115]. Polymeric micelles with a diameter less than 100 nm, for example, are capable of penetrating into the tumors. This ability of polymer micelles is attributed to the enhanced permeation and retention effect [116].

Polymeric micelles have a very low critical micelle concentration (CMC) value and show a very slow rate of dissociation in comparison to low-molecular surfactants, resulting in a higher stability for the development of drug delivery systems [117].

In fact, polymeric segments, containing block or graft copolymers, reduce the high exchange rate between micelles and monomers and, therefore, enhance micelle stability [118]. On of the main strategies for synthesis of polymeric micelles is based on secondary supramolecular interactions, such as host-guest interactions. Biocompatible CDs with a hydrophobic cavity have been extensively used as host unit to form polymeric micelles. Recently, Zhang et al., for example, synthesized a nanoassemblies based on host-guest interaction between cyclodextrin-polyethyleneimine conjugates (PEI-CD) and benzyl groups of poly(β-benzyl L-aspartate) (PBLA) [119].

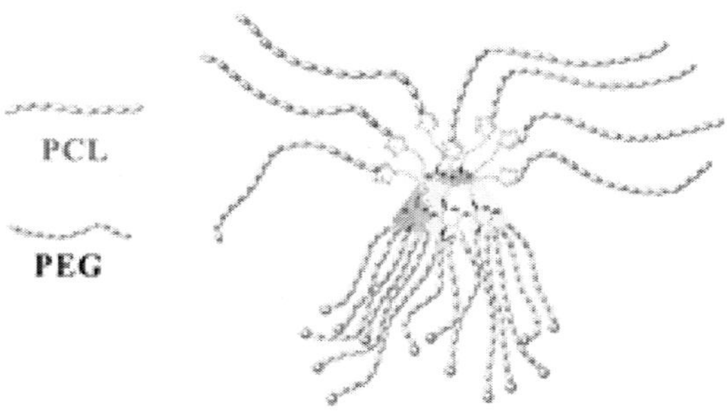

Figure 1. Schematic representation of amphiphilic star copolymer contain of PCL and PEG arms with β-CD core. Reprinted with the permission of Ref [120a].

Amphiphilic star copolymers with novel architecture can also provide promising route for synthesis of polymeric micelles. Star polymers are special types of branched polymers and possess some advantages in gene/drug delivery applications in comparison to linear polymers. CDs with many hydroxyl groups are used as initiator to induce the amphiphilic star copolymers consisting of several linear chains at primary and secondary positions of the CDs [120]. For example, Gou et al. reported a amphiphilic star copolymer composed of 14 poly (ε-caprolactone) (PCL) arms and 7 PEG arms with β-CD as core moiety (figure 1). These amphiphilic copolymers formed self assembled aggregates in aqueous solution. The hydrophilic PEG arms serve as the corona surrounding and PCL arms form the core domain [120a].

4. CD-Polymers in Drug Delivery

Although the development of pharmaceutical biotechnologies have led to an increasing number of new therapeutic agents, these products still possess many intrinsic disadvantages such as low stability *in vivo*, poor solubility, short half-life and immunogenicity to large-scale applications [121]. On the other hand, all of the intrinsic properties of a drug are fixed after synthesis, thus, the design of an appropriate delivery system can be used as a promising way to overcome such problems [122].

CDs and their derivatives with many unique properties have been widely used in drug delivery systems to improve the solubility, stability and bioavailability of various drugs.

CD-polymers can be used as drug delivery systems in at least three ways:

(1) Drug molecules can be physically delivered by CD-polymers.
(2) Drug molecules can be chemically delivered by CD-polymers.
(3) Drug molecules can be delivered using CD-polymers based on a combination of first and second routes.

The main strategy for the physical delivery of drug molecules by CD-polymers is the formation of inclusion complex. The major non-covalent forces for the encapsulation of drug molecule or its aromatic moiety in to the cavity of CD and thereby form the CD/drug inclusion complex are hydrogen bonding, dipole-dipole and van der waals interactions between drug molecule and CD. Therefore no covalent bonds are formed during formation of the inclusion complex. Formation of a CD inclusion complex can significantly improve the solubility, stability and bioavailability of drugs as discussed in section 2.

Naproxen as a non-steroidal anti-inflammatory drug (NSAID) are often applied for the reduction of moderate to severe pain, fever, inflammation and stiffness [123], but it has low aqueous solubility. Li et al. prepared a range of novel cationic β-cyclodextrin polymers (CP*β*CDs) containing quaternary ammonium groups via condensation polymerization of *β*-CD, epichlorohydrin (EP) and choline chloride (CC). The results of this study indicated that the water solubility of naproxen upon encapsulation in the CP*β*CDs was significantly increased 120-fold; from 27 to 3.2 ± 10^3 mg/l at 25 °C. Extraction of cholesterol from cell membrane, particularly through inclusion complexation, leads to hemolysis. CP*β*CDs also showed relatively low hemolytic activity, compared with parent *β*-CD because structure hindrance of cationic P*β*CDs decreased the inclusion ability of their hydrophobic cavities to include membrane cholesterol [124].

The other strategy for the physical delivery of drug molecules by CD-polymer is based on metal coordination. In this strategy, hydroxyl groups of CD are converted to the functional groups which are able to form favorable coordination complexes. Liu et al. synthesized a supramolecular assembly, bis(molecular tube)s composed of complexes of organoselenium-bridged *β*-cyclodextrins and platinum(IV) ion. In this work, *β*-CD was first converted to mono[6-*O*-(*p*-toluenesulfonyl)]-*β*-cyclodextrin and then reacted with 1,2-diselenacyclopentane to yield organoselenium-bridged bis(*β*-cyclodextrin). The resulting dimer formed a coordination complex with Pt(IV) via selenium groups. The complexation of *β*-CD dimer and Pt(IV) caused a suitable orientation for the *β*-CD to form a pseudorotaxane with PPG, poly(propylene glycol). The pseudorotaxane was converted to rotaxane by the esterification of the terminal hydroxyl groups of PPG axis with 3, 5-dinitrobenzoic acid. Finally, cross-linking of adjacent CD rings with epichlorohydrin and removal of the polymeric chain through the hydrolysis of the terminal ester groups led to formation of bis(molecular tube)s. It is known that organoselenium compounds act as repressors of human immunodeficiency virus (HIV) transcription [125]. On the other hand, some *cis*-platinum complexes are extensively used for treatment of a wide spectrum of cancers such as lung, ovarian, head and neck cancer [126]. Cisplatin exerts its antitumor activity by the formation of stable DNA–cisplatin complexes via intrastrand crosslinks [123]. This results in interference with normal transcription and DNA replication mechanisms leading to apoptosis [126]. Therefore, the reported nano assembly can have application in drug delivery systems.

Polymeric micelles can also be used for the physical delivery of drug molecules. For example, Quan et al. synthesized a polymeric micelle for active drug delivery [127]. Cancer is now the number one cause in worldwide mortality. Most anticancer drugs have no tumor selectivity and poison normal tissues [128]. Therefore, the primary challenge in cancer therapy is to deliver anticancer drugs into the disease site without harming healthy tissues. A number of polymeric carriers have been developed to transport drugs to their intended targets [129]. Polymeric carriers can be targeted to tumor cells through passive or active targeting [130, 131].

Passive targeting occurs due to the higher affinity of polymeric drug delivery systems for accumulation in tumor tissue as a result of enhanced permeability and retention (EPR) effect [132]. In active targeting, the surface of polymeric carrier is modified with antibodies, peptides and ligands such as folic acid that can specifically recognize the tumor cells via receptors that are present on these cells [129, 133].

Quan et al. prepared three components to form the polymeric micelle: 1. Hydrophilic component containing *N*-isopropylacrylamide (NIPAAm) and *N*-acroyloxysuccinimide (NAS) units, P(NIPAAm-*co*-NAS), with a phenyl termination group. A peptide including the Arg-Gly-Asp (RGD) sequence was prepared as a target ligand to enhance the cell uptake efficacy due to the presence of RGD receptors on the surface of tumor cells. On the other hand, a modified PEG was also produced. Modified PEG and RGD was conjugated to the P(NIPAAm-*co*-NAS) via an amide condensation reaction. It is also worth mentioning that, the modified PEG side chains are attached to the P(NIPAAm-*co*-NAS) by using benzoic-imine bonds. 2. Hydrophobic component containing poly(ε-caprolactone) with a terminal adamantyl group. 3. α-β Cyclodextrin dimmer component. The core-shell assemblies were formed based on host-guest interactions. In general, terminal phenyl and adamantyl groups were included into the cavity of α-CD and β-CD, respectively (Figure 2a). In the certain aqueous concentration of the self-assembly system (CMC), the PCL hydrophobic segments self-assembled and hydrophobic core of micelles was formed (Figure 2b). This hydrophobic core was used as nanocontainers for the doxorubicin (DOX) drug, an anthracyclinic antibiotic. Investigation of endocytosis behavior of the resulting micelle showed that at pH 7.4, very few nanoparticles could be endocytosed by tumor cells because of the stability of benzoic-imine bonds and therefore the shielding provided by PEG corona for the target ligands. However, at pH 6.8, the endocytosis of nanoparticles was greatly improved. In fact, the hydrolysis of benzoic-imine bonds and dissociation of PEG chains from the outer layer of the nanoparticles at pH 6.8 resulted in the exposure of target ligands. With the exposed target ligands, the nanoparticles would be easily endocytosed by tumor cells. It should be noted that pH in malignant cells (< 6.8) is slightly less than that of normal cells (7.4) [127].

The second way is based on covalent interactions between CD-polymers and drugs. In this way, drug molecules are covalently bound to the functional groups of CDs or polymeric segment of delivery systems. In addition to functional groups of polymeric segment, CDs have many active hydroxyl groups which could be modified by a large number of chemical reactions, allowing the attachment of drugs to the CD [134]. Ooya et al. synthesized theophylline–polyrotaxane conjugates by coupling theophylline, as a model drug, with α-CD in the polyrotaxane end-capped with L-phenylalanine (L-Phe). In this study, hydroxyl groups of the α-CDs in the backbone of polyrotaxane were first activated by 4-nitrophenyl chloroformate and then coupled with *N*-aminoethyl-theophylline-7-acetoamide derivative via amide and urethane linkages to obtain the theophylline–polyrotaxane conjugates. In vitro degradation of the conjugates showed that theophylline-immobilized α-CDs were completely released by the terminal peptide cleavage of the L-Phe moiety in the polyrotaxanes [135].

In another work, polyrotaxanes consisting α-CD rings, PEG axis and cadmium selenide quantum dots (CdSe QDs) with cysteine capping agent as stoppers was synthesized (Figure 3a) by our research group. Then amino group of DOX drug were conjugated to the carboxylate groups of QDs (Figure 3b) and subjected to the endocytosis and release inside the cancer cells. MTT assay showed a high toxicity for anticancer drug delivery systems against L929 cell line.

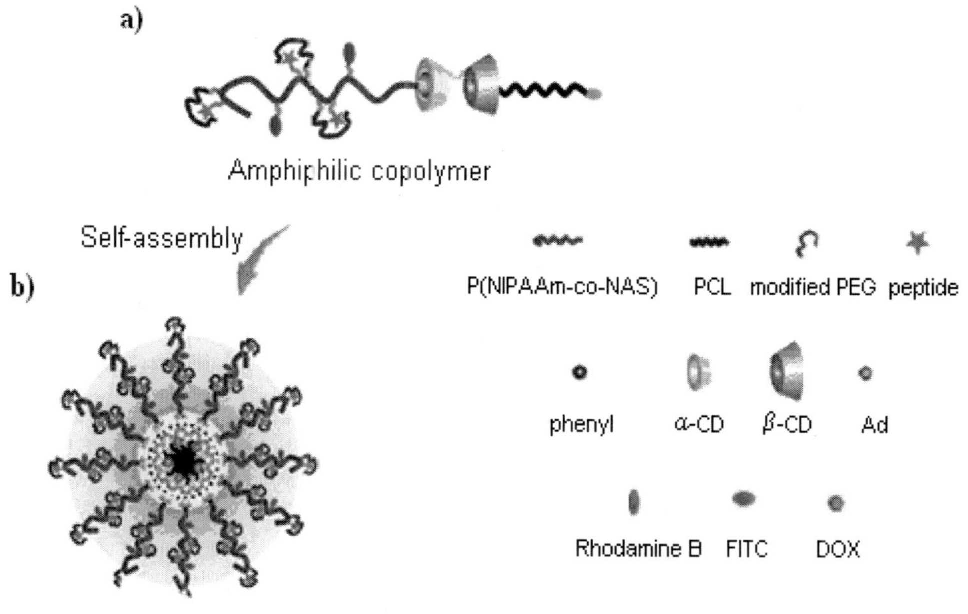

Figure 2. (a) Supramolecular diblock copolymer connected by host-guest interactions and (b) Micelles formed by assembly of this copolymer. Reprinted with the permission of Ref [127].

In this study fluorescence microscopy was used to observe the rate of transferring of drug delivery systems from the cell membrane. It was found that the rate of transfer of CdSe QDs through the cell membrane increased upon conjugation to polypseudorotaxane containing α-CD rings and PEG axis [136 a]. We also used quantum dots with conjugated cyclodextrins onto their surface as drug delivery systems with a potential application as diagnosis system [136 b].

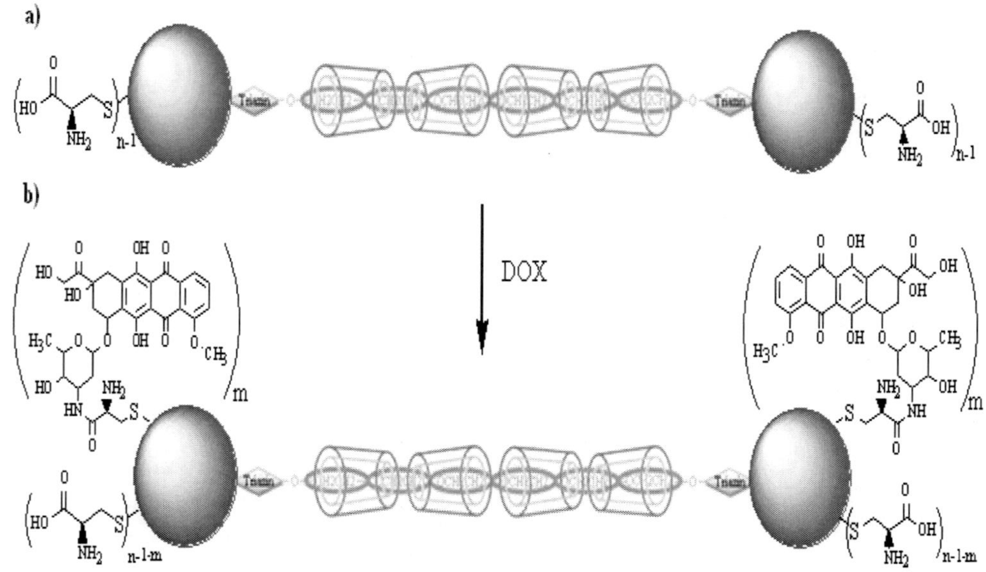

Figure 3. (a) Polyrotaxanes consisting α-CD rings, PEG axis and CdSe QDs stoppers and (b) The attachment of DOX to the carboxylate groups of QDs.

In the third way, drug molecules are covalently attached to the functional groups of CD-polymers. If conjugated drug molecule is capable of forming an inclusion complex with CD, then inclusion complexation between drug and CD (i.e., intermolecular inclusion complexes) may lead to the formation of self-assembles. In this route, therefore, drug delivery is based on both covalent and non-covalent interactions.

Davis synthesized a linear, water-soluble and highly biocompatible cyclodextrin-containing polymer conjugate of camptothecin (CPT). The CD-polymer was synthesized by grafting a diaminoacid-β-CD monomer to poly(ethylene glycol) dipropanoic succinimide (MW=3400), as a difunctionalized PEG. Anticancer drug camptothecin (CPT) was then conjugated to the carboxylate groups of the difunctionalized PEG via an ester bond. Lactone form of the CPT was maintained in the resulting CPT-conjugated polymers because CPT was coupled to the polymeric backbone by forming an ester bond at its 20-hydroxyl group. In water, the CPT-conjugated polymers formed self-assembles into ca. 30 nm nanoparticles which suggested that self-assembles formation was mainly the result of inclusion complexation between CPT and CD. When the CPT is released, the nanoparticle disassembles. Assembled nanoparticles are large enough to avoid renal clearance, but the disassembled nanoparticles can give individual polymer chains that can exit via the kidney. The results of animal studies and clinical trials show that CPT-conjugated polymers have long circulation time, which allows for significant accumulation in tumors. This process results in prolonged plasma half-life and enhanced distribution to tumor tissue in comparison to free CPT [137 a].

Recently we have synthesized star polymers consisting of cyclodextrin core and polyoxazoline, POX, arms with end aromatic groups, aniline groups, (Figure 4a) that are able to form inclusion complex with the cyclodextrin core [137 b]. The synthesized star polymers are able to form dendritic molecular self-assemblies in aqueous solutions (Figure 4b). The molecular self-assemblies encapsulate and deliver nano-objects easily.

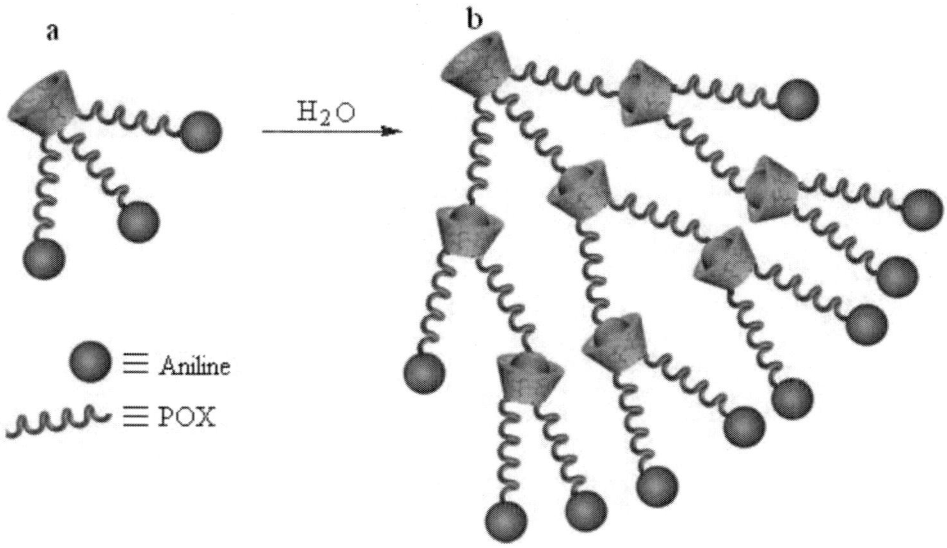

Figure 4. (a) Star polymers consisting of cyclodextrin core and polyoxazoline arms with end aromatic groups and (b) Dendritic molecular self-assemblies in aqueous solutions.

5. CD-Polymers in Gene Delivery

Gene therapy has long sought to treat genetic-based diseases by delivering exogenous, therapeutic genes to diseased cells [138]. Sickle cell anemia, HIV, Parkinson's disease, Huntington disease, Alzheimer's disease, for example, have been given a genetic identity and for this reason, gene therapy may be a possible prescription [138-142]. However, the success of gene therapy is largely dependent on the design of gene delivery systems with low cytotoxicity and high transfection efficiency. There are two groups of gene therapy vectors: viral vectors and nonviral vectors. Viral vectors, clinical tests by using adenoviruses, adeno-associate viruses, retroviruses, etc, have high gene expression, but their side effects such as severe pathogenicity restricted further development for the gene therapy. In comparison with viral vectors, nonviral vectors possess many advantages such as lower toxicity, non-immunogenicity and convenient handling [143]. Cationic polymers are one of the main types of nonviral gene therapy vectors [144-148]. They are able to deliver plasmid DNA into cells via electrostatic interactions between their cationic groups and anionic DNA. Transfection efficiencies of cationic polymers differ from one polymer to another [149]. A great number of polycations, containing polyethylenimine (PEI) [150], poly(tertiary amine methacrylate) [151-153], poly(L-lysine) [154, 155], polyamidoamine [156], chitosan,[157, 158], poly(L-glutamic acid) [159], and polyphosphoester [160, 161] have been synthesized as gene carriers. Although nonviral vectors are effective for gene delivery, they have relatively lower transfection efficiency in comparison to viral vectors. Recently, CD-containing cationic polymers and CD-containing cationic polyrotaxanes have been applied to effect gene transfection. The use of CD-containing cationic polymer in the field of gene delivery was started in 1999 [162].

Arima et al. synthesized polyamidoamine dendrimer conjugates with α-, β-, and γ cyclodextrins, CDE conjugates, (Figure 5). In these CDE conjugates, α-, β-, and γ-CDs were covalently bound to the dendrimer (generation 2) in a molar ratio of 1:1. In these compounds, dendrimer are able to form the complex with plasmid DNA (pDNA) and to increase the cellular uptake of pDNA and CDs bear a disrupting effect on biological membranes via the complexation with membrane constituents such as phospholipids and cholesterols. Dendrimer conjugate with α-CD enhanced gene transfection activity (approximately 100 times higher than that of dendrimer alone) in NIH3T3 and RAW264.7 cells. Although the exact mechanism for the enhancing gene transfer effect of α-CDE conjugate was unclear, intracellular distribution of FITC-Labeled pDNA showed that conjugate affected the intracellular trafficking of pDNA [163].

PEI homopolymers with a molecular weight higher than 25K are considered for nonviral gene delivery because of their high transfection efficiency. However, the rather high toxicity of these polymers restricts their applications in gene therapy. On the other hand PEI homopolymers with a molecular weight of less than 1.8K exhibit low gene delivery ability but have less toxicity effects. In this regard, Yang et al. synthesized a series of cationic star polymers as nonviral gene delivery vectors. In this study, oligoethylenimine (OEI) arms of different lengths were bound to primary hydroxyl groups of α-CD core (α-CD-OEI). All α-CD-OEI star polymers formed complexes with pDNA. The transfection efficiency of α-CD-OEI in HEK293 and Cos7 cells enhanced with an increase in the OEI arm length. α-CD-OEI with the longest OEI arms revealed the highest transfection efficiency which was comparable to or even higher than that in branched PEI (25K). In addition, in vitro cytotoxicity in α-CD-OEI was much lower than that in branched PEI (25K) [164].

In another study by Xu et al., functional hydroxyl groups on the outside surfaces of CDs was used as initiation sites for growing cationic branches. In this work, bromoisobutyryl-terminated β-CD was prepared and used to polymerize 2-(dimethylamino)ethyl methacrylate via atom transfer radical polymerization (ATRP). This star-shaped cationic polymer containing the CD core and poly(2-(dimethylamino)ethyl methacrylate) (P(DMAEMA)) arms formed complexes with pDNA. In comparison with P(DMAEMA), the star-shaped cationic polymer showed lower cytotoxicity and higher gene transfection efficiency [165].

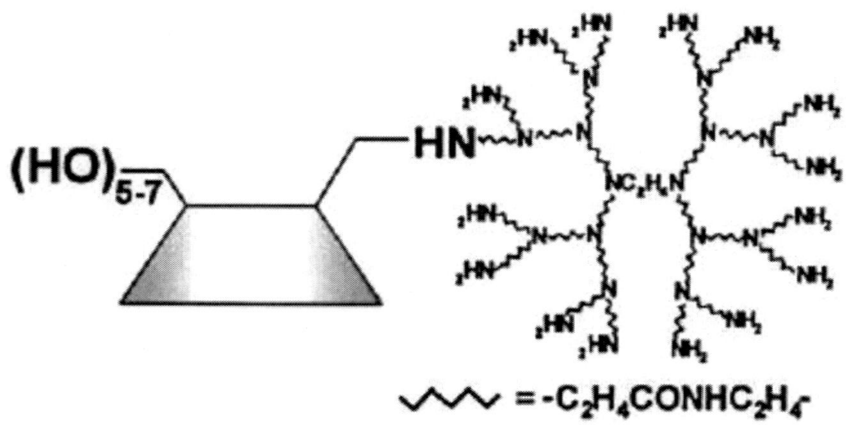

Figure 5. Chemical structure of CDE conjugates. Reprinted with the permission of Ref [163].

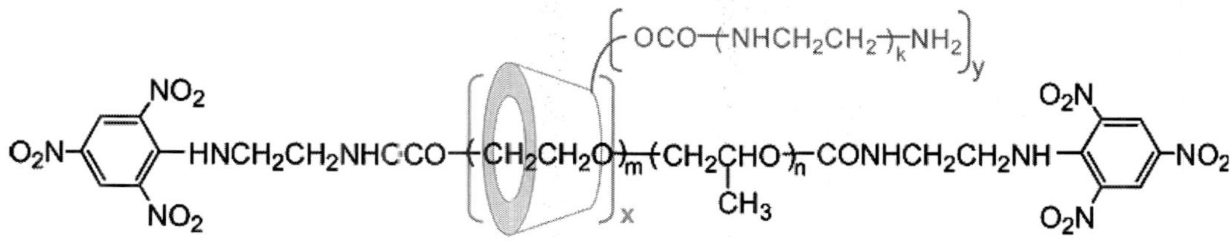

Figure 6. Cationic polyrotaxanes containing OEI-grafted α-CD rings and poly[(ethylene oxide)-*ran*-(propylene oxide)] chain. Reprinted with the permission of Ref [166].

In all of the above examples, CDs reduced the cytotoxicity and enhanced the gene transfection efficiency of cationic polymers. In fact, these effects will lead to the further application of CDs in gene therapy.

In comparison to the common cationic polymers containing long sequences of covalently bonded repeating units [127], cationic polyrotaxanes (Figure 6) have been designed for gene delivery by threading multiple cationic CDs upon a polymer chain. These cationic supramolecules show DNA binding ability, low cytotoxicity, and high gene transfection efficiency.

Oligoethylenimine-grafted *β*-CDs threaded on a PEO–PPO–PEO triblock copolymer, for example, were synthesized by Li et al. In this polyrotaxane, poly(propylene oxide) (PPO) parts were covered with *β*-CD molecules, while poly(ethylene oxide) (PEO) parts were free of complexation. This concept provided some free space for *β*-CD rings to move along both PPO and PEO parts in solution, allowing more efficient grafting of oligoethylenimine (OEI) to *β*-CD because a dense coverage of *β*-CD on the polymer might be unfavorable to the grafting reaction. Resulting cationic polyrotaxane showed high gene transfection efficiency because the system has a lot of OEI chains including many primary and secondary amines [167].

Conclusion

Recent progresses in construction of CD-polymers have opened new opportunities for designing novel drug and gene delivery systems with improved properties compared to conventional polymeric systems. Hydrogels with CDs as building blocks have attracted considerable attention for their promising application in drug delivery systems. CD-hydrogels are capable of forming complex with peptides and proteins such as cyclosporin, insulin, human growth hormone and other drug molecules. Polyrotaxanes with several CD rings threaded on a polymer chain capped with cleavable chain stoppers can be used as multivalent carrier for drug and biological active molecules. Each CD in the backbone of polyrotaxane has several hydroxyl or other functional groups that drug molecules can be conjugated to them. CD containing cationic polymers as gene delivery vectors showed reduced cytotoxicity and enhanced gene transfection efficiency than cationic polymeric systems without CD. In addition to CD containing cationic polymers, cationic polyrotaxanes composed of multiple cationic CDs threaded upon a polymer chain have been designed as new gene delivery vectors. These cationic supramolecules revealed DNA binding ability, low cytotoxicity, and high gene transfection efficiency.

References

[1] Jazkewitsch, O.; Ritter, H. *Macromolecules* 2011, 44, 375–382.

[2] Xing, H.; Zhou, H-T.; Yu, H-Q.; Gou, Z-M.; Xiao, J-X. *J. Chem. Eng. Data* 2011, 56, 1423–1432.

[3] Tsai, C-C.; Leng, S.; Jeong, K-U.; Horn, R M. V.; Wang, C-L.; Zhang, W-B.; Graham, M. J.; Huang, J.; Ho, R-M.; Chen, Y.; Lotz, B.; Cheng, S Z. D. *Macromolecules* 2010, 43, 9454–9461.

[4] Chen, X.; Parker, S. G.; Zou, G.; Su, W.; Zhang, Q. *Acs. Nano* 2010, 4, 6387–6394.

[5] Fernandez-Garcia, E.; Carvajal-Lerida, I.; Rincon, F.; Rios, J. J.; Perez-galvez, A. *J. Agric. Food Chem.* 2010, 58, 3213–3221.

[6] Szejtli, J. *Chem. Rev.* 1998, 98, 1743-1753.

[7] Yuan, H-N.; Yao, S-J.; Shen, L-Q.; Mao, J-W. *Ind. Eng. Chem. Res.* 2009, 48, 5070–5078.

[8] Zou, C-J.; Wu, H-m.; Ma, L. *J. Chem. Eng. Data* 2010, 55, 2935–2937.

[9] Crupi, V.; Majolino, D.; Venuti, V. *J. Phys. Chem. A* 2010, 114, 6811–6817.

[10] Arun, R.; Ashok, K C. K.; Sravanthi, V. V. N. S. S. *Sci Pharm.* 2008, 76, 567–598.

[11] Hashemianzadeh, S M.; A. Rafati, A.; B. Nojini, Z. *Monatsh Chem.* 2008, 139, 763–771.

[12] Masson, M.; Loftsson, T.; Masson, G.; Stefansson, E. *Journal of Controlled Release.* 1999, 59, 107–118.

[13] Kralova, J.; Kejık, Z.; Brıza, T.; Pouckova, P.; Kral, A.; Martasek, P.; Kral, V. *J. Med. Chem.* 2010, 53, 128–138.

[14] Wenz, G.; Krauter, I.; Sackmann, E. *Journal of Polymer Science: Part A: Polymer Chemistry* 2009, 47, 6229–6230.

[15] Hedges, AR. *Chem Rev.* 1998, 98, 2035–2044.

[16] L. Carrier, R.; A. Miller, L.; Ahmed, I. *Journal of Controlled Release* 2007, 123, 78–99.

[17] Higuchi, T.; Connors, KA. *Adv. Anal. Chem. Instrum.* 1965, 7, 117–212.

[18] Del Valle, E.M M. *Process Biochemistry.* 2004, 39, 1033–1046.

[19] Mura, P.; Corti, G.; Maestrelli, F.; Cirri, M. *J. Incl. Phenom. Macrocycl. Chem.* 2007, 59, 307–313.

[20] Loftssona, T.; Jarvinen, T. *Advanced Drug Delivery Reviews* 1999, 36, 59–79.

[21] L. Loukas, Y.; Vraka, V.; Gregoriadis, G. *International Journal of Pharmaceutics* 1998, 162, 137–142.

[22] Shimpi, S.; Chauhan, B.; Shimpi, P. *Acta Pharm.* 2005, 55, 139–156.

[23] K. Roy, A.; Guillory, J. K. *International Journal of Pharmaceutics* 1996, 138, 37-43.

[24] Challa, R.; Ahuja, A.; Ali, J.; Khar, R.K. *AAPS Pharm. Sci. Tech.* 2005, 6, 329-357.

[25] Fox, M. E.; Guillaudeu, S.; Frechet, J M. J.; Jerger, K.; Macaraeg, N.; Szoka, F. C. *Molecular Pharmaceutics* 2009, 6, 1562–1572.

[26] Bugreev, D. V.; Nevinsky, G. A. *Biochemistry* (Moscow) 2009, 74, 1467-1481.

[27] P. Rivory, L.; Chatelut, E.; Canal, P.; Mathieu-BouÃ, A.; Robert, *J. Cancer Res.* 1994, 54, 6330-6333.

[28] Kang, J.; Kumar, V.; Yang, D.; Roy Chowdhury, P.; J. Hohl, R. *European Journal of Pharmaceutical Sciences* 2002, 15, 163–170.

[29] Utsuki, T.; Hirayama, F.; Uekama, K. *J. Chem. Soc.*, Perkin Trans. 1993, 2, 109-114.
[30] Nagase, Y.; Hirata, M.; Wada, K.; Arima, H.; Hirayama, F.; Irie, T.; Kikuchi, M.; Uekama, K. *Int. J. Pharm.* 2001, 229, 163-172.
[31] Kang, J.; Kumar, V.; Yang, D.; Chowdhury, PR.; Hohl, RJ. *Eur. J. Pharm. Sci.* 2002, 15, 163-170.
[32] Ma, DQ.; Rajewski, RA.; Velde, DV.; Stella, VJ. *J. Pharm. Sci.* 2000, 89, 275-287.
[33] Singla, AK.; Garg, A.; Aggarwal, D. *Int. J. Pharm.* 2002, 235, 179-192.
[34] Makoid, M. C. *Basic Pharmacokinetics*. http://kiwi.creighton.edu/pkinbook/. 1996-1999.
[35] Gamsiz, E D.; Miller, L.; G. Thombre, A.; Ahmed, I.; Lyn Carrier, R *Biotechnology and Bioengineering* 2010, 105, 409-420.
[36] Klein, S. *ACS Symp. Ser.* 2010, 1017, 13-30.
[37] Ajavon, A. D.; Taft, D. R. *Preclinical Drug Development* 2009, 187, 71-116.
[38] Loftsson, T.; E. Brewster, M.; Masson, M. *Am. J. Drug Deliv.* 2004, 2, 1-15.
[39] Szejtli, J. *Pure Appl. Chem.* 2004, 76, 1825-1845.
[40] Manakker, F v d.; Vermonden, T.; Nostrum, C F. v.; E. Hennink, W. *Biomacromolecules* 2009, 10, 3157-3175.
[41] Auzely-Velty, R.; Djedaini-Pilard, F.; Desert, S.; Perly, B.; Zemb, Th. *Langmuir* 2000, 16, 3727-3734.
[42] Silva, O. F.; A. Fernandez, M.; L. Pennie, S.; R. Gil, R.; H. de Rossi, R. *Langmuir* 2008, 24, 3718-3726.
[43] Adeli, M.; Zarabi, A.; Vosoughi, M. *Macromolecular Bioscience* 2011, 11, 383-390.
[44] Chen, J.; Rong, L.; Lin, H.; Xiao, R.; Wu, H. *Materials Chemistry and Physics* 2009, 116, 148–152.
[45] Li, J.; Li, X.; Ni, X.; Wang, X.; Li, H.; W. Leong, K. *Biomaterials* 2006, 27, 4132–4140.
[46] Peppas, N.A.; Khare, A.R. *Advanced Drug Delivery Reviews* 1993, 11, 1–35.
[47] Deligkaris, K.; Tadele, T S.; Olthuis, W.; van den Berg, A. *Sensors and Actuators* B 2010, 147, 765–774.
[48] Moya-Ortega, M. D.; Alvarez-Lorenzo, C.; H. Sigurdsson, H.; Concheiro, A.; Loftsson, T. *Carbohydrate Polymers* 2010, 80, 900–907.
[49] Uekama, K. *Chem. Pharm. Bull.* 2004, 52, 900–915.
[50] Liu, Y -Y.; Fan, X.-D. *Biomaterials* 2005, 26, 6367–6374.
[51] dos Santos, J.-F.R.; Couceiro, R.; Concheiro, A.; Torres-Labandeira, J-J.; Alvarez-Lorenzo, C. *Acta Biomaterialia* 2008, 4, 745–755.
[52] Cesteros, L. C.; Ramırez, C. A.; Pecina, A.; Katime, I. *Macromol. Chem. Phys.* 2007, 208, 1764–1772.
[53] Salmaso, S.; Semenzato, A.; Bersani, S.; Matricardi, P.; Rossi, F.; Caliceti, P. *Int. J. Pharm.* 2007, 345, 42–50.
[54] Xu, J.; Li, X.; Sun, F. *Acta Biomaterialia* 2010, 6, 486–493.
[55] Yao, W-J.; Sun, K-X.; Liu, Y.; Liang, N.; Mu, H-J.; Yao, C.; Liang, R C.; Wang, A-P. *Biol. Pharm. Bull.* 2010, 33, 1371-1377.
[56] A. Zawko, S.; Truong, Q.; E. Schmidt, C. *Journal of Biomedical Materials Research Part A* 2008, 87A, 1044-1052.
[57] Fraser, J. R. E.; Laurent, T. C.; Laurent, U. B. G. *Journal of Internal Medicine* 1997, 242, 27-33.

[58] Wang, H-D.; Chu, L-Y.; Yu, X-Q.; Xie, R.; Yang, M.; Xu, D.; Zhang, J.; Hu, L. *Ind. Eng. Chem. Res.* 2007, 46, 1511-1518.

[59] Komori, K.; Takada, K.; Tatsuma, T. *Anal. Sci.* 2005, 21, 351-353.

[60] Chu, L. Y.; Li, Y.; Zhu, J. H.; Chen, W. M. *Angew. Chem., Int.* Ed. 2005, 44, 2124-2127.

[61] Xiao, X. C.; Chu, L. Y.; Chen, W. M.; Wang, S.; Xie, R. *Langmuir* 2004, 20, 5247-5253.

[62] Chu, L. Y.; Niitsuma, T.; Yamaguchi, T.; Nakao, S. *AIChE J.* 2003, 49, 896-909.

[63] Chu, L. Y.; Park, S. H.; Yamaguchi, T.; Nakao, S. *Langmuir* 2002, 18, 1856-1864.

[64] Chu, L. Y.; Park, S. H.; Yamaguchi, T.; Nakao, S. *J. Membrane Sci.* 2001, 192, 27-39.

[65] Ogawa, K.; Wang, B.; Kokufuta, E. *Langmuir* 2001, 17, 4704-4707.

[66] Choi, Y. J.; Yamaguchi, T.; Nakao, S. *Ind. Eng. Chem. Res.* 2000, 39, 2491-2495.

[67] Dincer, S.; Turk, M.; Piskin, E. *Gene Therapy* 2005, 12, S139–S145.

[68] Yoshinari, E.; Furukawa, H.; Horie, K. *Polymer* 2005, 46, 7741-7748.

[69] Kato, N.; Sakai, Y.; Shibata, S. M*acromolecules* 2003, 36, 961-963.

[70] Xiao, X. C.; Chu, L. Y.; Chen, W. M.; Wang, S.; Li, Y. *AdV. Funct. Mater.* 2003, 13, 847-852.

[71] Chu, L. Y.; Li, Y.; Zhu, J. H.; Wang, H. D.; Liang, Y. J. *Controlled Release* 2004, 97, 43-53.

[72] Marshall, A. J.; Blyth, J.; Davidson, C. A. B.; Lowe, C. R. *Anal. Chem.* 2003, 75, 4423-4431.

[73] Hamidi, M.; Azadi, A.; Rafiei, P *Advanced Drug Delivery Reviews* 2008, 60, 1638–1649.

[74] Liu, Y-Y.; Fan, X-D. *Polymer* 2002, 43, 4997–5003.

[75] Nozaki, T.; Maeda, Y.; Kitano, H. *J. Polym. Sci. A, Polym. Chem.* 1997, 35, 1535–1541.

[76] Nozaki, T.; Maceda, Y.; Ito, K.; Kitano, H. *Macromolecules* 1995, 28, 522–524.

[77] Hirasawa, T.; Maeda, Y.; Kitano, H. *Macromolecules* 1998, 31, 4480–4485.

[78] Abu Hashim, I. I.; Higashi, T.; Anno, T.; Motoyama, K.; Abd-ElGawad, A-E H.; H. El-Shabouri, M.; Borg, T M.; Arima, H. *International Journal of Pharmaceutics* 2010, 392, 83–91.

[79] van de Manakker, F.; Vermonden, T.; Morabit, N.; F. van Nostrum, C.; E. Hennink, W. *Langmuir* 2008, 24, 12559-12567.

[80] Huh, K M.; Ooya, T.; Lee, W K.; Sasaki, S.; Kwon, I C.; Jeong, S Y.; Yui, N. *Macromolecules* 2001, 34, 8657-8662.

[81] Koopmans, C.; Ritter, H. *Macromolecules* 2008, 41, 7418-7422.

[82] Mislovicova, D.; Kogan, G.; Gosselet, N. M.; Sebille, B.; Soltes, L. *Chem. BiodiVersity* 2007, 4, 52-57.

[83] Amiel, C.; Moine, L.; Sandier, A.; Brown, W.; David, C.; Hauss, F.; Renard, E.; Gosselet, M.; Sebille, B. *ACS Symp. Ser.* 2001, 780, 58-81.

[84] Sandier, A.; Brown, W.; Mays, H.; Amiel, C. *Langmuir* 2000, 16, 1634-1649.

[85] Wenz, G.; Weickenmeier, M.; Huff, J. *ACS Symp. Ser.* 2000, 765, 271-283.

[86] Weickenmeier, M.; Wenz, G.; Huff, J. *Macromol. Rapid Commun.* 1997, 18, 1117-1123.

[87] Harada, A.; Hashidzume, A.; Yamaguchi, H.; Takashima, Y. *Chem. Rev.* 2009, 109, 5974–6023.

[88] Yin, J.; Dasgupta, S.; Wu, *J. Org. Lett.* 2010, 12, 1712-1715.

[89] Fang, L.; Olson, M. A.; Benitez, D.; Tkatchouk, E.; Goddart, W. A.; Stoddart, J. F. *Chem. Soc. Rev.* 2010, 39, 17–29.

[90] Wenz, G.; Han, B-H.; Muller, *A. Chem. Rev.* 2006, 106, 782-817.

[91] Okada, M.; Harada, A. *Macromolecules* 2003, 36, 9701-9703.

[92] He, L.; Huang, J.; Chen, Y.; Liu, L. *Macromolecules* 2005, 38, 3351-3355.

[93] Davis, M.; Belloco, N. *Journal of Inclusion Phenomena and Macrocyclic Chemistry* 2002, 44, 17-22.

[94] Li, J.; Loh, X-J. *Advanced Drug Delivery Reviews* 2008, 60, 1000–1017.

[95] Ooya, T.; Mori, H.; Terano, M.; Yui, N. *Macromol. Rapid Commun.* 1995, 16, 259–263.

[96] Chen, y.; Dong, C-M. *J. Phys. Chem.* B 2010, 114, 7461–7468.

[97] Nasongkla, N.; Shuai, X.; Ai, H.; Weinberg, BD.; Pink, J.; Boothman, DA.; Gao, J. *Angew. Chem. Int. Ed.* 2004, 43, 6323–6327.

[98] Shuai, X.; Ai, H.; Nasongkla, N.; Kim, S.; Gao, J. *J. Control Release* 2004, 98, 415–426.

[99] Yoo, HS.; Park, TG. *J. Control Release* 2004, 100, 247–256.

[100] Lee, ES.; Na, K.; Bae, YH. *J. Control Release* 2005, 103, 405–418.

[101] Kim, SY.; Lee, YM. *Biomaterials* 2001, 22, 1697–1704.

[102] Cho, Y.W.; Lee, J.; Lee, S.C.; Huh, K.M.; Park, K. *J. Control. Release* 2004, 97, 249–257.

[103] Shuai, X.; Merdan, T.; Schaper, AK.; Xi, F.; Kissel, T. *Bioconjug. Chem.* 2004, 15, 441–448.

[104] Liu, S.; Tong, Y.; Yang, Y. *Mol. Biosyst.* 2005, 1, 158–165.

[105] Han, L.; Guo, J.; Zhang, L.; Wang, Q.; Fang, X. *Acta Pharm. Sinica* 2006, 6, 747–756.

[106] Huh, K.M.; Min, H.S.; Lee, S.C.; Lee, H.J.; Kim, S.; Park, K. J. *Control. Release* 2008, 126, 122–129.

[107] Zhang, C.; Qu, G.; Sun, Y.; Wu, X.; Yao, Z.; Guo, Q.; Ding, Q.; Yuan, S.; Shen, Z.; Ping, Q.; Zhou, H. *Biomaterials* 2008, 29, 1233–1241.

[108] Forrest, M.L.; Yanez, J.A.; Remsberg, C.M.; Ohgami, Y.; Kwon, G.S.; Davies, N.M. *Pharm. Res.* 2008, 25, 194–206.

[109] Musacchio, T.; Laquintana, V.; Latrofa, A.; Trapani, G.; Torchilin, V.P. *Molecular Pharmaceutics* 2008, 6, 468–479.

[110] Yang, X.; Deng, W.; Fu, L.; Blanco, E.; Gao, J.; Quan, D.; Shuai, X. *J. Biomed. Mater Res. A.* 2008, 86, 48-60.

[111] Nasongkla, N.; Bey, E.; Ren, J.; Ai, H.; Khemtong, C.; Guthi, J S.; Chin, S-F.; Sherry, A. D.; Boothman, D.A.; Gao, J. *Nano Lett.* 2006, 6, 2427-2430.

[112] Lavasanifar, A.; Samuel, J.; Kwon, G. S. *Advanced Drug Delivery Reviews* 2002, 54, 169–190.

[113] Hu, Z.; Luo, F.; Pan, Y.; Hou, C.; Ren, L.; Chen, J.; Wang, J.; Zhang, Y. *J. Biomed. Mater Res. A.* 2008, 85, 797-807.

[114] Gillies, E. R.; Frechet, J.M.J. *Bioconjugate Chem.* 2005, 16, 361-368.

[115] Wu, X L.; Kim, J H.; Koo, H.; Bae, S M.; Shin, H.; Kim, M S.; Lee, B-H.; Park, R-W.; Kim, I-S.; Choi, K.; Kwon, I C.; Kwangmeyung, K.; Lee, D S. *Bioconjugate Chem.* 2010, 21, 208–213.

[116] Danhier, F.; Magotteaux, N.; Ucakar, B.; Lecouturier, N.; Marcus, B.; Préat, V. *European Journal of Pharmaceutics and Biopharmaceutics* 2009, 73, 230–238.
[117] Kim, J-H.; Emoto, K.; Iijima, M.; Nagasaki, Y.; Aoyagi, T.; Okano, T.; Sakurai, Y.; Kataoka, K. *Polym. Adv. Technol.* 1999, 10, 647-654.
[118] Svenson, S. *ACS Symp. Ser.* 2006, 923, 2-11.
[119] Zhang, J.; Sun, H.; X. Ma, P. *ACS NANO* 2010, 4, 1049–1059.
[120] (a) Gou, P-F.; Zhu, W-P.; Shen, Z-Q. *Biomacromolecules* 2010, 11, 934–943. (b) Adeli, M.; Zarnegar, Z.; Kabiri, R. *Eur. Polym. J.* 2008, 44, 1921-1930.
[121] Pasut, G.; Veronese, F.M. *Prog. Polym. Sci.* 2007, 32, 933–961.
[122] Moon, C.; Kwon, Y M.; Lee, W K.; Park, Y J.; Chang, L-C.; C. Yang, V. *J. Biomed. Mater Res. A.* 2008, 84, 238-246.
[123] Svenson, S. *European Journal of Pharmaceutics and Biopharmaceutics* 2009, 71, 445–462.
[124] Li, J.; Xiao, H.; Li, J.; Zhong, Y. *International Journal of Pharmaceutics* 2004, 278, 329–342.
[125] Liu, Y.; You, C-C.; Zhang, H-Y.; Kang, S-Z.; Zhu, C-F.; Wang, C. *Nano Lett.* 2001, 1, 613-616.
[126] Ndinguri, M. W.; Solipuram, R.; Gambrell, R. P.; Aggarwal, S.; Hammer, R. P. *Bioconjugate Chem.* 2009, 20, 1869–1878.
[127] Quan, C-Y.; Chen, J-X.; Wang, H-Y.; Li, C.; Chang, C.; Zhang, X-Z.; Zhuo, R-X. *Acs. Nano* 2010, 4, 4211–4219.
[128] Sunderland, C. J.; Steiert, M.; Talmadge, J. E.; Derfus, A. M.; Barry, S. E. *Drug Development Research* 2006, 67, 70–93.
[129] Gullotti, E.; Yeo, Y. *Molecular Pharmaceutics* 2009, 6, 1041–1051.
[130] Shi, J.; Votruba, A. R.; Farokhzad, O. C.; Robert, L. *Nano Lett.* 2010, 10, 3223–3230.
[131] Adair, J. H.; Parette, M. P.; Altınoglu, E. I.; Kester, M. *Acs. Nano* 2010, 4, 4967–4970.
[132] Singh, P.; Gupta, U.; Asthana, A.; Jain, N. K. *Bioconjugate Chem.* 2008, 19, 2239–2252.
[133] Duncan, R. Nature Publishing Group 2006, 6, 688–701.
[134] Li, J.; Loh, X. J. *Advanced Drug Delivery Reviews* 2008, 60, 1000–1017.
[135] Ooya, T.; Yui, N. *Journal of Controlled Release* 1999, 58, 251–269.
[136] (a) Adeli, M.; Kalantari, M.; Sadeghi, E.; Mahmoudi, M. *Nanomedicine: Nanotechnology, Biology and Medicine* 2011, In Press. (b) Adeli, M.; Hakimpour, F.; Sagvand, M.; Jaafari, M. R.; Kabiri, R.; Moshari, Z. *Supramolecular Chemistry* 2011, 23, 411-418.
[137] (a) Davis, M.E. *Advanced Drug Delivery Reviews* 2009, 61, 1189–1192. (b) Adeli, M.; Kalantari, M. *Polymer* 2011, Submitted.
[138] Wong, S.Y.; Pelet, J.M.; Putnam, D. *Prog. Polym. Sci.* 2007, 32, 799–837.
[139] Pawliuk, R.; Westerman, KA.; Fabry, ME.; Payen, E.; Tighe, R.; Bouhassira, EE. *Science* 2001, 294, 2368–2371.
[140] Burton, EA.; Glorioso, JC.; Fink, DJ. *Gene Ther.* 2003, 10, 1721–1727.
[141] von, Laer D.; Hasselmann, S.; Hasselmann, K. *J. Gene Med.* 2006, 8, 658–667.
[142] Wong, LF.; Goodhead, L.; Prat, C.; Mitrophanous, KA.; Kingsman, SM.; Mazarakis, ND. *Hum. Gene. Ther.* 2006, 17, 1–9.
[143] Menuel, S.; Fontanay, S.; Clarot, I.; Duval, R. E.; Diez, L.; Marsura, A. *Bioconjugate Chem.* 2008, 19, 2357–2362.

[144] Yang, C.; Li, H.; Goh, S H.; Li, *J. Biomaterials* 2007, 28, 3245–3254.
[145] Luo, D.; Saltzman, WM. *Nat. Biotechnol.* 2000, 18, 33–37.
[146] Smedt, S. C. D.; Demeester, J.; Hennink, W. E. *Pharm. Res.* 2000, 17, 113-126.
[147] Niidome, T.; Huang, L. *Gene Ther.* 2002, 9, 1647–1652.
[148] Pack, DW.; Hoffman, AS.; Pun, S.; Stayton, PS. *Nat. Rev. Drug Discov.* 2005, 4, 581–593.
[149] Hwang, S.J.; Bellocq, N.C.; Davis, M.E. *Bioconjugate Chem.* 2001, 12, 280-290.
[150] Bisht, H. S.; Manickam, D. S.; You, Y.; Oupicky, D. *Biomacromolecules* 2006, 7, 1169–1178.
[151] Wetering, P. V. D.; Moret, E. E.; Nieuwenbroek, N. M. E.; Steenbergen, M. J. V.; Hennink, W. E. *Bioconjugate Chem.* 1999, 10, 589–597.
[152] Agarwal, A.; Unfer, R.; Mallapragada, S. K. *J. Controlled Release* 2005, 103, 245–258.
[153] Xu, F. J.; Li, H. Z.; Li, J.; Zhang, Z. X.; Kang, E. T.; Neoh, K. G. *Biomaterials* 2008, 29, 3023–3033.
[154] Wagner, E.; Ogris, M.; Zauner, W. *AdV. Drug DeliVery ReV.* 1998, 30, 97–113.
[155] Dimitrova, M.; Arntz, Y.; Lavalle, P.; Meyer, F.; Wolf, M.; Schuster, C.; Haıkel, Y.; Voegel, J. C.; Ogier, *J. AdV. Funct. Mater.* 2007, 17, 233–245.
[156] Kukowska-Latallo, J. F.; Bielinska, A. U.; Johnson, J.; Spindler, R.; Tomalia, D. A.; Baker, J. R., Jr. *Proc. Natl. Acad. Sci. U.S.A.* 1996, 93, 4897–4902.
[157] Roy, K.; Mao, H. Q.; Leong, K. W. *Nat. Med.* 1999, 5, 387–391.
[158] Thanou, M.; Florea, B. I.; Geldof, M.; Junginger, H. E.; Borchard, G. *Biomaterials* 2002, 23, 153–159.
[159] Dekie, L.; Toncheva, V.; Dubruel, P.; Schacht, E. H.; Barrett, L.; Seymour, L. W. *J. Controlled Release* 2000, 65, 187-202.
[160] Wang, J.; Mao, H. Q.; Leong, K. W. *J. Am. Chem. Soc.* 2001, 123, 9480-9481.
[161] Wang, J.; Zhang, P.-C.; Lu, H.-F.; Ma, N.; Wang, S.; Mao, H.-Q.; Leong, K. W. *J. Controlled Release* 2002, 83, 157-168.
[162] Gonzalez, H.; Hwang, S.J.; Davis, M.E. *Bioconjug. Chem.* 1999, 10, 1068–1074.
[163] Arima, H.; Kihara, F.; Hirayama, F.; Uekama, K. *Bioconjugate Chem.* 2001, 12, 476-484.
[164] Yang, C.; Li, H.; Goh, S H.; Li, J. *Biomaterials* 2007, 28, 3245–3254.
[165] Xu, F. J.; Zhang, Z. X.; Ping, Y.; Li, J.; Kang, E. T.; Neoh, K. G. *Biomacromolecules* 2009, 10, 285–293.
[166] Yang, C.; Wang, X.; Li, H.; Goh, S H.; Li, J. *Biomacromolecules* 2007, 8, 3365-3374.
[167] Li, J.; Yang, C.; Li, H.; Wang, X.; Goh, S H.; Ding, J L.; Wang, D Y.; Leong, K. W. *Adv. Mater.* 2006, 18, 2969–2974.

In: Hybrid Nanostructures in Cancer Therapy
Editor: Mohsen Adeli
ISBN: 978-1-62100-517-9
© 2012 Nova Science Publishers, Inc.

Chapter III

Dendrimers and Cancer Therapy

Mohsen Adeli[1,2] and Masoumeh Hamid[1]
[1]Department of Chemistry, Faculty of Science, Lorestan University, Khoramabad, Iran
[2]Department of Chemistry, Sharif University of Technology, Tehran, Iran

Abstract

Dendrimers are generally described as macromolecules that are characterized by their extensively branched three dimensional structures which provide a high degree of surface functionality and versatility. The unique properties associated with dendrimers such as uniform size, high degree of branching, water solubility, multivalency, well-defined molecular weight and available internal cavities makes them attractive to use in nanomedicine.

Nanomedicine is explained as the application of nanotechnology to health. It exploits the improved and frequently novel physical, chemical, and biological properties of materials at the nanometric scale. Nanomedicine has potential impact on the prevention, early and reliable diagnosis and therapy of diseases. Nanomedicine encompasses the three interrelated subjects of:

- nanodiagnostics including imaging
- targeted drug delivery and controlled release
- regenerative medicine

Cancer is one of the most intricate diseases including a multitude of molecular and cellular processes, arising as the final result of a gradual accumulation of genetic changes caused by different factors in specific cells. A useful drug carrier system should have a high drug loading and suitable release properties together with long shelf-life and low toxicity [1].

Dendrimers are ideal delivery systems for unambiguous study of the effects of polymer properties including size, charge, and composition on the biologically relevant properties such as lipid bilayer interactions, cytotoxicity, internalization, blood plasma-retention time, biodistribution, and filtration [2].

1. Introduction

Dendrimers are a new generation of the nanosized, highly branched and three-dimensional polymers with compact spherical geometry in solution. Their name is taken from the Greek word "dendron", that means "tree" and refers to the distinctive tree-like organization of polymer units.

The unique properties associated with dendrimers such as monodisperse size, high functionality, water solubility, multivalency, well-known molecular weight and internal cavities make them suitable candidates for biomedical applications. The first works on the synthesis of dendrimers were started in the 1970s by Vögtle and co-workers, who studied the synthesis of dendritic arms initiated from a central core by repetitive reactions of mono- and diamines to obtain polymeric branching units with molecular cavities, but the first real dendrimer was synthesized and developed by Tomalia and his group, who explained the synthesis of polyamidoamines (PAMAMs) by iterative Michael reactions between methyl acrylate and ethylenediamine initiated from a central ammonia core to produce sequences of branched macromolecules named "starburst dendrimer" [3].

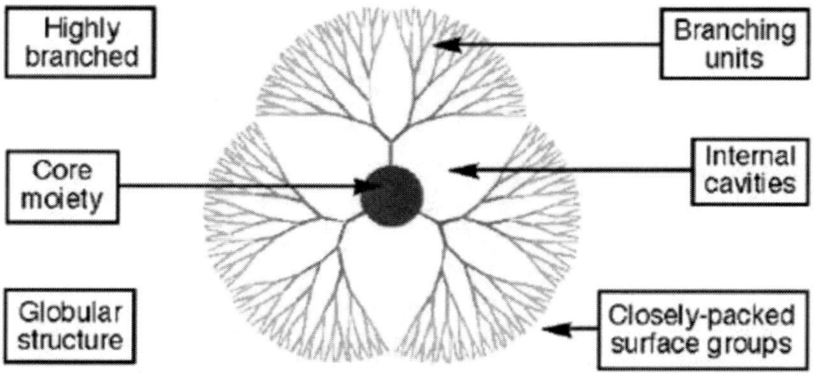

Figure 1. Structural characteristics of a dendritic macromolecule.

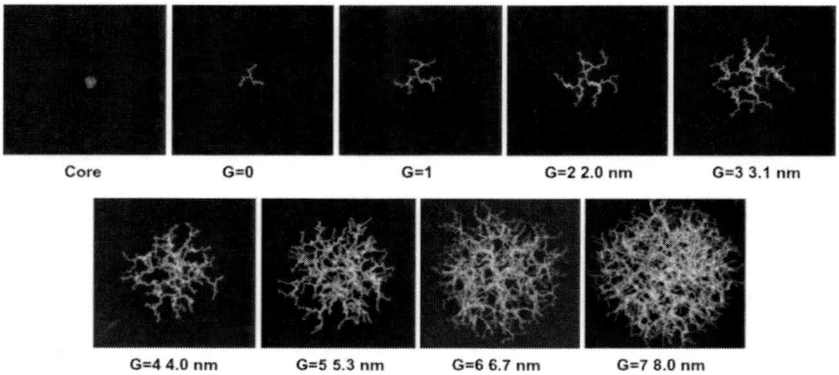

Figure 2. Graphical presentation of PAMAM dendrimers from core to generation G = 7 showing the linear increase in diameter and exponential growth of the number of surface groups. Reprinted with the permission of Ref. [2].

Dendrimers are created from several "wedges" or dendrons that are conjugated to a central core where each layer of branching units constitutes one complete generation (G) [2].

The type of synthesis strategy and structure leads to a controlled increase in a dendrimer's molarmass, size, and number of functional groups. Over the past four decades, several synthetic methods were developed to prepare dendrimers having special properties required for a variety of applications [2].

2. Dendrimers Chemistry,

Structure and Some Properties

The three classes of traditional macromolecular architectures including linear, cross-linked, and branched polymers are useful materials with polydispersity in their molecular weights and indefinite properties. In contrast, the synthesis of dendrimers suggests the opportunity to generate monodisperse, well-known structure similar to those observed inbiological systems or small molecules [2].

2.1. Types of Dendrimers

In the 1980s and 1990s research works were focused on the synthetic strategies of dendrimers and dendrimers with different designed functionalities and structures were become goals of particular academic and practical interest because of their unique super-branched architectures, high densities of external functionalities, symmetrical shapes, and monodispersity [4]. Some of the dendrimers having different functionalities are:

1. Liquid crystalline dendrimers
2. Tecto dendrimers
3. Chiral dendrimers
4. Hybrid dendrimers
5. Peptide dendrimers
6. Glycodendrimers
7. PAMAM dendrimer

2.2. Architecture and Composition

Grate different characteristics between dendrimers and linear polymers or their analogues come back to their synthetic procedures. As above mentioned the synthetic procedures of dendrimers result in macromolecules with nearly monodisperse molecular weight, tree-like shape, high functionality and other structural characteristics that cannot be found in linear polymers. Dendrimers are commonly synthesized by one of two strategies. A dendrimer can be grown outwards from a central multifunctional core, a process known as the divergent method developed by Tomalia and Newkome, or it can be synthesized by Fréchet's convergent method in which the dendrimer is synthesized from the periphery inwards, terminating at the core [5-8].

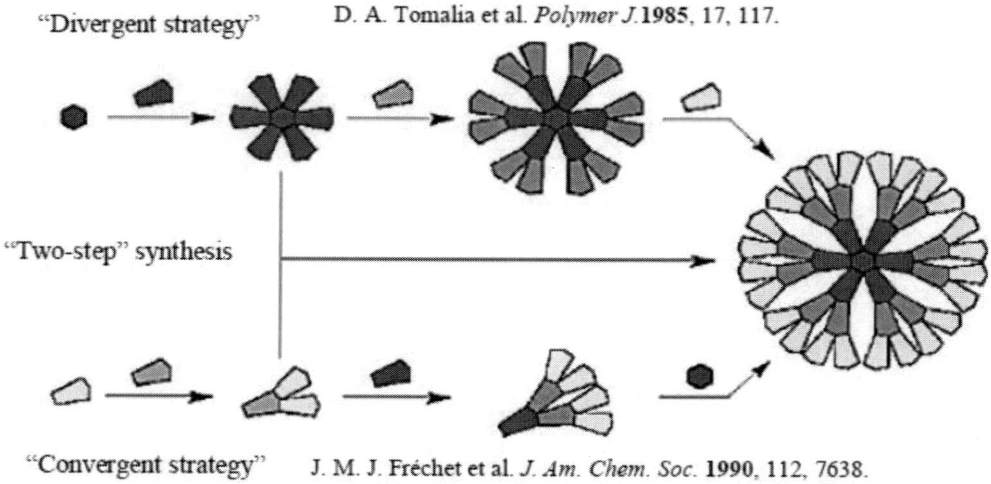

Figure 3. Two main strategies for synthesis of dendrimers.

Numerous research work recorder as patents and articles are performed on the characterization, modification and applications of PAMAM dendrimer, because PAMAM generations 0 through 10 (G_0-G_{10}) havinga broad number of peripheral groups (4 to 4096), variety of functional groups e.g. amine, carboxylic acid, hydroxyl with a wide range of molecular weights (657 to 935,000 g/mol) are commercially available now. Other dendritic molecules under active investigation are poly(propylene imine), poly(glycerol-co-succinic acid), poly(L-lysine), poly(glycerol), poly(2,2bis(hydroxymethyl)propionic acid), polycitric acid and melamine dendrimers.

2.3. Dendrimer-Membrane Interactions

It has been shown that large and cationic macromolecules can interact with the cell membranes to facilitate transport of biomolecules into cells. The interaction of a dendrimer or a dendritic structure with the memberane lipidic bilayer includes the formation of a vehicle with a lipidic bilayer hole around this structure. This mechanism was investigated for PAMAMs and it was also broadened to some linear and dendritic polycationic macro-moelcules that were applied for drug delivery applications, including poly-L-lysine (PLL), polyethylene imine (PEI) and diethylaminoethyl-dextran (DEAE-DEX) and it was compared with neutrally-charged polymers, involving polyvinyl alcohol (PVA) and polyethylene glycol (PEG). The enhanced permeability of the cell membrane against PAMAMs was assigned to their spherical structure promoting interactions between the dendrimer and lipid molecules. However all above cationic polymers were able to transfer through the cell membrane effectively and finally lead to the cell death.

Although membrane permeability may play a function in the cellular uptake of certain dendrimers, conventional styles of endocytotic internalization are attributed to the uptake of many dendrimers. Recently the effect of the structure of polymers with a potential application in the drug delivery systems on the rate and mechanism of cellular uptake of linear and branched PEIs and PAMAM (G_2, G_3, and G_4) dendrimers was investigated. It was shown that all three type polymers were internalized into the B16f10 melanoma cells through an adsorptive endocytosis pathway. The rate of uptake was as below:

PAMAM (G_4) > branched PEI> linear PEI> PAMAM (G_3) > PAMAM (G_2). Clearly the rate of internalization depends on the degree of branching in the PAMAM series [9].

The PAMAM (G_4) uptake rate was 130 fold greater than that for FITC-dextran. Branched PEI had the highest extracellular binding whereas for the linear PEI it was much lower. Unlike FITC-dextran, all cationic polymers didn't show a significant exocytosis over the time period studied. The PAMAM (G_4) and the branched PEI were predominately internalized by cholesterol-dependent pathways but internalization of linear PEI appeared to be independent of clathrin and cholesterol [10].

2.4. Properties of Dendrimers

2.4.1. Physicochemical Properties

As above described, compared to traditional classes of polymers including linear, branched and crosslinked types, dendrimers have unique chemical properties.

(1)Dendrimers generally have a molecular weight with narrow molecular weight distribution.

(2)Dendrimers have a controllable tree-like architecture and at higher generations they have a densely packed surface region surrounded by a large number of surface functional groups.

(3)There is a direct relationship between the size and generation number of dendrimers.

(4)There is a control on the structure and functionality of dendrimers.

(5)Dendrimers with low generation number are flexible and are not able to encapsulate small molecules while those with middle generation numbers have accessible cavities to encapsulate and transfer small molecules. In dendrimers with high generation number the internal cavity is not accessible due to the packed surface.

(6)Generally, the solubility property of dendrimers depends on their surface functional groups strongly.

2.4.2. Biological Properties

In order to use dendrimers for biomedical applications, they should achieve a minimum level of biological safety including low toxicity, biocompatibility, and immunogenicity testing. Using them as drug or gene delivery systems and upon administration they should also cross variety of barriers from blood stream to nucleolus. Structural characteristics dominate the biological properties of carrier systems. For example the surface functional groups dominate the water solubility and surface charge of dendrimers and therefore have a deep effect on their biodistribution, tolerance to enzymatic attack and their circulation time in the blood stream.

In the case of dendrimers, cytotoxicity has been found to be dose-and generation-dependent so that there is a direct relationship between their generation and toxicity. The type of functional groups has also a significant effect on the toxicity of dendrimers for example PAMAMs with primary amines are more toxic than secondary or tertiary amines or those having negative surface charge, anionic surface functional groups, significantly show lower cytotoxicity against Caco-2 cells than cationic dendrimers [11]. Loading capacity and interactions between dendrimers as host molecules and drugs as guest molecules strongly depends on the structure of dendrimers and specifically their core. It even affects the rate and type of release of drugs from dendrimers [12, 13]. Uptake mechanisms of nanostructures from the gastrointestinal area includes per sorption, endocytosis by enterocytes, paracellular transport, uptake by intestinal macrophages, and route through the break down associated lymphoid tissue. It has been found that uptake of lipidic dendrimers throughout the gastrointestinal tract is not uniform but there was a preferential uptake in the small intestine [14].

3. Nanomedicine Application

Dendrimers are the result of a synthetic strategy which is so called the "bottom-up" approach in nanotechnology. They have well-defined and tailored structure with a high versatility for different applications. Due to their high water solubility, in most cases, and high functionality and also their ability to transport small molecules through encapsulation or conjugation routes, dendrimers have been used for the deliveryof anticancer drugs and imaging agents in order to early cancer therapy or diagnosis [11, 13, 15].

3.1. Drug and Gene Delivery

A drug carrier candidate should have several advantages such as high loading capacity, well-defined size and structure, water solubility, high functionality and non-immunogenicity to be considered for *in vitro* and *in vivo* experiments. Dendrimers offer most of these advantages and can be considered as unique drug carrier agents. These advantages include: (1) Their nanosize range; (2) Monodispersity; (3) High number of functional groups with a high reactivity which can be modified by different molecules easily; (4) Rigid globular structure with high physical stability; (5) Well-defined structure that ensure reproductive pharmacokinetics; (6) Controllable size leading to versatility in biomedical applications; (7) High transport capacity due to their high ability to cross cell membranes;(8) High loading capacity which is the result of their high functionality; (9) Low immunogenicity compared tothe synthesized peptide carriers and natural protein carriers; (10) Ability for passive targeting of anticancer drugs to tumors due to the enhanced penetration and retention (EPR) effect of dendrimers; (11) Versatility of functional groups of dendrimers has caused well-established methodologies proposed to construct nanodevices with several functional moieties provide miscellaneous biomedical applications of these promising materials, like for example cancer targeting therapy, magnetic response imaging, photodynamic therapy, neutron capture therapy; (12) Perfectly programmed release of drugs or other bioactive agents from dendrimers leads to decreased toxicity, increased bioavailability and simplified dosing schedule; (13) Controllable surface charge leading to control on interactions between dendrimers and biomolecules; (14) Biodegradability and break down to the biocompatible materials in the destination organelles; (15) Favorable retention and biodistribution characteristics; (16) Appropriate bioavailability. In the case of dendrimers, the loading ability of drug molecules and other bioactive agents can be altered by varying dendrimer generations, the water solubility, biodistribution, circulation time in blood and therapeutic efficiency of drugs in dendrimer-based formulations can be tuned by varying dendrimer surface components, the release of drugs from dendrimer scaffolds can be controlled by using different degradable linkers between dendrimers and drugs, and the specific accumulation of the dendrimer-based therapeutics can be achieved by further modifying the dendrimers with targeting moieties. These properties together prove dendrimer perfect candidates in the design of new drug delivery systems [2, 11, 16-20].

Dendrimer-based transfection agents have become usual tools for many molecular and cell biologists but therapeutic delivery of nucleic acids remains a challenge. Recently it has been shown that dendrimer based gene delivery system also have significant potential in clinical trials [4]. Positive charged dendrimers interact with all forms of nucleic acids like for example DNA, RNA, and antisense oligonucleotides by electrostatic interaction to form complexes that condense/compact the nucleic acid. Upon complexation, the opened or extended configuration of the nucleic acid changed to a closed and a more compact configuration and the cationic dendrimer amines and the anionic nucleic acid phosphates reach the local charge neutralization resulting in the making of dendrimer–nucleic acid complexes ("dendriplexes"). The nature of the complex is not only depends on the stoichiometry and concentration of the DNA phosphates and dendrimer-amines but also on the bulk solvent properties (e.g. pH, salt concentration, buffer strength) and even the dynamics of mixing.

Due to the more fluid structure of smaller dendrimers such as PAMAM (G_2), it has been shown that they bind to nucleic acids better than the larger dendrimers such as PAMAM (G_6) with a more rigid and wrapped structure. In all cases, the formation of toroidal structures with a size around 45 nm was observed and dendriplexes consisting of intact PAMAM dendrimer and DNA, in particular higher generations, were found to have an affinity to create clusters rather than distinct units, in opposite of those complexes observed for the PEI and fractured PAMAMs. Size of dendriplexes was reduced with increasing the dendrimer/DNA ratios for the fractured PAMAMs [21].

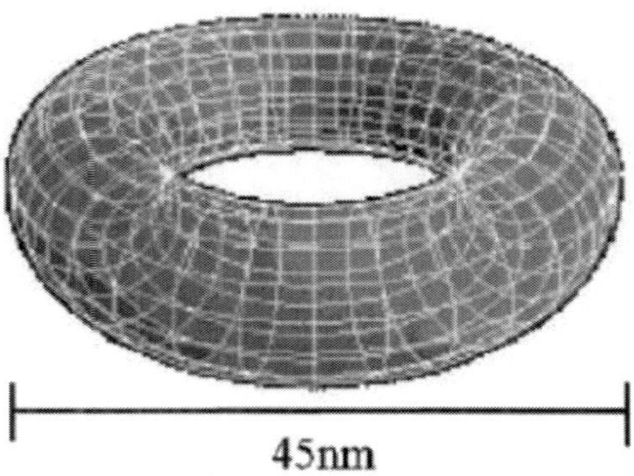

Figure 4. A "coiled globule" or "toroid" particle formed after multivalent cation–caused DNA condensation. Reprinted with the permission of Ref. [21].

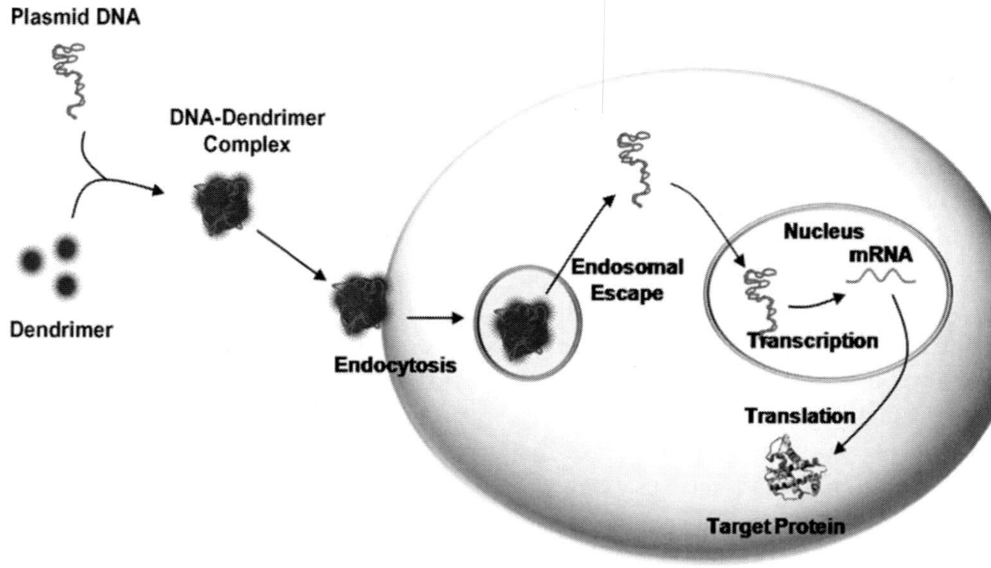

Figure 5. Proposed mechanism of gene transfection with dendritic gene carrier. Reprinted with the permission of Ref. [11].

A proposed mechanism for the gene transfection by non-viral vectors have been shown in figure 5. In the case of dendrimer carriers, the first step is the complexation of positively charged dendrimer and DNA with a negative charge and preparation of dendriplexes. Then dendriplexes cross the cell membrane and internalize into the cells through an endocytotic route. After passing the cell membrane and cytoplasm, they finally internalize into the cell nucleus which is the target compartment of the non-viralgene transfection [11, 22, 23, 24].

Therapeutic agents are delivered by dendrimers using noncovalent or covalent approaches. Noncovalent interactions between dendrimer and drugs such as encapsulation, hydrophobic-hydrophobic and electrostatic interactions dominate the quality of the first approach while in the second approach drugs conjugated to the functional groups covalently. Dendrimer-based drug delivery systems are designed to make better the pharmacokinetics and biodistribution of a drug and/or supply controlled release kinetics to the intended target.

3.1.1. Encapsulation of Drugs by Dendrimers

In the most cases encapsulation of anticancer drugs by dendrimers is performed to raise their water solubility and control their release in the target tumors. In a research work poly(glycerol succinic acid) dendrimers (PGLSA) were used to encapsulate and deliver camptothecins, a group of naturally-derived hydrophobic compounds having anticancer activity. PGLSA (G_4) with hydroxyl (G4-PGLSA-OH) or carboxylate (G4-PGLSA-COONa) functional groups were used to complex 10-hydroxycamptothecin (10-HCPT) for delivery to cancer cells.

Multi arm star block copolymers containing poly(γ-caprolactone) and PEG arms based on PAMAM dendrimers were synthesized and their micelles in aqueous solution was used to encapsulate anticancer drugs such as doxorubicin.

Medium-generation melamine-based dendrimers (i.e., G_4–G_6) have been shown to both enhance solubility and increase toxicity (lower IC50) of hydrophobic anti-cancer drugs by way of non-covalent encapsulation [9].

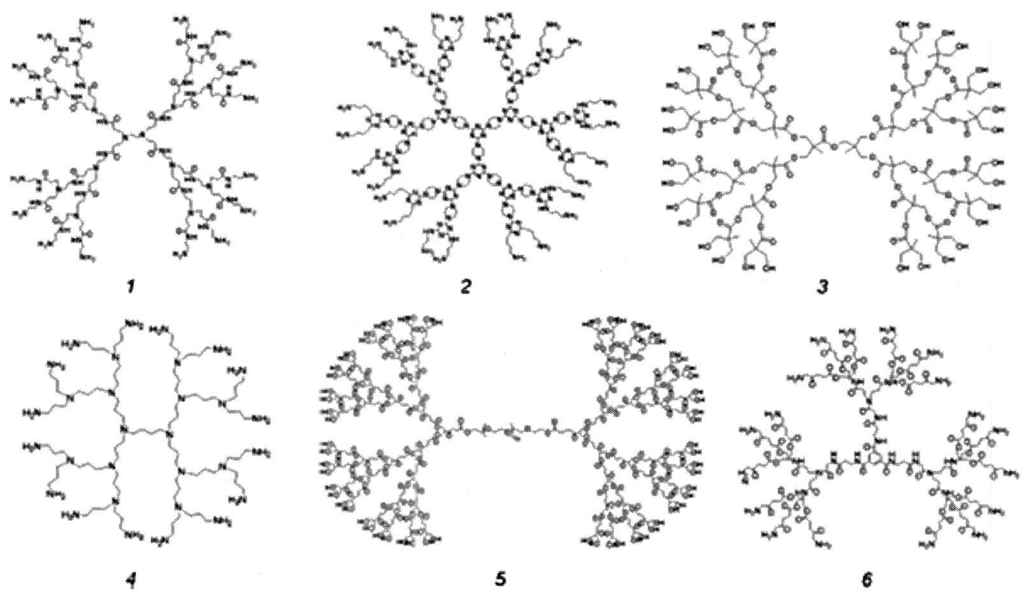

Figure 6. Most uses dendrimers as anticancer drug delivery systems. (1) PAMAM, (2) melamine-based dendrimer, (3) dendrimer based on 2, 2-bis (hydroxyl methyl) propionic acid, (4) polypropylene imine (PPI), (5) dendrimer based on glycerol and succinic acid with a PEG core, and (6) dendrimer based on 5-aminolaevulinic acid. Reprinted with the permission of Ref. [9].

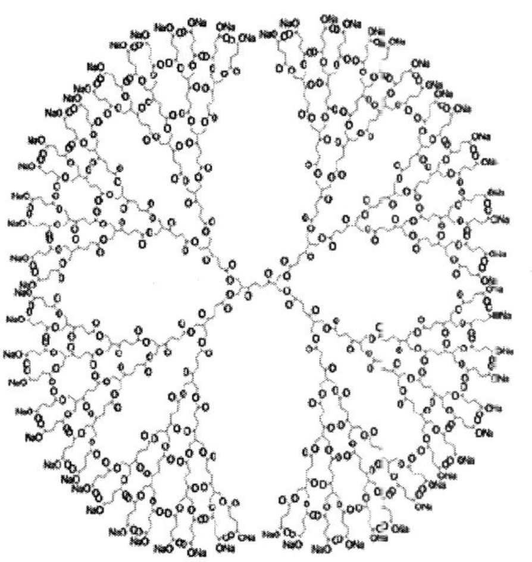

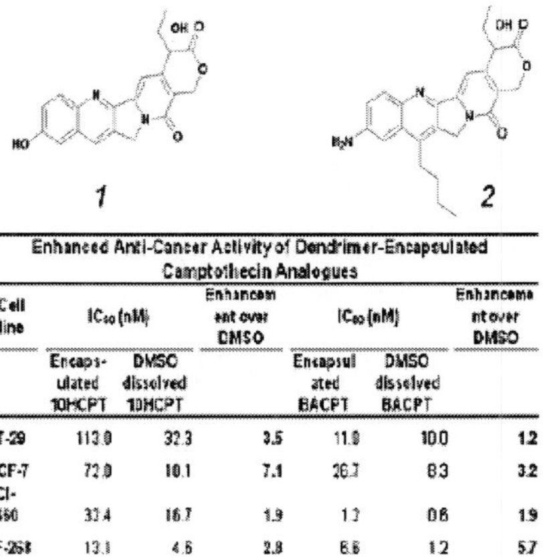

Enhanced Anti-Cancer Activity of Dendrimer-Encapsulated Camptothecin Analogues

Cell line	IC_{50} (nM) Encapsulated 10HCPT	IC_{50} (nM) DMSO dissolved 10HCPT	Enhancement over DMSO	IC_{50} (nM) Encapsulated BACPT	IC_{50} (nM) DMSO dissolved BACPT	Enhancement over DMSO
HT-29	113.0	32.3	3.5	11.8	10.0	1.2
MCF-7	72.0	10.1	7.1	26.3	8.3	3.2
NCI-H460	33.4	16.7	1.9	1.3	0.6	1.9
SF-268	13.1	4.6	2.8	6.6	1.2	5.7

Figure 7. Drug delivery via a dendrimer based on glycerol and succinic acid. Left, chemical structure of G4.5-PGLSA-COONa dendrimer. Right, chemical structures of (1) 10-hydroxycamptothecin, and (2) 7-butyl-10-aminocamptothecin with IC50 values for HT-29 colorectal adenocarcinoma, MCF-7 breast carcinoma, NCI-H460 large cell lung carcinoma, and SF-268 astrocytoma human cancer cell lines. Reprinted with the permission of Ref. [32].

Complexes of PAMAM dendrimers and poly(styrenesulfonate) (PAMAM/PSS) were prepared and used to selective encapsulation of drug into the dendrimers which are the core of these core/shell structures and therefore providing a dual release system of either two different drugs (i.e., drug cocktail) or of one drug released following two different time protocols (i.e., fast and sustained release). Doxorubicin hydrochloride was encapsulated by these systems and its release was studied [2, 25]. However due to the short age of the controlled drug release kinetics of these drug delivery systems, they are not suitable to inject in the blood vessels and active targeting to tumors.

PAMAM dendrimers with end hydroxyl functional groups with a lower cytotoxicity than those with end amino functional groups have been synthesized and used to complex small guest molecules with carboxyl functional groups. For example benzoic acid and 2, 6-dibromo-4-nitrophenol in 1/1 and 2/1 (drug/dendrimer) ratios were complexed by these systems while non-acidic drug tioconazole were not complexed [2]. A promising system that has been prepared and reported is PAMAM dendrimers/cisplatin complexes in which cisplatin has been complexed by PAMAM dendrimers. These systems exhibited slower release, higher accumulation in solid tumors, and lower toxicity compared to free cisplatin [26].

Adriamycin, methotrexate and 5-fluorouracil anticancer drugs were encapsulated and transferred by PEG functionalized PAMAMs (G_3 and G_4) [2, 27].

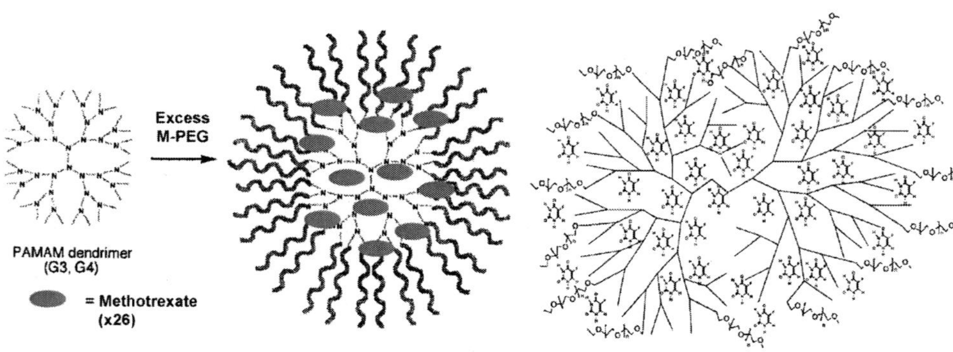

Figure 8. Schematic presentation of the encapsulation of anticancer drugs methotraxate (left) and 5-fluorouracil (right) into PEGylated generation 3 and 4 PAMAM dendrimers. Reprinted with the permission of Refs. [88, 89].

PEGylated PAMAMs revealed reasonable drug loading, and reduced release rate and hemolytic toxicity compared to the non-PEGylated dendrimer. It has been found that PAMAM dendrimers enhance the bioavailability of indomethacin in transdermal delivery applications [28]. Branched poly(l-glutamic acid) chains were centered around PAMAM dendrimers generations 2 and 3 and poly(ethylene imine) (PEI) cores to generate new biodegradable polymers with enhanced biodistribution and targeting ability.

They were terminated by PEG to enhance their biocompatibility, and conjugated with folic acid receptors to introduce cells specific targeting [2, 3, 29-37].

3.1.2. Drug-Dendrimer Conjugates

Due to the high functionality of dendrimers, they are able to deliver drugs with a high loading capacity through conjugation method. In this approach drugs are conjugated to the functional groups of dendrimers usually by esteric bonds. High loading capacity and partially controlled the release of the drugs by the nature of the covalent attachment are most important advantages of this method over the encapsulation method. Methotrexate has been conjugated to the carboxylic acid-terminated PAMAM ($G_{2.5}$) and amine-terminated PAMAM (G_3) and its activity against CCRF-CEM human leukemia and CHO Chinese hamster ovary cell lines has been investigated. Then it has been found that these conjugates reduce interactions with proteases and diminished drug release. It has been found that dendrimer-drug conjugates are promising materials for the treatment of cancer cells, particularly those that have demonstrated resistance to chemotherapeutics [9, 38].

An asymmetric doxorubicin-functionalized bow-tie dendrimeras a controlled release drug delivery system was synthesized by PEGylation of a 2, 2-bis(hydroxyl methyl)propionic acid dendrimer (G_3) in one side and conjugation of the drug via an pH sensitive acyl hydrazone linkage to the other side (G_4) leading to 8–10 wt.% doxorubicin content in drug delivery system. The drug content was release inside the cell through cleavage the pH sensitive linkage abruptly [9, 37].

A bow-tie structure in which two polyester dendrons are covalently conjugated together is also use as anticancer drug delivery system. In this system one dendron is highly functionalized and is used to deliver anticancer drugs with a high loading capacity while another is utilized for the attachment of PEG chains to increase the solubility and bioavailability of system. Linear-dendritic systems of PAMAM (G_4) and poly (styrenesulfonate) (PSS) are used to synthesize microcapsules as drug delivery systems [2, 15, 16, 35, 58, 59, 93].

In a research work paclitaxel was conjugated to PEG and PAMAM (G_4) and anticancer activity of conjugates was compared to evaluate the role of a linear and highly branched macromolecule in these systems [4, 35].

Clearly dendrimer-drug conjugates are promising systems to deliver anticancer drugs with a high loading capacity and with a sufficient bioavailability to achieve a therapeutic goal. The kinetic of the release of conjugated drugs depends on the nature of the chemical linkage binding the agent to the carrier. Dendritic structures and systems are created and evaluated to control of the release kinetics of conjugated drugs [3, 9, 29-37].

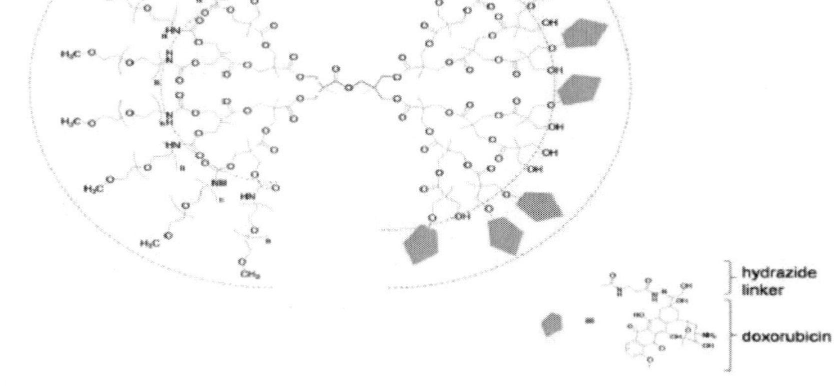
PEG Chains
• Increase plasma circulation time
• Sterically shield drug payload
• Enhances tumor uptake due to EPR effect
Conjugated Doxorubicin (DOX)
• Lower IC50 than free DOX
• Gradual hydrolytic release
• Increased DOX elimination half-life
hydrazide linker
doxorubicin

Figure 9. Doxorubicin-functionalized bow-tie dendrimer.PEGylated polyester dendrimer with tunable molecular weight, drug-loading, water solubility, pharmacokinetics, and biodistribution cures C-26 colon carcinomas in mice with one dose. Reprinted with the permission of Ref. [40].

3.2. Targeted Drug Delivery Systems Based on Dendrimers

Nowadays anticancer chemotherapeutics are not effective sufficiently in their ability to cure tumors and patients are not satisfied with them because of their nonspecific action leading to variety of the side effects. Delivery of the therapeutic agents to tumor cells selectively by suitable carriers has achieved credence as a promising way for treating cancer and offers a new strategy to both increased therapeutic index and reduced drug resistance. A carrier system has to have high functionality to couple multiple components like targeting molecule, drug and cancer imaging agent in order to be an effective targeting drug-delivery system [4].

The aim of drug delivery and targeting systems is to minimize drug nonspecific interactions, diminish side effects and killing healthy cells and increase the accumulation of the drug at the tumor site.

Targeting of the drugs to the tumor cells can be achieved by two mechanisms including "passive" or "active" targeting. An example passive targeting is the preferential accumulation of the chemotherapeutic agents in tumors due to the differences in the vascularization of the tumor tissue compared with healthy tissue. Active targeting includes the conjugation of the drug delivery systems by ligands enabling them to be selectively attached to the membrane of the cancer cells [1, 41].

3.2.1. Passive Targeting

Drug delivery systems based on dendrimers and dendritic polymers preferentially extravasate and accumulate in tumor tissue in a process so called enhanced permeability and retention (EPR) effect using the pathophysiological patterns of solid tumors, specifically their leaky vasculature. Several factors such as conformation, overall size, molecular weight, and also functional groups of dendrimers and dendritic polymers dominate the circulation time, transport beyond the endothelial barrier and uptake by RES and consequently determine the amount of accumulated drugs in the tumor tissue. El-Sayed et al. studied the effect of structural parameters such as size, molecular weight, and surface charge on the permeability of amino functionalized polyamidoamine, PAMAM-NH2 (G_0-G_4), dendrimers across epithelial and endothelial barriers [3].

Subsequently biodistribution of Gadolinium-functionalized dendrimers, G_2-NH_2 to G_{10}-NH_2, administered intravenously into normal mice was also studied [41, 42, 43].

3.2.2. Active Targeting

Polymer or dendrimer prodrugs can be targeted to tumor sites actively by means of conjugation of tumor-specific targeting ligands including vitamins, carbohydrate residues, peptides, or antibodies to their functional groups to mediate them to selectively bind to receptors over expressed on the surface of cancer cells and to bypass the nonspecific uptake with the RES systems and increase their net accumulation in cancer cells.

Folic acid (FA) has been extensively utilized as a targeting ligand for dendrimers-based drug delivery systems.

Dendrimer-based drug delivery systems with conjugated FA molecules to their functional groups show substantially higher accumulation and toxicity in tumor sites compared to nontargeted dendrimers and free anticancer drugs [44, 45, 46].

Variety of targeting ligands has been used to target dendrimers-based drug delivery systems to tumor sites and bond them to cancer-specific receptors. Neurotensin (NT) peptides are conjugated to dendrimers to produce NT-targeted dendrimers for targeting chlorin e6 (Che6) and MTX chemotherapeutic agents to different malignancies expressing the neurotensin receptor, that involve colon, pancreatic, prostate, and small-cell lungcarcinomas. Polyether-copolyester (PEPE) dendrimer-MTX inclusion complexes have been targeted to brain tumors using D-glucosamine ligands [48]. Tetramericavidin glycoproteins have been conjugated to the functional groups of dendrimers to bond them to target lectins differentially expressed on the surface of ovarian carcinoma cells [3]. For example J591 antibodies have been used to direct PAMAM dendrimers to the prostate-specific membrane antigen (PSMA), that is a glycoprotein expressed by all prostate cancer cells and supporting vasculature [9, 49].

Kinetics and quality of binding of dendrimers with conjugated cyclic Arg-Gly-Asp (RGD) ligands to the integrin receptors expressed solely during angiogenesis and there by present in high numbers in rapidly growing tumor capillaries has been studied. The same study was performed for dendrimers having FA ligand on their surface. Result of these studies suggests that dendrimers having targeting ligands are preferentially taken up with targeted cancer cells not as aresult of any increase in the endocytic rate but rather due to longer residence times of the conjugates on the cell surface [3, 9, 40, 49, 50-57].

However it was well found that the conjugation of special targeting ligands to dendrimers can lead to preferential distribution of the cargo in the targeted tissue or cells [50-58].

3.3. Imaging

Imaging of target tissues in body plays an increasingly significant role in disease detection and arrangement of therapy and surgery. Additionally, clinical works depend on imaging data to supply noninvasive and effective therapy [49]. Imaging is a promising way to be used in oncology to diagnose, locate, stage, plan treatment, and potentially find recurrence. Nanomaterials have been recognized as one of the most important tools for a successful imaging. Imaging using the advantages of the nanoscale carriers is a promising way to early recognize of tumors and cancer. In vivo imaging of these nanoscale systems can be achieved using various types of imaging techniques including single photon emission computed tomography (SPECT), positron emission tomography (PET), magnetic resonance imaging (MRI), fluorescence microscopy, computed tomography, and ultrasound.

Magnetic resonance imaging (MRI) and Computed tomography (CT) are two standard techniques of imaging associated with cancer diagnoses [9]. Although these methods are used to detect tumor sites abundantly but they are not effective to early detection of cancer cells and they are not able to detect tumors with a size less that a millimeter. Modification of these techniques using dendrimers has been led to promising results in the case of cancer diagnosis and therapy.

Complexes of Gadolinium (Gd) and different generations of dendrimers have been synthesized and used as contrast agents to recognize tumors and study their physiological behaviors. PAMAM dendrimers labeled by Gd have been used for investigating tumor vasculature and lymphatic involvement. Magnetic resonance imaging using G_8-Gd-PAMAM contrast agents showed that the permeability of vessel of SCCVII tumors increase after a single large dose of radiation treatment. The increased permeability of vessels of tumors is probably the result of reduced tumor interstitial pressure or increases in vascular permeability factor or vascular endothelial growth factor. The result of this study could be used to enhance the permeability of tumor vasculature to anti-cancer drug delivery systems [60, 61, 62].

The functional anatomy of the lymphatic system could be three-dimensionally imaged, explaining both normal and abnormal lymphatic and distinguishing between intra-lymphatic and extra-lymphatic involvement, using dendrimer based contrast agents leading to improved care as extralymphatic involvement may change during the chemotherapy regime. Gd-labeled G_6-PAMAM was accumulated in the sentinel lymph nodes, therefore it was used to recognize them that are generally imaged before surgery for breast cancer and melanoma [63]. Dendrimer-based Gadolinium MRI contrast agents with a low molecular weight (<60 kd) have been developed to overcome the prolonged retention times and toxicity of larger dendrimer and albumin MRI products [49].

Another type of Gd-dendrimer systems have been prepared through conjugation of Gadolinium contrast agents to different generations of polypropylene imine (PPI). Then these systems have been evaluated as macromolecular magnetic resonance contrast agents and it has been found that Gd-PPI systems with higher generations of PPI (G_3 and G_5) have lower limits of detection compared to those with lower generations of PPI (G_0 and G_1) but showed more slow diffusion into tumors. Blood vessels that their sizes was lower that a millimeter were imaged using these systems. Assemblies of polydiamidoproponoate and nucleic acid which is the complementary of oncogene mRNAs in tumor cells have been used as contrast agent for detection tumors. Complexation of several contrast paramagnetic ions to these assemblies enhanced their ability for imaging a signal generated from cells even with a few oncogene mRNAs [64].

As above mentioned Computed tomography (CT) has been developed by dendrimers as targeted delivery systems to improve retention times. Linear-dendritic copolymers consist of polyethylene glycol (PEG) with different molecular weights as linear block and different generations of poly(lysine) dendrimers (G_3–G_5) as dendritic blocks have been synthesized and used as iodinated contrast agents for possible tumor microvasculature CT imaging. Contrast agent based on linear-dendritic copolymer consist of G_4-poly(lysine) and PEG_{12000} showed good visualization in vivo of normal rat vasculature by a mono exponential blood half life of about 35 min, compared to more typical exhaustion times of 5 min for small molecule CT contrast agents.

In addition to above methods, fluorescent probes are usually used to recognize tumors as invasive procedure. In order to increase the efficacy of these fluorescent probes and also influence of their emission through the tissues they are delivered to tumors using targeted delivery systems such as G5-PAMAM dendrimers conjugated to folic acid [9].

As a result, dendritic polymers and copolymers have been found as promising agents in the area of molecular imaging having clear leads and many opportunities yet to be explored [2, 40, 63, 65-72].

4. Biocompatibility

The first characteristic for systems to be used in body is their biocompatibility. These systems should be non-toxic, non-immunogenic (except for vaccines), biopermeable (through barriers such as the intestines, the blood–tissue barriers and cell membranes), circulate in blood for a long time and able to target to desirable sites.

Like all other agents who are used in biological systems, the toxicity, biocompatibility and potential dangers of dendrimers should be examined. The toxicity and fate of all species of a drug delivery system based on dendrimer including drug molecules, antibody and dendrimer should be investigated by in vivo tests and final degradation or clearing from the body should be evaluated. PAMAMs are a type of dendrimers which their biocompatibility and cytotoxicity have been investigated better than other dendrimers. Short and long term experiments have been conducted to different cell lines and organs to find the bio-ompatibility of PAMAM dendrimers. In a comprehensive research work, the cytotoxicity and biocompatibility of different generations of PAMAM dendrimers with positive and negative surface charges were investigated [47]. In this research work human lung adenocarcinoma A549 cells were treated with G_1, G_2, G_3, G_4, G_5, G_6, G_7, G_8, $G_{3.5}$, $G_{4.5}$, $G_{5.5}$, and $G_{7.5}$ of PAMAMs having negative surface charge and G_3, G_4, G_5, G_6, G_7 and G_8 of this dendrimer with positive surface charge. Dendrimers with positive surface charge caused cell death while those with negative surface charge did not damage cells. In order to investigate the mechanism of the cell death, G_3 dendrimers with positive and negative surface charges were chose and tested for caspase activity and DNA fragmentation which are two main symptoms for apoptosis. It was found that the cell death was not due to apoptosis process but was the result of an alternate pathway called autophagic cell death [47]. This type of cell death is different from other mechanisms such as apoptotic pathway and come back to the excess autophagy, separating organelles and other proteins into a double- layer membrane vesicle called anautophagosome [17].

The cytotoxicity of these dendrimers was directly depended on the generation so that higher generations showed higher toxicity. Other structural factors including rigidity, type of functional groups (for example primary amines being more toxic than secondary or tertiary amines), skeletal backbone and type of the core influence the toxicity of dendrimers. Dendrimers with an aromatic polyether skeletal backbone and negative surface charge have shown haemolytic activity against rat blood cells. A suggested mechanism for haemolytic activity of this type of dendrimers (with hydrophobic core or moiety inside) is their hydrophobic-hydrophobic interactions with the cell membrane. As rigidity and generation of dendrimers increase influence of the hydrophobic core or moiety decrease because a thick shell around core and interior moieties do not allow contact between them and cell surface. Dendrimers with similar structures show similar toxicity, for example poly(propylene imine) (PPI) dendrimers with end amino functional groups have shown cytotoxicity and haemolytic effects similar to those observed for PAMAMs with the same functional groups. A well-known way to modify and diminish the toxicity of dendimers is the modification of their surface. Conjugation of PEG and fatty acid molecules onto the surface of PAMAM dendrimers decrease their non-specific interactions with the proteins and biological systems and consequently diminish their toxicity. For example conjugation of six lipid chains or four PEG chains onto the surface of PAMAM dendrimer (G_4) increases its biocompatibility substantially. Absorption of the proteins of fetal calf serum onto the surface of PAMAM dendrimers could decrease their toxicity [13, 74-81].

N-(2-hydroxypropyl)methacrylamide (HPMA) is a copolymer which anticancer drug delivery system based on it is completely studied and its safety concerns are well documented. This anticancer drug delivery system is the first synthetic system to enter clinical test and a good guide for other dendrimer-based drug delivery systems to enter this stage and real usage in cancer therapy [73, 82-88]. The immunological and haemocompatibility properties of HPMA copolymers were completely investigated and a molecular weight range amenable to renal elimination and therefore safe for clinical use was found [89-92].

5. Release of Therapeutic Agents from Dendrimer-Based Delivery Systems

When a drug delivery system arrives to target site, it should release drug efficiency. The time and place of release is very important and it affects the biocompatibility and efficiency of system. For example the release of drug from the endosomal compartment is a limiting factor for some of targeted drug delivery systems. These requirements impose the need for the development of systems that can release drugs in a controllable manner. Controlled release of drugs from delivery systems is either sustain or pulsatile. In sustained release, a polymer-based drug delivery system release drug continuously and at a controlled rate with diffusion out of the polymer or with degradation of the polymer over the time. Second type of release is achieved using stimuli-responsive drug delivery systems [1, 2, 4, 22, 93].

PAMAM dendrimers with conjugated PEG molecules on their surface have used to encapsulate drugs and release them in a controlled manner. While drug molecules release from dendrimer slowly in low ionic strength aqueous solution, they release in isotonic solutions quickly which is not desirable. Changes in the structure of dendrimers upon changes in the medium conditions such as pH or temperature are factors which are interested to release the encapsulated drugs or those that are delivered by non-covalent interactions [93, 94].

Citric acid-polyethylene glycol-citric acid (CPEGC) triblock linear-dendritic copolymers are used as drug delivery systems. The quantity of trapped molecules and drugs such as 5-amino salicylic acid (5-ASA), pyridine, mefenamic acid, and diclofenac by CPEGC are measured. The drug/dendrimer complexes were stable at room temperature for about 10 months and release of drug was not observed. The controlled release of drugs from these systems was investigated. The comparison of the data has shown that in different pH's the drugs release in different rates. It has been found that the rate of release of polar drugs is slower than the others. In pH7.4 the rate of release of drugs has been lower than pH 1 and 10. Interestingly, in all cases after approximately 350 min, the release of drugs from the complexes has been approximately completed. A distinct relationship between the rate of release and the size of drugs has not been found in these systems [95].

Release of encapsulated guest molecules (Rose Bengal) from organic to water phase by dendritic core-shell architectures containing poly(glycerol) and poly(ethylene imine) cores and poly(lactide) shell (PG-PLA and PEI-PLA respectively) and their analogues containing the same cores but poly(L-lactide) shell (PG-PLLA and PEI-PLLA, respectively) has been investigated. Rate of release of guest molecules from these core-shell architectures (nanocarriers) depends on the type of the core, shell and solvent.

Nanocarriers containing PLLA shell release guest molecules faster than those containing PLA shell. Dispersion of aggregates in the presence of several drops of acetone increase the rate of release of guest molecules from nanocarriers (Figure 11) [96].

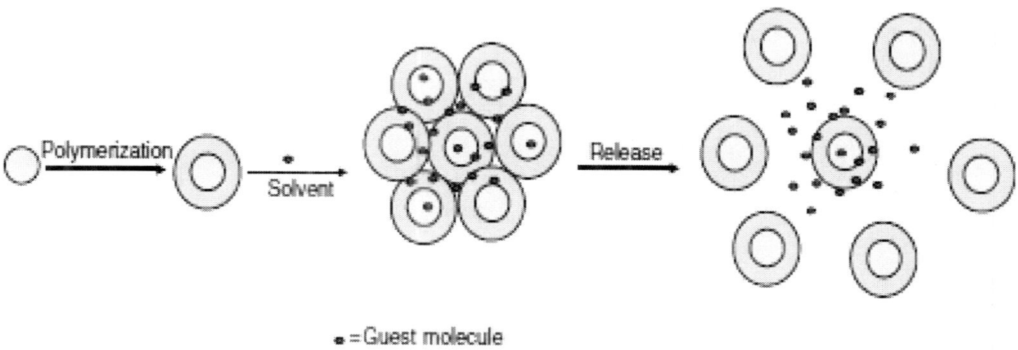

Figure 11. Schematic representation of preparation of core–shell architectures, encapsulation and release of the guest molecules.

Dendritic unimolecular micelles from polyaryl ether dendrimers containing both PEG and hydrophobic moieties (including cholesterol, phenyl alanine and tryptophan) conjugated on their surface are synthesized and used to encapsulate hydrophobic drug molecules. A micelle consisting of third-generation dendrimer with 24 surface chains has entrapped indomethacin, loading up to approximately 9-10 drug molecules per micelle. *In vitro* release of drug molecules from these micelles was slow and sustained type [15].

Methotrexate has been delivered by dendrimers through both encapsulation and conjugation methods. It has been shown that encapsulated methotrexate molecules release from dendrimers in a solution of phosphate buffered saline quickly, while conjugated ones release slower in the same conditions. *In vitro* toxicity of encapsulated methotrexate molecules was similar to that for free drug molecules against cancer cells while conjugated drug molecules accompanied by conjugated folic acid molecules specifically killed receptor-expressing cells with intracellular delivery of the drug through receptor-mediated endocytosis. Therefore drug delivery system with conjugated methotrexate molecules is a promising candidate to specifically targeted drug delivery [2, 73].

pH sensitive drug delivery systems based on PPI dendrimers in order to encapsulate and controlled release of pyrene as a guest molecule have been prepared [15]. In addition to pH, rate of release of drug molecules depended on the solubility and functionality of PPI strongly [22, 73].

Conclusion

Several structural characteristics of dendrimers including high functionality, small size, spherical shape, cavity, narrow polydispersity and well-know structure beside their physiological properties such as enhanced uptake of dendrimer-drug complexes, endosomal escape capability of cationic dendrimers, extra-vasate across tumor's leaky vasculature and controlled release of encapsulated or conjugated drugs promises them as efficient future drug delivery systems.

References

[1] (a) Tomellini, R.; Faure, U.; Panzer, O. *European Technology Platform on NanoMedicine- Nanotechnology for Health*. 2005. (b) Cerroni, B.; Chiessi, E.; Margheritelli, S.; Oddo, L.; Paradossi, G. *Biomacromolecules*. 2011, *12* (3), 593.

[2] (a) Svenson, S.; Donald, A. T. *Advanced Drug Delivery Reviews*. 2005, *57*, 2106. (b) Yuan, H.; Luo, K.; Lai, Y.; Pu, Y.; He, B.; Wang, G.; Wu, Y; Gu, Z. *Mol. Pharmaceutics*. 2010, *7* (4), 953.

[3] Medina, S. H.; Elsayed, M. *Chem. Rev*. 2009, *109*, 3141.

[4] (a) Nanjwade, B.K.; Bechra, H. M. *European Journal of Pharmaceutical Sciences*. 2009, *38*, 185. (b) Namazi, H.; Adeli, M.; Zarnegar, Z.; Jafari, S.; Dadkhah, A.; Shukla, A. *Journal of Applied Polymer Science*. 2007,*285*, 1527. (c) Adeli, M.; Zarnegar, Z. *Journal of Applied Polymer Science*. 2009, *113*, 2072. (d) Namazi, H.; Adeli, M. *Polymer*. 2005,*46*, 10788. (e) Namazi, H.; Adeli, M. *European Polymer Journal*. 2003, *39*, 1491.

[5] Maraval, V.; Pyzowski, J.; Caminade, A.M.; Majoral, J.P. *J. Org. Chem.* 2003, *68*, 6043.

[6] Launay, N.; Caminade, A. M.; Lahana, R.; Majoral, J. P. *Angew. Chem., Int. Ed.* 1994, *33*, 1589.

[7] Adeli, M.; Zarnegar, Z. *Journal of Applied Polymer Science*. 2009, *115*, 9.

[8] Namazi, H.; Adeli, M. *Iranian Polymer Journal*. 2005, *14*, 942.

[9] Wolinsky, J. B.; Grinstaff, M. W. *Advanced Drug Delivery Reviews*. 2008, *60*, 1037.

[10] Philipp, S. F.; Jones, A. T.; Duncan, R. *Journal of Controlled Release*. 2007, *117*, 291.

[11] (a) Jang, W. D.; KamruzzamanSelim, K. M. *Progress in Polymer Science*. 2009, *34*, 1. (b) Santos, J. L.; Pandita, D.; Rodrigues, J.; Pêgo, A. P.; Granja, P. L.; Balian G.; Tomás, H. *Mol. Pharmaceutics*. 2010, *7* (3), 763.

[12] (a) Gupta, U.; Pharm, B. *Nanomedicine: Nanotechnology, Biology, and Medicine*. 2006, *2*, 66. (b) Feng, X.; Cheng, Y.; Yang, K.; Zhang, J.; Wu, Q.; Xu, T.*J. Phys. Chem. B*. 2010, *114* (34), 11017.

[13] (a) Svenson, S. *European Journal of Pharmaceutics and Biopharmaceutics*. 2009, *71*, 445. (b) Yang, K.; Weng, L.; Cheng, Y.; Zhang, H.; Zhang, J.; Wu, Q.; Xu, T. *J. Phys. Chem. B*. 2011, *115* (10), 2185.

[14] Al-Jamal, K. T.; Chandrasekaran, R. *Advanced Drug Delivery Reviews*. 2005, *57*, 2238.

[15] (a) Patri, A. K.; Majoros, I. J.; Baker, R. J. *Current Opinion in Chemical Biology*. 2002, *6*, 466. (b) Astruc, D.; Boisselier E.; Ornelas, C. *Chem. Rev*. 2010, *110* (4), 1857.

[16] Cheng, Y.; Xu, T. *European Journal of Medicinal Chemistry*. 2008, *43*, 2291.

[17] Astruc, D.; Boisselier, E.; Ornelas, C. *Chem. Rev*. 2010, *110*, 1857.

[18] (a) Hawker, C. J.; Fréchet, J. M. *J. Am. Chem. Soc.* 1990, *112*, 7638. (b) Natali, S.; Mijovic, J. *Macromolecules*. 2010, *43* (6), 3011.

[19] Tomalia, D. A.; Baker, H.; Dewald, J.; Hall, M.; Kallos, G.; Martin, S.; Roeck, J.; Ryder, J.; Smith, P. *Macromolecules*. 1986, *19*, 2466.

[20] (a) Newkome, G. R.; Yao, Z.; Baker, G. R.; Gupta, V.K. *J. Org.Chem.*1985, *50*, 2003. (b) Kaminskas, L. M.; Kelly, B. D.; McLeod, V. M.; Gian Sberna, Boyd, B. J.; Owen, D. J.; Porter, C. J. H. *Mol. Pharmaceutics*. 2011, *8* (2), 338.
[21] Dutta, T.; Jain, N. K. *Nanomedicine: Nanotechnology, Biology, and Medicine*. 2010, *6*, 25.
[22] Paleos, C. M.; Tsiourvas, D.; Sideratou, Z. *Reviews*. 2006, *10*, 71.
[23] Choi, J. S.; Ko, K. S. *International Journal of Pharmaceutics*. 2006, *320*, 171.
[24] Dufes, Ch.; Uchegbu, I. F. *Advanced Drug Delivery Reviews*. 2005, *57*, 2177.
[25] Khopade, A. J.; Caruso, F. *Biomacromolecules*. 2002, *3*, 1154.
[26] Malik, N.; Evagorou, E. G.; Duncan, R. *Anticancer Drugs*. 1999, *10*, 767.
[27] Bhadra, D.; Bhadra, S.; Jain, S.; Jain, N. K. *Int. J.Pharm*. 2003, *257*, 111.
[28] Guillaudeu, S. J.; Fox, M. E.; Haidar, Y. M.; Dy, E. E.; Szoka, F. C.; Frechet, J. M. *Bioconjugate Chem*. 2008, *19*, 461.
[29] (a) Allen, T.M.; Cullis, P. R. *Science*. 2004, *303*, 1818. (b) Zhang, Y.; Thomas, T. P.; Desai, A.; Zong, H.; Leroueil, P. R.; Majoros I. J.; Baker, J. R. Jr. *Bioconjugate Chem*. 2010, *21* (3), 489.
[30] Morgan, M. T.; Carnahan, M. A.; Finkelstein, S.; Prata, C. A.; Degoricija, L.; Lee, S. J.; Grinstaff, M. W. *Chem. Commun*. 2005, *34*, 4309.
[31] Wang, F.; Bronich, T. K.; Kabanov, A. V.; Rauh, R. D.; Roovers, J. *Bioconjug. Chem*. 2005, *16*, 397.
[32] Ooya, T.; Lee, J.; Park, K. *Bioconjug. Chem*. 2004, *15*, 1221.
[33] Neerman, M. F.; Chen, H. T.; Parrish, A. R.; Simanek, E. E. *Mol. Pharm*. 2004, *1*, 390.
[34] Gurdag, S.; Khandare, J.; Stapels, S.; Matherly, L. H.; Kannan, R. M. *Bioconjug. Chem*. 2006, *17*, 275.
[35] Khandare, J. J.; Jayant, S.; Singh, A.; Chandna, P.; Wang, Y.; Vorsa, N.; Minko, T. *Bioconjug. Chem*. 2006, *17*, 1464.
[36] Papagiannaros, A.; Dimas, K.; Papaioannou, G.T.; Demetzos, C. *Int. J. Pharm*. 2005, *302*, 29.
[37] (a) Lee, C. C.; Gillies, E.R.; Fox, M. E.; Guillaudeu, S. J.; Fréchet, J. M.; Dy, E. E.; Szoka, F. C. *Proc. Natl. Acad. Sci. U. S. A*. 2006, *103*, 16649. (b) Fant, K.; K. Esbjorner, E.; Jenkins, A.; Grossel, M. C.; Lincoln, P.; Norden, B.*Mol. Pharmaceutics*. 2010, *7* (5), 1734.
[38] Gurdag, S.; Khandare, J.; Stapels, S.; Matherly, L. H.; Kannan, R. M. *Bioconjug. Chem*. 2006, *17*, 275.
[39] Klutz, K. Y.; Klutz, A. M. *Bioconjugate Chem*. 2008, *19*, 1660.
[40] Patri, A. K.; Kukowska-Latallo, J. F. *Advanced Drug Delivery Reviews*. 2005, *57*, 2203.
[41] El-Sayed, M.; Ginski, M.; Rhodes, C.; Ghandehari, H. J. *Controlled Release*. 2002, *81*, 355.
[42] El-Sayed, M.; Ginski, M.; Rhodes, C. A.; Ghandehari, H. J. *Bioact. Compat. Polym*. 2003, *18*, 7.
[43] El-Sayed, M.; Kiani, M. F.; Naimark, M. D.; Hikal, A. H.; Ghandehari, H. *Pharm. Res*. 2001, *18*, 23.
[44] Majoros, I. J.; Thomas, T. P.; Mehta, C. B.; Baker, J. R. *J. Med. Chem*. 2005, *48*, 5892.
[45] Nigavekar, S. S.; Sung, L. Y.; Lanes, M.; El-Jawahri, A.; Lawrence, T. S.; Becker, C. W.; Balogh, L.; Khan, M. K. *Pharm. Res*. 2004, *21*, 476.

[46] Kukowska-Latallo, J. F.; Candido, K. A.; Cao, Z.; Nigavekar, S. S.; Majoros, I. J.; Thomas, T. P.; Balogh, L. P.; Khan, M. K.; Baker, J. R. *Cancer Res*. 2005, *65*, 5317.
[47] Dhanikula, R. S.; Argaw, A.; Bouchard, J. F.; Hildgen, P. *Mol. Pharm*. 2007, *5*, 105.
[48] Patri, A. K.; Myc, A.; Beals, J.; Thomas, T. P.; Bander, N. H.; Baker, J. R. *Bioconjug. Chem*. 2004, *15*, 1174.
[49] Koo, O. M.; Rubinstein, I.; Onyuksel, H. *Nanomedicine: Nanotechnology, Biology, and Medicine*. 2005, *1*, 193.
[50] Iyer, A. K.; Khaled, G.; Fang, J.; Maeda, H. *Drug Discov*. 2006, *11*, 812.
[51] (a) Wiener, E. C.; Konda, S.; Shadron, A.; Brechbiel, M.; Gansow, O. *Invest. Radiol*. 1997, *32*, 748. (b) Barz, M.; Canal, F.; Koynov, K.; Zentel, R.; Vicent, M. J. *Biomacromolecules*. 2010, *11* (9), 2274.
[52] Hong, S.; Leroueil, P. R.; Majoros, I. J.; Orr, B.G.; Baker, J. R.; BanaszakHoll, M. M. *Chem. Biol*. 2007, *14*, 107.
[53] Patri, A. K.; Kukowska-Latallo, J. F.; Baker, J. R. *Adv. Drug Deliv. Rev*. 2005, *57*, 2203.
[54] (a) Majoros, I. J.; Thomas, T. P.; Mehta, C. B.; Baker, J. R. *J. Med. Chem*. 2005, *48*, 5892. (b) Cao, W.; Zhou, J.; Wang, Y.; Zhu, L. *Biomacromolecules*. 2010, *11* (12), 3680.
[55] Thomas, T. P.; Majoros, I. J.; Kotlyar, A.; Kukowska-Latallo, J. F.; Bielinska, A.; Myc, A.; Baker, J. R. *J. Med. Chem*. 2005, *48*, 3729.
[56] Majoros, I. J.; Myc, A.; Thomas, T.; Mehta, C. B.; Baker, J. R. *Biomacromolecules*. 2006, *7*, 572.
[57] Myc, A.; Majoros, I. J.; Thomas, T. P.; Baker, J. R. *Biomacromolecules*. 2007, *8*, 13.
[58] Yang, W.; Cheng, Y. *European Journal of Medicinal Chemistry*. 2009, *44*, 862.
[59] Singh, P.; Gupta, U. *Bioconjugate Chem*. 2008, *19*, 2239.
[60] Kobayashi, H.; Reijnders, K.; English, S.; Yordanov, A. T.; Milenic, D. E.; Sowers, A. L.; Citrin, D.; Krishna, M. C.; Waldmann, T. A.; Mitchell, J. B.; Brechbiel, M. W. *Clin. Cancer Res*. 2004, *10*, 7712.
[61] Dvorak, H. F. *J. Clin. Oncol*. 2002, *20*, 4368.
[62] Znati, C. A.; Rosenstein, M.; Boucher, Y.; Epperly, M. W.; Bloomer, W. D.; Jain, R. K. *Cancer Res*. 1996, *56*, 964.
[63] Kobayashi, H.; Kawamoto, S.; Bernardo, M.; Brechbiel, M. W.; Knopp, M. V.; Choyke, P. L. *J. Control. Release*. 2006, *111*, 343.
[64] Amirkhanov, N. V.; Wickstrom, E. *Nucleosides Nucleotides Nucleic Acids*. 2005, *24*, 423.
[65] (a) Wiener, E. C.; Konda, S.; Shadron, A.; Brechbiel, M.; Gansow, O. *Invest. Radiol*. 1997, *32*, 748. (b) Fleming, C. J.; Yin, N.; Riechers, S. L.; Chu, G.; Liu, G. *ACS Nano*. 2011, *5* (3), 1685.
[66] Backer, M. V.; Gaynutdinov, T. I.; Patel, V.; Bandyopadhyaya, A. K.; Thirumamagal, B. T. S.; Tjarks, W.; Barth R. F.; Claffey, K.; Backer, J. M. *Mol. Cancer Ther*. 2005, *4*,1423.
[67] Kobayashi, H.; Kawamoto, S.; Brechbiel, M. W.; Bernardo, M.; Sato, N.; Waldmann, T. A.; Tagaya, Y.; Choyke, P. L, *Neoplasia*. 2005, *7*, 984.
[68] Langereis, S.; Lussanet, Q. G.; Genderen, M. H.; Meijer, E. V.; Beets-Tan, R. G.; Griffioen, A. W.; Engelshoven, J. M. van.; Backes, W. H. *NMR Biomed*. 2006, *19*, 133.

[69] Amirkhanov, N. V.; Zhang, K.; Aruva, M. R.; Thakur, M. L.; Wickstrom, E. *Bioconjugate Chem.* 2010, *21*, 731.
[70] Fu, Y.; Nitecki, D. E.; Maltby, D.; Simon, G. H.; Berejnoi, K.; Raatschen, H. J.; Yeh, B. M.; Shames, D. M.; Brasch, R. C. *Bioconjug. Chem.* 2006, *17*, 1043.
[71] (a) Thomas, T. P.; Myaing, M. T.; Ye, J. Y.; Candido, K.; Kotlyar, A.; Beals, J.; Cao, J.; Keszler, B.; Patri, A. K.; Norris, T. B.; Baker, J. R. *Biophys. J.* 2004, *86*, 3959. (b) Singh, A.; Dilnawaz, F.; Mewar, S.; Sharma, U.; Jagannathan, N. R.; Sahoo, S. *ACS Appl. Mater. Interfaces.* 2011, *3* (3), 842.
[72] Duncan, R.; Izzo, L. *Advanced Drug Delivery Reviews.* 2005, *57*, 2215.
[73] (a) Boas, U.; Heegaard, P. M. H. *Chem. Soc. Rev.* 2004, *33*, 43. (b) Sadekar, S.; Ray, A.; Janat-Amsbury, M.; Peterson, C. M.; Ghandehari, H. *Biomacromolecules.* 2011, *12* (1), 88.
[74] (a) Domanski, D. M.; Klajnert, B.; Bryszewska, M. *Bioelectrochemistry.* 2004, *63*, 189. (b) Patil, M. L.; Zhang, M ; Minko, T. *ACS Nano.* 2011, *5* (3), 1877.
[75] Duncan, R. *Nat. Rev. Drug Discov.* 2003, *2*, 347.
[76] Jevprasesphant, R.; Penny, J.; Jalal, R.; Attwood, D.; McKeown, N. B.; Emanuele, A. D. *Int. J. Pharm.* 2003, *252*, 263.
[77] (a) Fischer, D.; Li, Y.; Ahlemeyer, B.; Krieglstein, J.; Kissel, T. *Biomaterials.* 2003, *24*, 1121. (b) Lee, H.; Larson, R. G. *J. Phys. Chem. C.* 2011, *115* (13), 5316.
[78] Zinselmeyer, B. H.; Mackay, S. P.; Schatzlein, A. G.; Uchegbu, I. F. *Pharm. Res.* 2002, *19*, 960.
[79] (a) Padilla De Jesús, O. L.; Ihre, H. R.; Gagne, L.; Fréchet, J. M. J.; Szoka, F. C. *Bioconjug. Chem.* 2003, *13*, 453. (b) Yuan, Q.; Yeudall, W. A.; Yang, H. *Biomacromolecules.* 2010, *11* (8), 1940.
[80] Kobayashi, H.; Kawamoto, S.; Saga, T.; Sato, N.; Hiraga, A.; Ishimori, T.; Konishi, J.; Togashi, K.; Brechbiel, M. W. *Magn. Reson. Med.* 2001, *46*, 781.
[81] (a) Rihova, B. *Adv. Drug Deliv. Rev.* 1996, *21*, 157. (b) Fant, K.; Esbjörner, E. K.; Jenkins, A.; Grossel, M. C.; Lincoln, P.; Nordén, B. *Mol. Pharmaceutics.* 2010, *7* (5), 1734.
[82] Rihova, B.; Ulbrich, K ; Kopecek, J.; Mancal, P. *Folia Microbiol.* 1983, *28*, 7.
[83] (a) Rihova, B.; Kopecek, J.; Ulbrich, K.; Pospisil, J.; Mancal, P. *Biomaterials.* 1984, *5*, 143. (b) Kopeček, J. *Mol. Pharmaceutics.* 2010, *7* (4), 922.
[84] Rihova, B.; Kopecek, J.; Ulbrich, K.; Chytry, V. *Makromol. Chem.* 1985, *9*, 13.
[85] [85] Flanagan, P.A.; Duncan, R.; Rihova, B.; Subr, V.; Kopecek, J. *J. Bioact. Compat. Polym.* 1990, *5*, 151.
[86] [86] (a) Simeckova, J.; Plocova, D.; Rihova, B.; Kopecek, J. *J. Bioact. Compat. Polym.* 1986, *1*, 20. (b) Rihova, B.; Etrych, T.; Sirova, M.; Kovar, L.; Hovorka, O.; Kovar, M.; Benda, A.; Ulbrich, K. *Mol. Pharmaceutics.* 2010, *7* (4), 1027.
[87] Rihova, B.; Ulbrich, K.; Strohalm, J.; Vetvicka, V.; Bilej, M.; Duncan, R.; Kopecek, J. *Biomaterials.* 1989, *10*, 335.
[88] Seymour, L.; Duncan, R.; Strohalm, J.; Kopecek, J. *J. Biomed. Mater. Res.* 1987, *21*, 1341.
[89] (a) Goddard, P.; Williamson, I.; Brown, J.; Hutchinson, L.; Nicholls, J.; Petrak, K. *J. Bioact. Compat. Polym.* 1996, *6*, 4. (b) Sadekar, S.; Ray, A.; Janát-Amsbury, M.; Peterson, C. M.; Ghandehari, H. *Biomacromolecules.* 2011, *12* (1), 88.

[90] Duncan, R, Polymer-drug conjugates, in: Budman D, Calvert H, Rowinsky E (Eds.), Handbook of Anticancer Drug Development, Lippincott, Williams and Wilkins, 2003, 239.

[91] Duncan, R.; Coatsworth, J. K.; Burtles, S. *Human Exp. Toxicol.* 1998, *17*, 93.
[92] (a) Yeung, T. K.; Hopewell, J. W.; Simmonds, R. H.; Seymour, L. W.; Duncan, R.; Bellini, O.; Grandi, M.; Spreafico, F.; Strohalm, J.; Ulbrich, K. *Cancer Chemother.Pharmacol.* 1991, *29*, 105. (b) Paul, A.; James, C.; Heenan, R. K.; Schweins, R. *Biomacromolecules.* 2010, *11* (8), 1978.
[93] Gillies, E. R.; Frechet, J. M. J. *Reviews.* 2005, *10,* 35.
[94] Ashootosh, V. A.; Elamprakash, N. S.; Thayumanavan, S. *Reviews.* 2005, *2*, 4.
[95] Namazi, H.; Adeli, M. *Biomaterials.* 2005, *26*, 1175.
[96] Adeli, M.; Haag, R.; Zarnegar, Z. *Journal of Nanoparticle Research.* 2007, *9*, 1057.

In: Hybrid Nanostructures in Cancer Therapy
Editor: Mohsen Adeli
ISBN: 978-1-62100-517-9
© 2012 Nova Science Publishers, Inc.

Chapter IV

Biomedical Applications of Carbon Nanotube's Supramolecules

Mohsen Adeli[1,2], Masoumeh Ashiri[1], Siamak Beyranvand[1], and Masooumeh Parsamanesh[1]

[1]Department of chemistry, Faculty of Science, Lorestan University, Khoramabad, Iran
[2]Department of chemistry, Sharif University of Technology, Tehran, Iran

Abstract

Among diverse classes of hybrid nanomaterial-based drug delivery systems (HNDDSs) those based on the carbon nanotubes have attracted particular attention as carriers for the biologically relevant molecules due to their unique properties such as ability to cross the cell membranes and high surface area per unit weight for the high drug loading. Varity of HNDDSs based on the carbon nanotubes have been prepared and tested in vitro and in vivo for delivery of the drugs recently.

Poor water solubility and low functionality are two critical factors that influence the performance of the CNTs for biomedical applications. Therefore, in order to make HNDDSs based on CNTs these factors should be improved. Solubility of CNTs can be developed by treatment with polymers either covalently or noncovalently. Non-covalent method is based on the supramolecular interactions between CNTs and polymers and includes polymer wrapping or adsorption. In this method the structure of the CNTs does not change as much as the covalent method, but its disadvantage is the low functionality of the final product.

1. Introduction

Unique mechanical, thermal and electrical properties make carbon nanotubes (CNTs) as attractive candidates for various applications including field emission devices [1], sensors [2], transistors [3] and polymer composites [4-6]. Early diagnosis of the diseases such as cancer is possible using CNTs-based nanodevises. Cell membrane permeability of carbon nanotubes due to their hydrophobicity and subcellular size would also expand medical applications to therapeutic as carriers in gene and drug delivery systems [7]. However, agglomeration, entanglement and poor water solubility of CNTs originated from their high aspect ratio and van-der Waals interactions between individual CNTs would limit their biomedical application. Thus increased water solubility and distribution of the CNTs bundles are under investigation to obtain CNTs-based nanomaterials with desirable properties [7]. Polymers are used to improve the water solubility and biological properties of CNTs abundantly. Polymeric modifiers can be bound to CNTs via two general synthetic strategies. The first include noncovalent attachment of polymer chains (a ‘‘polymer wrapping” process) [8-11], and the other is based on covalently attachment of polymer to the side walls of CNTs [12]. An optimized modifier for coating carbon nanotubes and conferring biological properties to them via noncovalent interactions should have several characteristics.

i) The coating molecules should be biocompatible and nontoxic. ii) Since in biological solutions, especially in serum having high salt and protein contents, detachment of polymer from the nanotube surface can occur easily, coating molecules should have strong interaction with the surface of CNTs. iii) Water solubility and functionality of carbon nanotubes should improved upon noncovalent interactions with polymers or coating molecules. iv) Noncovalent interactions between polymers and carbon nanotubes should be lead to the developed biological properties. v) CNTs/polymer hybrid nanomaterials should cross the biological barriers successfully and rich to the targeted places and finally degraded to the safe materials.

Suitable functional groups of the used polymer in the ‘‘polymer wrapping” process that can specifically interact with the surface of CNT may include aromatic and diene segments such as pyrene [12-15] that have π–π stacking interaction with the graphitic structure of CNTs. Various natural and synthetic polymers including polypeptides, amylase, DNA, chitosan (CTS), poly(acrylic acid), poly(N-isopropyl acrylamide), poly (ethylene glycol) [16], polyethylene (PE), nylon 6,6 [17], α-pyrene functionalized polymers [18], phospholipids [19], etc. have been used to disperse CNTs in different solutions. However polymers that can have strong noncovalent interactions with the CNT’s surface are generally limited due to complication synthetic procedures [12-15]. Strength of the noncovalent interactions between polymers and CNTs depend on several factors such as molecular weight, functional groups, hydrophobicity, hydrophilicity and three dimensional structure of polymer. With the thermodynamic view, conformational degrees of freedom of polymers and thus chains entropy reduced upon interaction with the surface of CNTs and since all systems trends to the increased entropy, this lead to a repulsive interaction between polymers and CNTs. However enthalpic factor compensate the decreased entropy and lead to attractive interactions between CNTs and polymers.

2. Synthesis and Characterization of Carbon Nanotube/Polymer Supramolecules

General methods to produce CNT’s supramolecules in organic or aqueous media involves ultrasonication of carbon nanotubes with interacting objects and then filtration or centrifugation of the mixture to separate the graphitic or other types of impurities. Noncovalent interactions leading to supramolecules includes

i) hydrophobic interactions between the surface of carbon nanotubes and long chain hydrophobic polymers, ii) π–π interactions between the π system of CNTs and polymers or molecules containing several π bonds such as pyrene, ferrocene and other aromatic containing molecules [20] (this type of interaction in some cases is so called "π–π stacking"), iii) electrostatic, zwitterionic or hydrogen bond interactions between acid treatment CNTs (CNT-COOH) and macromolecules or polymers with polar functional groups such as poly(ethylene glycol)-polycitric acid linear-dendritic copolymers or ionic macromolecules such as sodium alginate and chitosan [21, 22].

Efficiency of the functionalization through zwitterionic interaction often taken place in harsh condition and needs long reaction time. On the other hand existence of the limited sites for interaction with CNTs, sometimes failed to disperse bundles to individual tubes. Application of a polymer or macromolecule containing several types of functional groups or several blocks such as amphiphilic macromolecules can effectively addressed this problem, because it is able to interact with CNTs through more than one type of above noncovalent interactions [23]. Mild experiment conditions, non toxic solvent involved, ambient temperature, shorter reaction time and free of sonication make this method more favorable than other approaches. Since by noncovalent functionalization, structure of CNTs change less than covalent approaches (where defects sites with SP^3 hybridized carbons are created) and therefore their electronic, optical, thermal and other intrinsic properties remain almost intact, this approach is desirable to produce nanodevices for biomedical applications [24-28].

However among different types of noncovalent interactions π–π staking is more effective and well studied interaction than other types [29, 30]. Ferrocene or pyrene functionalized polymers are used to disperse CNTs, leading to hybrid nanomaterials that can be processed to make biosensors (Figure 1). [31, 32].

Cyclodextrins are well-known cyclic molecules to form inclusion complex with the especial small molecules. However the size of cavity of α, β and γ,-CDs is so small (less than one nanometer) to host CNTs with several nanomateter (1-100nm). η- CD with a 12-membered ring structure and 1.8 nm inner cavity is able to encapsulate SWNT with a diameter less than their cavity size [33]. DNA and proteins make supramolecules with CNTs through different interactions including especial inclusion complexes, [34, 35], electrostatic interactions, hydrogen bonding and other mechanisms [36, 37].

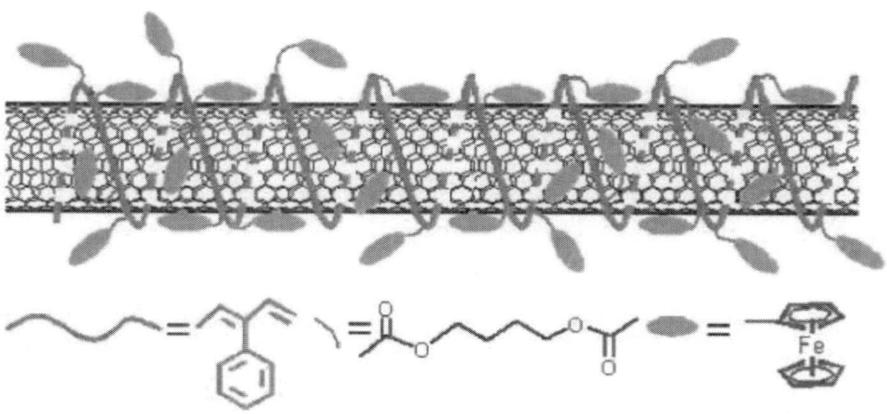

Figure 1. Functionalization of CNTs by ferrocene functionalized polymers. Reprinted with the permission of Ref. [31].

3. Biomedical Applications of Carbon Nanotube/Polymer Supramolecules

3.1. Imaging Devices

The best technique which is highly used to diagnosis unusual and damaged tissues in body and is also used to evaluate the function and structure of biological systems in clinical medicine is "Magnetic resonance imaging" (MRI) [38, 39]. This technique is based on the stimulation of the hydrogen nuclei of water by a strong external magnetic field followed by their resonance between the energy levels by applying a radio frequency pulses and magnetic field gradients which resulted in the nucleus reorientation in the first manner and finally create an image based on the density of water in different places. Quality and resolution of the MRI images can be enhanced by paramagnetic contrast agents that reduce the T_1 and T_2 relaxation times of the exited and radiated protons of water [40]. A well-studied type of contrast agents that has been frequently used to develop the ability of the MRI technique are Gd^{3+} complexes. Hybridization of the desirable properties of CNTs and contrast agents such as Gd^{3+} complexes by construction of their hybrid nanomaterials leads to powerful agents to improve the brightness of the MRI images [41]. Lipids with head polar groups that are able to form complex with Gd^{3+} have been prepared and then used to functionalize CNTs noncovalently. In these supramolecules surface of CNTs is fully covered by lipid-Gd^{3+} complexes, hence they are accessible to water molecules and thus create brighter images (Figure 2) [42]. Toxicity related to the Gd^{3+} complexes is also reduced in the CNTs/lipid-Gd^{3+} supramolecules.

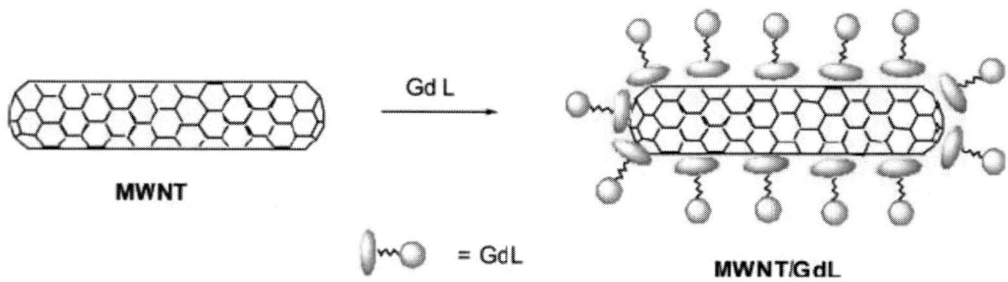

Figure 2. CNTs/lipid-Gd3+ supramolecules used to enhance the brightness of MRI images. Reprinted with the permission of Ref. [42].

Poly(ethylene glycol) (PEG) functionalized by fluorescein isothiocyanate (FITC) is also used to form supramolecules with CNTs through π-π staking interactions between the aromatic fluorescein segment of PEG and π system of CNTs. The resulted supramolecule is promising system in order to image the subcellular systems [43]. On the other hand, having small band gaps on the order of ~1 eV make individual semiconducting SWNTs favorable for photoluminescence imaging of the subcellular systems in the near-infrared (NIR) range (900-1600 nm) in which autofluorescence from proteins of biological systems is minimal that is a result of large separation between the excitation (550-850 nm) and emission bands (900-1600 nm) in SWNTs. Due to its high water solubility, protein resistance property, high biocompatibility and low toxicity PEG is the best candidate to produce the CNTs/PEG supramolecules for biomedical applications. Variety of PEG functionalized (PEGylated) CNTs attached to therapeutic agents, antibodies and fluorescent tags have been prepared and used as probes or nanocarriers [44]. PEG functionalized SWNT attached to herceptin as NIR fluorescent tag for selective probing of cell surface receptors has been synthesized and characterized. Figure 3 shows NIR fluorescence images of BT-474 (which is HER2/neu positive) and MCF-7 (which is HER2/neu negative) treated with PEG functionalized SWNT attached to herceptin. The high and low level of the fluorescence signal in BT-474 and MCF-7 cell fluorescence images indicates the selective and receptor mediated surface binding of the SWNT-herceptin conjugate to these cells [44].

Cyclic arginine-glycine-aspartic acid (RGD) peptide is also conjugated to the PEGylated SWNTs and the obtained hybrid nanomaterial is used as Raman probes for *in vivo* tumor imaging in live mice (Figure 4) [45,46]. Accumulation of PEGylated SWNTs attached to RGD (as a Raman probe) in the tumor site of living mice bearing a tumor xenograft upon injection this system causes a stronger SWNT Raman signals rather than a system without RGD [47].

Carbon nanotubes are used as photoacoustic imaging tolls in which sound generation takes place through local heating by laser light. Due to the strong light absorption of SWNTs that generates an acoustic signal, this technique has higher spatial resolution than traditional ultrasound and deeper tissue penetration than fluorescence imaging. PEGylated SWNTs attached to RGD are used as the contrast agent for photoacoustic molecular imaging of cancer in a mouse tumor model [43]. As it can be seen in figure 4 the resolution of the image of cancer cells treated with PEGylated SWNTs attached to RGD is much higher than those treated with PEGylated SWNTs without RGD.

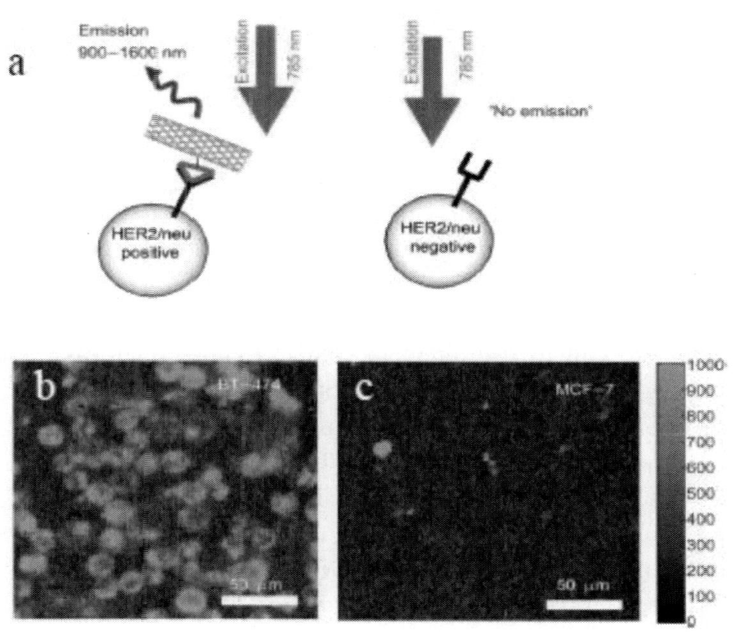

Figure 3. (a) Schematic representation of conjugating of SWNT-herceptin to BT-474 (HER2/neu positive) and MCF-7 (HER2/neu negative) cells. (b) NIR photoluminescence image of BT-474 cells treated with the SWNT-herceptin conjugate. (c) NIR photoluminescence image of MCF-7. Reprinted with the permission of Ref. [44b].

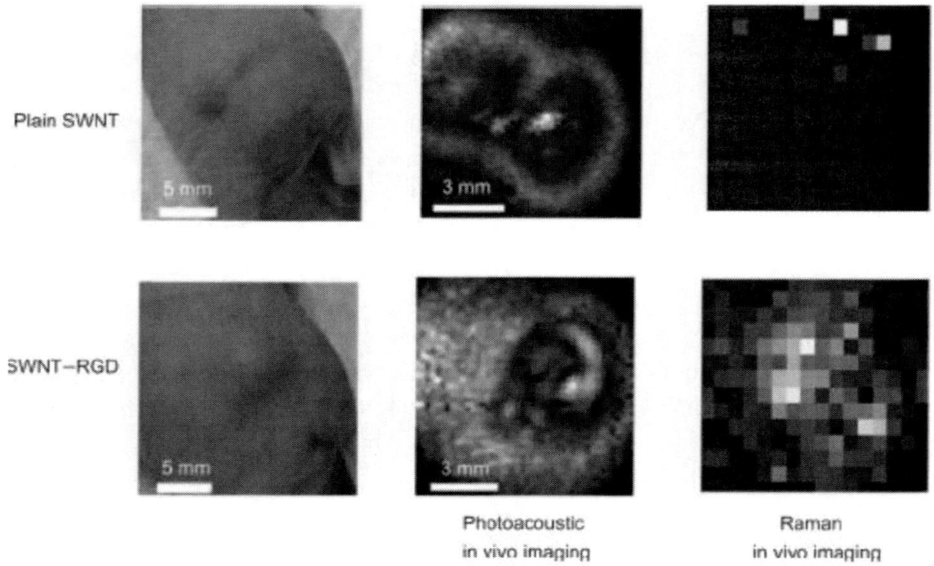

Figure 4. Comparison of the images of U87MG tumors in live mice after injecting the SWNT attached to RGD and without it for *In vivo* photoacoustic and Raman imaging. Strong tumor contrast induced by SWNT RGD was observed in both imaging techniques. Reprinted with the permission of Ref. [45].

3.2. Drug Delivery System Based on Carbon Nanotube/Polymer Supramolecules

The most studied biomedical application of CNTs is to target therapeutic agents to tumor sites or cancer cells. Two factors including poor water solubility and low functionality limit the biomedical applications of CNTs chemically. Linear polymers are able to wrap around CNTs through noncovalent interactions to soluble them in different solvents. Among variety of linear polymers that are used to solublize the CNTs in aqueous solutions, PEG is the most promising and well studied polymer that develops both their water solubility and biocompatibility [49]. Drug delivery systems based on PEGylated CNTs show prolonged blood circulation time, reduced RES uptake and accelerated excretion for long PEG. Moreover branched PEGs causes longer SWNT blood circulation half-life (~5 h) than that for linear PEGs (~2 h) of the same molecular weight [49]. Intravenously injection of SWNTs functionalized by PEGs with two different molecular weights conjugated with both RGD peptide as a targeting ligand and radiolabels (64Cu-DOTA)) into glioblastoma U87MG tumor-bearing mice and monitoring by micro-positron emission tomography (micro-PET) over time showed higher tumor uptake for RGD-conjugated SWNTs with a long PEG (SWNT PEG5400 RGD) than those without RGD. Highly efficient tumor targeting was achieved by SWNTs functionalized by long PEG (SWNT PEG5400 RGD) with long blood circulation time not those functionalized by short PEG (SWNT PEG2000 RGD) [50].

In the noncovalent approach therapeutic agents are either loaded on carbon nanotube directly or attached to a spacer and then loaded on carbon nanotube. Paclitaxel (PTX) and doxorubicin (DOX) are two anticancer drugs that their transferring to tumor sites or cancer cells by carbon nanotubes is well studied both *in vivo* and *in vitro*.

PTX as a commonly used cancer chemotherapy drug is a mitotic inhibitor. It has poor water solubility, therefore amphiphilic agents such as Cremophor EL are used to improve its water solubility but these agents usually causes side effects include hypersensitivity reactions, nephrotoxicity and neurotoxicity. Delivery of PTX by CNTs increases the efficacy of this drug in inhibiting tumor growth in mice noticeably [51]. Figure 5 show a drug delivery system based on CNTs to transfer PTX molecules. In this system PTX is conjugated to branched PEG chains having a phospholipids tail through ester bonds that are cleavable in biological environment. Noncovalent interactions between hydrophobic phospholipids tail of branched PEG and hydrophobic surface of CNT lead to the final drug delivery system. In this system PEG chains not only increase the water solubility of system and decrease the nonspecific interaction with the biological molecules but also carry the PTX molecules.

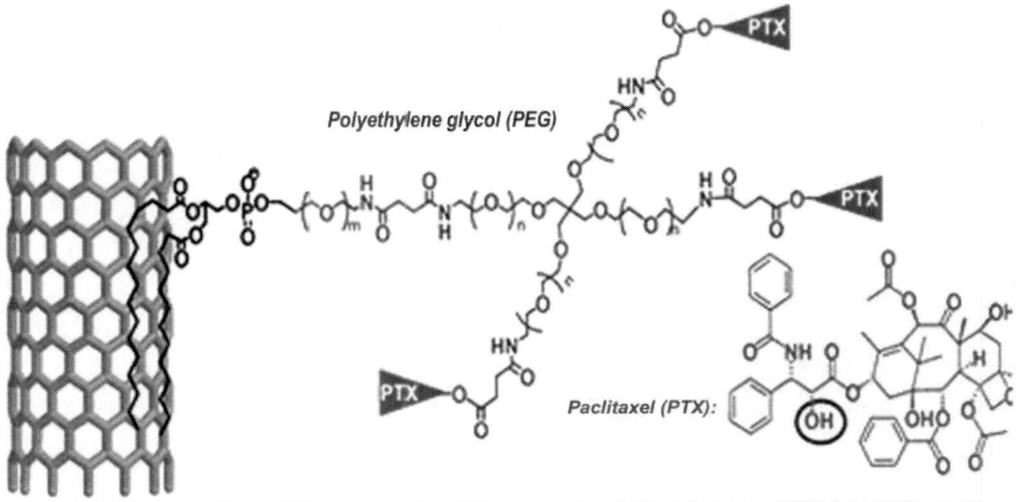

Figure 5. Schematic representation of a CNT based drug delivery system. While noncovalent interactions between phospholipids tail of branched PEG is led to CNT/polymer supramolecule, PTX molecules are conjugated to its end functional groups. The highlighted hydroxyl group with the blue circle indicates where the PTX molecules are attached to the PEG branches. Reprinted with the permission of Ref. [52].

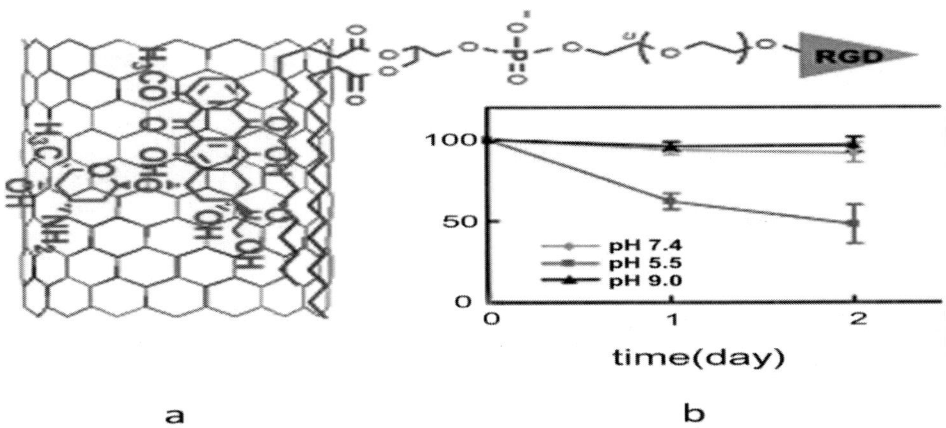

Figure 6. (a) π-π stacking of DCX molecule onto the surface of a CNT functionalized by PEG with phospholipids tail and RGD targeting ligand. (b) Release of the DOX molecules from the surface of functionalized SWNTs at different pHs. Faster release of the DOX molecules from the surface of SWNT in the acidic pH promise effective cancer therapy by this system with diminished side effects of DOX. Reprinted with the permission of Ref. [53a].

On the other hand CNT is responsible for fast transferring of system through the cell membrane. Higher tumor uptake of PTX and lower side effects are the most important advantages of this system [52]. DOX molecules have been directly loaded on the nanotube surface via π-π stacking. Loading capacity to transfer DOX molecules using this approach is high and resulted drug delivery system can be soluble in aqueous solution through noncovalent interactions with hydrophilic polymers. Targeting the obtained drug delivery system is possible by conjugation of the targeting molecules such as Arg Gly Asp (RGD) peptide to the functional groups of the CNT surface or the functional groups of the modifiers such as polymers (Figure 6a) [53]. Variety of targeting ligands including folic acid [54, 55], peptides [56, 57] and antibodies [58- 61] have been used to target CNTs to specific types of cells.

As above mentioned due to its aromatic rings and effective π-π stacking doxorubicin has remarkably high loading, up to 4 g of drug per 1 g of nanotube on the surface of PEGylated SWNTs. Interestingly the loading/binding interactions between DOX molecules and SWNTs surface is pH dependent and favorable for the controlled release of the drug in endosomes and lysosomes, as well as in tumor micro-environments with acidic pH (Figure 6b).

Chitosan (CHI) and Alginate (ALG) sodium have been used to functionalized and improve the water solubility and biocompatibility of loaded DOX molecules on SWNTs. Due to the cationic and anionic groups in the structure of chitosan and alginate respectively, their interaction with carbon nanotubes involves π-π stacking and electrostatic interactions. The red shift of two main absorptions of DOX molecules upon loading on SWNTs indicates their interactions with the surface of carbon nanotube (Figure 7a). Adsorption of the cationic DOX molecules onto the sidewalls of the modified SWNTs increased the zeta potentials of the nanotubes. The DOX loading efficiencies (defined as the weight ratio of DOX to the modified SWNTs) onto modified SWCNTs were found to be more than 120% (Figure 7b) and follow the order: DOX-ALG-SWNTs> DOX-SWNTs> DOX-CHI/ALG-SWNTs> DOX-CHI-SWNTs which corresponds to the ascending order of zeta potentials of the modified SWNTs. The release of the DOX molecules loaded on carbon nanotubes is pH-dependent.

The highest loading capacity and slowest rate of release of the loaded DOX molecules on the modified SWNTs is related to the ALG-SWNTs systems. In contrast, CHI-SWNTs has the lowest loading capacity but the rate of release of the loaded DOX molecules is high, therefore, the CHI/ALG-SWNTs systems are an ideal compromise in terms of loading and release of DOX [62].

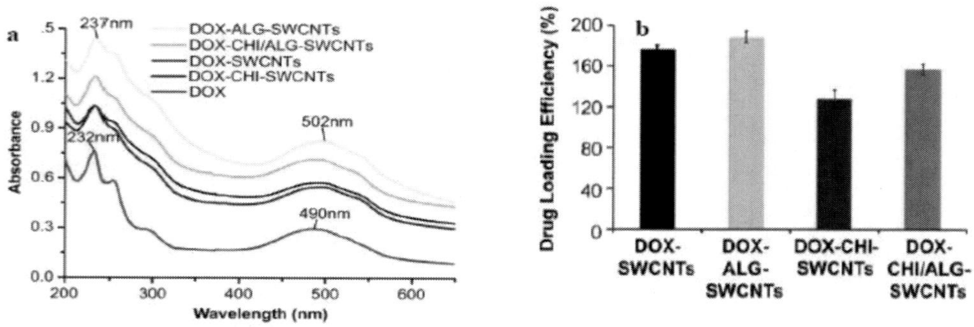

Figure 7. (a) UV-Vis absorption spectra of free DOX and DOX molecules loaded on functionalized and non-functionalized SWNTs. (b) Drug loading efficiency of functionalized and non-functionalized SWNTs. Reprinted with the permission of Ref. [62].

Platinum-based anticancer drugs are also transferred by carbon nanotubes that are functionalized noncovalently. SWNTs functionalized by phospholipids-poly(ethylene glycol) macromolecules (PL-PEG, *M*n~2000 Da) are used as a longboat delivery system to internalize a platinum(IV) complex into cancer cells also [63]. It has been found that platinum (IV) prodrug compounds do not have noticeable anticancer effects. After taking into cancer cells by endocytosis and reside in cell endosomes, where reduced pH induces reductive release of the platinum(II) core complex, they kill the cancer cells. The cytotoxicity of the platinum(IV) complex increases over 100-fold after attachment to SWNTs. Pt(IV) prodrugs attached to folic acid were conjugated to PEGylated SWNTs and used to kill the cancer cells [55]. An enhanced toxicity versus folate receptor (FR) positive cells but not to FR negative cells was observed by these systems.

Linear polymers such as PEG do not improve the functionality of CNTs as well as their water solubility and biocompatibility. Dendrimers and dendritic polymers are a type of tree-like polymers with a high functionality that should develop the functionality of CNTs, but a challenge is their weak non-covalent interactions with CNTs. Linear-dendritic copolymers such as PCA-PEG-PCA which are a hybrid of linear and dendritic polymers are the best candidates to develop the solubility and the functionality of CNTs by their linear and dendritic blocks respectively (Figure 8).

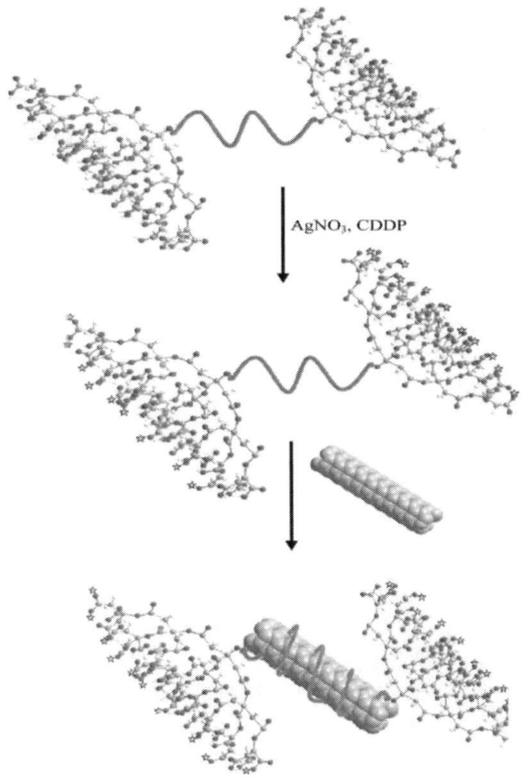

Figure 8. Noncovalent interactions between linear-dendritic copolymers and CNTs lead to hybrid nanomaterials with a high functionality. CNT/linear-dendritic hybrid materials are able to transfer a high number of anticancer drugs, due to their high functionality.

Noncovalent interactions between the PCA-PEG-PCA copolymers, synthesized using different ratios of poly(ethylene glycol)/citric acid (PEG/CA), and carbon nanotubes has led to the corresponding hybrid nanomaterials (CNT/PCA-PEG-PCA) that are completely soluble in water in different pHs and their aqueous solutions are stable over several months. Due to the high functionality of linear-dendritic copolymers, their noncovalent interactions with CNTs lead to highly functional hybrid materials with a high ability to transfer anticancer drugs such as cisplatin (CDDP) (Figure 8).

Various characterization methods have showed that both linear and dendritic blocks of linear-dendritic copolymers interact with the surface of CNTs [64].

These characterization shown that defects created on the sidewalls of carbon nanotubes, upon acid treatment, do not play an important role in the noncovalent interactions between the linear-dendritic copolymers and the CNTs and the π-π staking type of interactions between the carbonyl functional groups of dendritic blocks of linear-dendritic copolymers and π system of CNTs are the most significance interactions that attached these types of copolymers to CNTs noncovalently. Based on previous studies [65, 66] effective interactions between polymer and carbon nanotubes should lead to changes in their conformation.

Conformation and topology of CNT/PCA-PEG-PCA and CNT/PCA-PEG-PCA-CDDP hybrid nanomaterials has been investigated in solution and solid state by DLS, TEM and AFM.

DLS diagrams displayed unimodal size distributions with mean diameters of 237, 563 and 371 nm for PCA-PEG-PCA, CNT/PCA-PEG-PCA and CNT/PCA-PEG-PCA-CDDP hybrid nanomaterials respectively. The large size of the PCA-PEG-PCA linear-dendritic copolymers is ascribed to their self-assembly in aqueous solution [67].

While the length of carbon nanotubes is around several micrometres, the size (diameter) of the MWNT/PCA-PEG-PCA hybrid nanomaterials measured by DLS is 563 nm. Similar to linear polymers which are coiled in solution, the decreased diameter of the CNTs can be assigned to their looping due to the noncovalent interactions with the linear-dendritic copolymers (Figure 9).

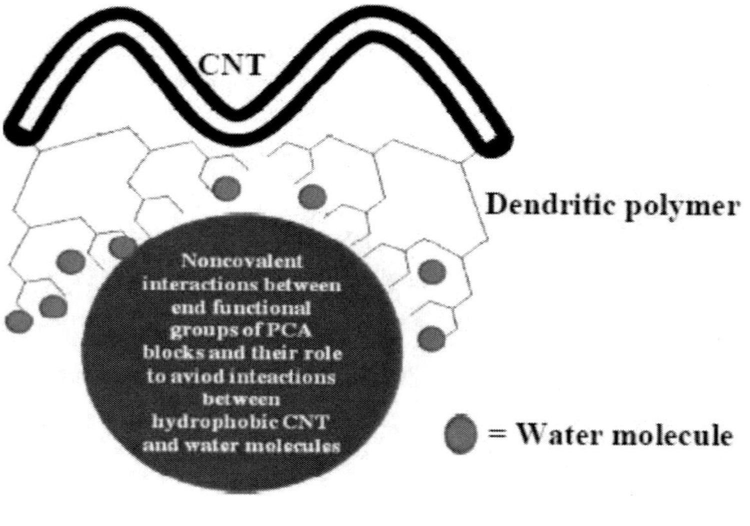

Figure 9. Noncovalent interactions between linear-dendritic copolymers and MWNTs change their conformation from extended to closed in the solution state.

Confirming the results obtained by IR and NMR spectroscopy, DLS show that the diameter of the CNT/PCA-PEG-PCA hybrid nanomaterials is even more decreased after the conjugation of CDDP molecules to the functional groups of linear-dendritic copolymers. Based on these results CNT/PCA-PEG-PCA-CDDP hybrid nanomaterials should have a very packed conformation or spherical structure in the solution state. AFM images show spherical topology with 200-350 nm diameter for CNT/PCA-PEG-PCA-CDDP hybrid nanomaterials (Figures 10a and c). Three phases relating to the three components of the hybrid nanomaterials can be clearly recognized in their phase contrast images (Figures 10b and d).

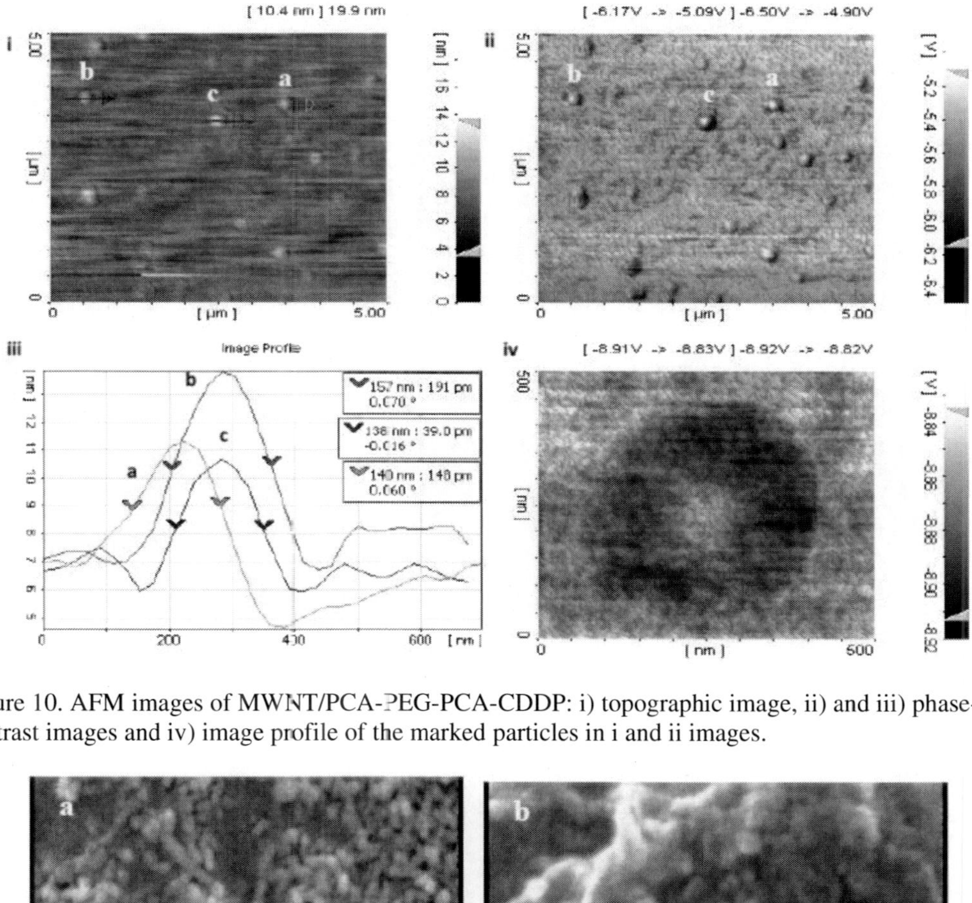

Figure 10. AFM images of MWNT/PCA-PEG-PCA-CDDP: i) topographic image, ii) and iii) phase-contrast images and iv) image profile of the marked particles in i and ii images.

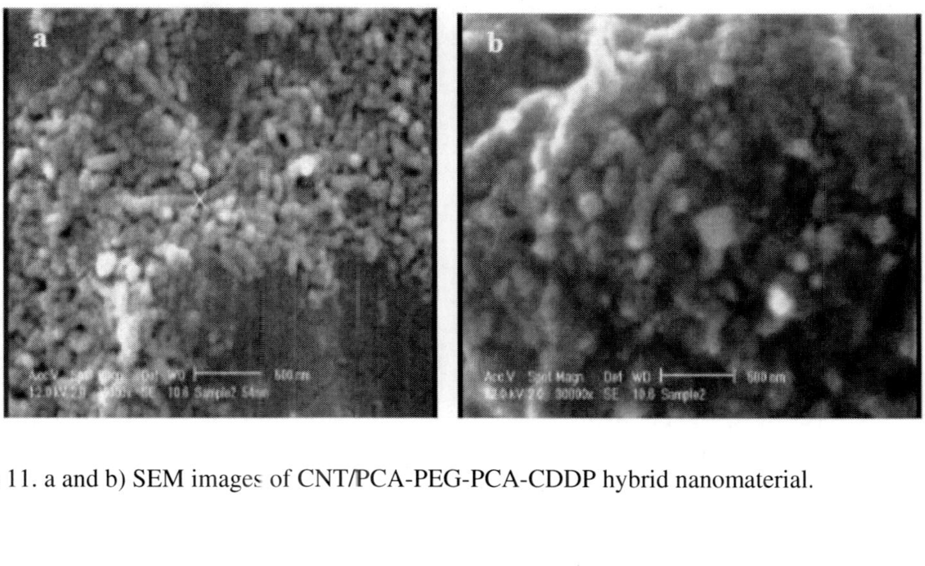

Figure 11. a and b) SEM images of CNT/PCA-PEG-PCA-CDDP hybrid nanomaterial.

According to the SEM images, MWNT/PCA-PEG-PCA-CDDP hybrid nanomaterials have a spherical topology and are in a packed conformation. The average size of the spherical objects is around 200-300 nm (Figure 11a and b).

This result is highly significant when carbon nanotubes are used for medical proposes, because their size is decreased to 200-300 nm which is desirable for an effective passive targeting. TEM images also show that noncovalent interactions between PCA-PEG-PCA linear-dendritic copolymer and CNT, causes a closed conformation and coiled shape for CNT (Figure 12 a).

As it is exhibited by TEM images, synthesized hybrid nanomaterials “transfer” CDDP moleculess not only by conjugation to linear-dendritic copolymers on their surface but also by their cavity (Figure 12 b).

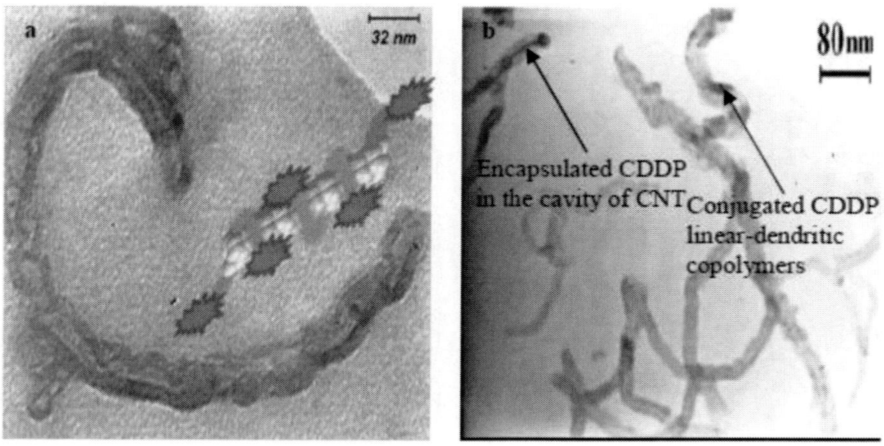

Figure 12. TEM images of a) MWNT/PCA-PEG-PCA and b) MWNT/PCA-PEG-PCA-CDDP.

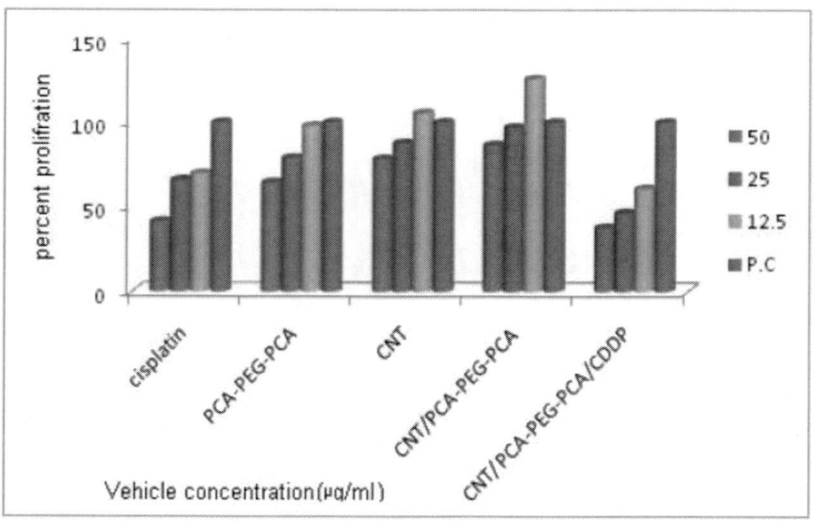

Figure 13. Percentage survival of C26 cancer cells, assessed by the MTT assay, after exposure to free CDDP, opened CNT, PCA-PEG-PCA, CNT/PCA-PEG-PCA and CNT/PCA-PEG-PCA-CDDP at 12.5, 25 and 50 μg/ml (n = 3). P.C is the positive control.

MTT (3-(4,5-dimethylthiazol-2-yl)-2,5-diphenyltetrazolium bromide) assay showed not only any toxicity, up to 12.5 μg/ml, for PCA-PEG-PCA linear-dendritic copolymers but also an increase in the growth of incubated cells against untreated control cells (Figure 13). Due to the citric acid backbone of linear-dendritic copolymers, probably it can be used as the source of energy by the cells and therefore it leads to an increase in the growth and division of the cells. Hence any object associated with the PCA-PEG-PCA linear-dendritic copolymers should insert in the cell metabolism and influence the viability of the cells extensively. MWNTs rise rate of the "transferring" of the linear-dendritic copolymers from the cell membrane leading to an increase in the cell growth (Figure 13).

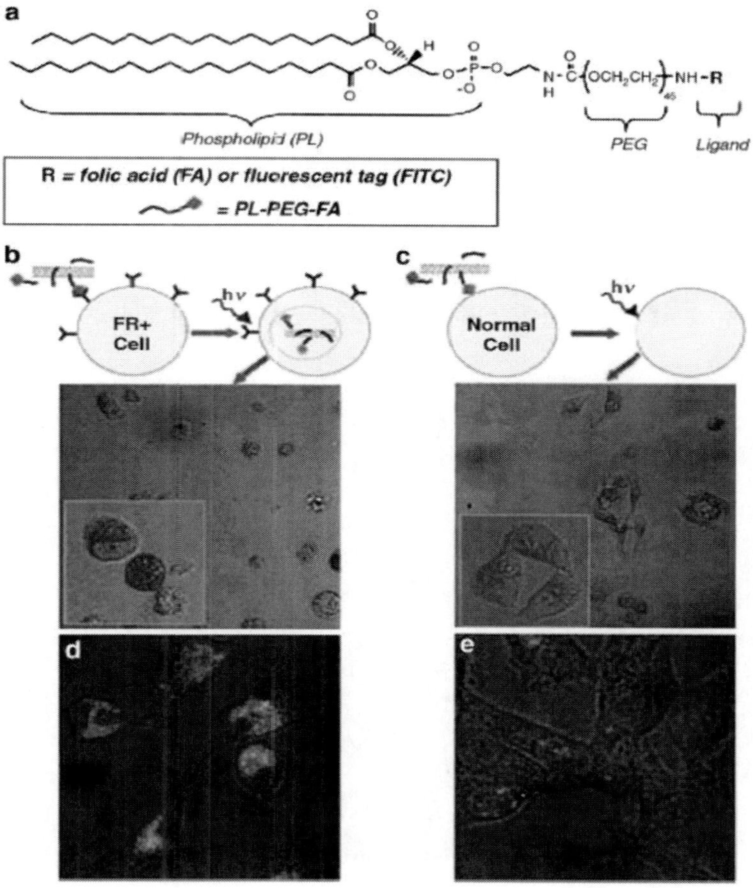

Figure 14. (a) Structure of PL-PEG-ligand (ligand is FA or fluorescine (FA)). PL-PEG–ligand spacers were used for solubilizing SWNTs, targeting them and (with the use of NIR radiation) killing tumor cells. (b) (upper) Schematic representation of SWNT/PL-PEG-FA hybrid materials entering tumor cells that have FR over-expressed (FR+) and (lower) killing the cells by NIR 808-nm laser radiation. Dead cells were identified as having a rounded morphology (inset, higher magnification image of dead cells). (c) (upper) Schematic representation of SWNT/PL-PEG-FA hybrid materials cultured with normal cells (no FR over-expressing). (lower) Normal cells remained intact after the same laser treatment as in (b). (inset) Higher magnification of a normal cell. (d) Confocal image of FR+ tumor cells showing the presence of SWNTs conjugated with PL-PEG-FA spacer and PL-PEG-marker (indicated by green FITC fluorescence). (e) Normal cells showed little uptake of SWNT/PL-PEG-marker (indicated by little green FITC fluorescence) under the same treatment condition as in (d). Reprinted with the permission of Ref. [72].

Due to their complementary roles, the toxicity of the CNT/PCA-PEG-PCA-CDDP is even higher than that for the free drug. Because MWNT increases the rate of the crossing of the cell membrane and PCA-PEG-PCA linear-dendritic copolymer improve the water solubility of the CNTs and probably inserts them in the cell metabolism.

CNTs can also be used for hyperthermia treatment of cancer cells and tumors [68]. Since SWNTs have a strong optical absorption in the near-infrared region (NIR, 700-1100 nm) [69] in which optical absorption by tissues and biological molecules is minimal and therefore penetration is optimal [70, 71], irradiation of SWNTs using NIR light can effectively heat up them in vivo. Attachment of several ligands to the surface of CNTs that can bind specifically to receptors over-expressed on cancer cells leads to assemblies of carbon nanotubes in these cells that upon irradiation kill the cancer cells. Functionalization of SWNTs with folic acid (FA) through phospholipids-PEG spacer to create SWNT/PL-PEG–FA supramolecules (Figure 14a), is an example of selective hyperthermia treatment of cancer cells. FA binds specifically to folate receptors (FR) that are over-expressed in many cancer cell types (such as ovarian, cervical, breast and lung cancers) and therefore dominate internalizing SWNT/PL-PEG-FA hybrid materials to tumor cells. Investigations have shown that SWNT/PL-PEG-FA hybrid materials accumulate inside FR-positive cancer cells but not inside normal cells (Figure 14b and c). Exposure cancer cells containing accumulations of SWNT/PL-PEG-FA hybrid materials to NIR radiation (808 nm laser) kill these cells (Figure 14d, e) [72].

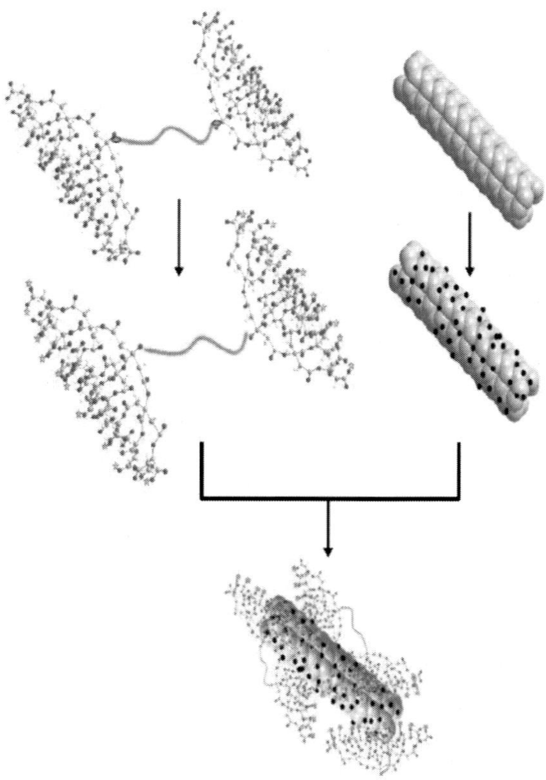

Figure 15. (a) Functionalization of carbon nanotubes by γ-Fe_2O_3 nanoparticles and PCA-PEG-PCA linear-dendritic prodrugs by noncovalent interactions.

However it is also possible to accumulate carbon nanotubes in tumors by passive targeting and without needing ligands, because blood vessels around cancer cells have an abnormal flow rather than healthy cells [73]. Therefore more heat increasing take place about cancer cells rather than healthy cells upon irradiation. Modifying of the carbon nanotubes by magnetic nanoparticles confer them magnetic properties so that they can response to an external magnetic field. Selective delivery of CNTs to tumor cells for minimizing their side effects can be achieved by simultaneously anchoring iron oxide nanoparticles and PCA-PEG-PCA copolymers to their surface followed by using an external magnetic field (Figure 15).

AFM images of PCA-PEG-PCA/CNT/γ-Fe_2O_3NP confirm that linear-dendritic copolymers are assembled onto the surface of CNTs. Non-continues molecular self-assemblies of linear-dendritic copolymers onto the surface of CNTs axis show that interactions between linear-dendritic copolymers and CNTs surface change regionally (Figures 16a and 16b). As it have been deduced from other characteristics data, dendritic parts are responsible for interactions between linear-dendritic copolymers and CNT/γ-Fe_2O_3NP surface. While dendritic parts have a large number of peripheral carboxyl functional groups they only interact with iron oxide nanoparticles on CNTs surface. Therefore in AFM images places where molecular self-assemblies are exist are regions of CNTs surface that defects are induced by acid treatments and other places are non-changed regions.

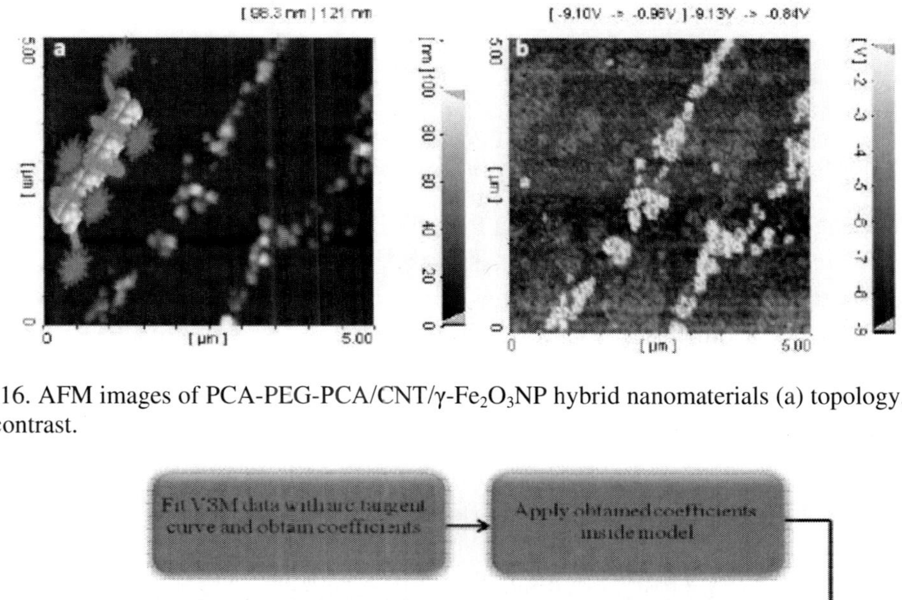

Figure 16. AFM images of PCA-PEG-PCA/CNT/γ-Fe_2O_3NP hybrid nanomaterials (a) topology, (b) phase contrast.

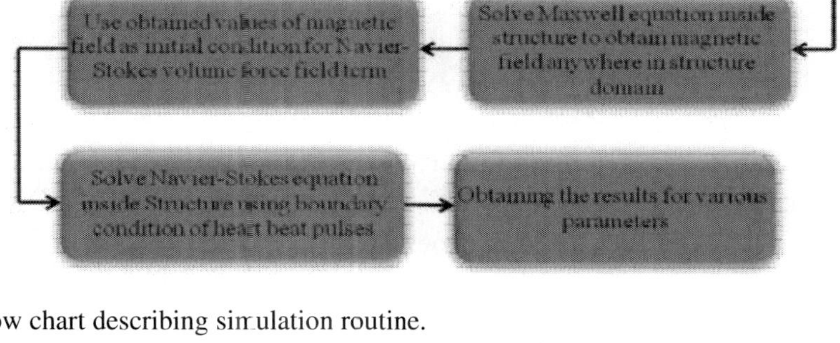

Figure 17. Flow chart describing simulation routine.

The main reason to anchor magnetic nanoparticles to functionalized CNTs was to target them to tumors using a magnetic field. In order to prove the efficacy of γ-Fe_2O_3 nanoparticles to target functionalized CNTs to tumors, interaction of an external magnetic field with magnetic fluid (blood containing PCA-PEG-PCA/CNT/γ-Fe_2O_3NP hybrid nanomaterials) was numerically simulated. The procedure to obtain the velocity of blood in the presence and absence of PCA-PEG-PCA/CNT/γ-Fe_2O_3NP hybrid nanomaterials has been illustrated in flow chart showed in figure 17.

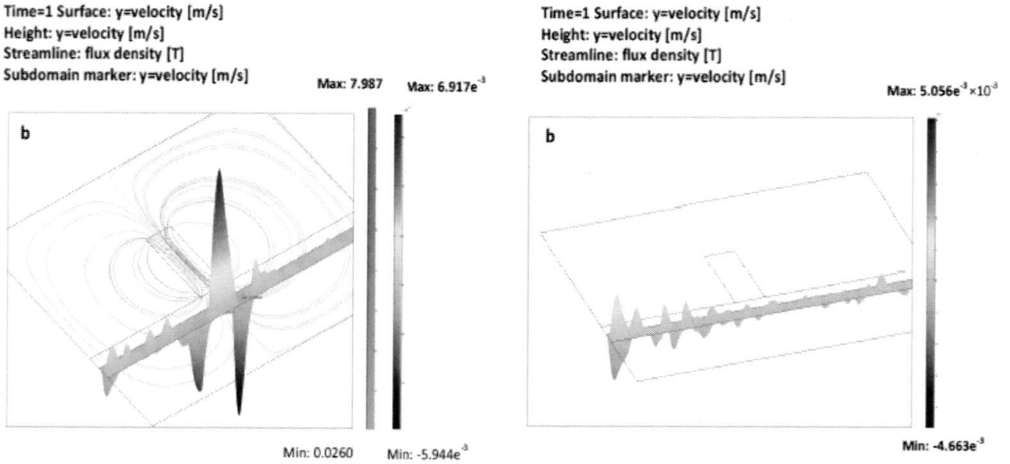

Figure 18. Velocity of fluid in y direction (perpendicular to vessel) for (a) PCA-PEG-PCA/CNT/γ-Fe_2O_3NP in the magnetic field and (b) PCA-PEG-PCA/CNT/γ-Fe_2O_3NP in the absence of the magnetic field.

Since changing the velocity of the blood from the "x" direction, along the blood vessel, to the "y" direction, perpendicular to the blood vessel, by PCA-PEG-PCA/CNT/γ-Fe_2O_3NP hybrid nanomaterials in a magnetic field show their efficacy to increase the diffusion of blood from blood vessel to tissues or tumors, the velocity of blood containing PCA-PEG-PCA/CNT/γ-Fe_2O_3NP hybrid nanomaterials in the presence and absence of a magnetic field was calculated. Results showed that there is a considerable difference between velocity of blood in the "y" direction in the presence and absence of a magnetic field. When blood was containing PCA-PEG-PCA/CNT/γ-Fe_2O_3NP hybrid nanomaterials, impacting of the blood to the vessel wall increased more than ten times upon switching the magnetic field on (Figures 18a and b) [74].

The magnetic CNTs prepared by filling them with iron oxides nanoparticles would apply for selective drug delivery to specific locations in the body, as well as for diagnostics without surgical interference [75]. Knowing the change in electronic properties of SWNT devices upon antibody adsorption scientists have reported detection of live breast cancer cells with a monoclonal antibody(mAb–SWNT) device in that they adsorbed mAb specific to insulin-like growth factor 1 receptor (IGF1R) onto interconnected SWNT networks placed between lithographically patterned electrode [76].

CNTs can be functionalized by DNA macromolecules noncovalently [77]. CNT/DNA supramolecules can be used to hyperthermia treatment of cancer cells and safely eradicate a tumor mass *in vivo*. The generated heat depends on irradiation time and laser power linearly. Irreversible protein denaturation or membrane damage at temperatures above 40 °C is responsible for the death of cancer cells [78, 79]. The mechanism of heat generation is based on enhanced vibrational modes due to excitation of optical transitions with relaxation.

3.3. Biosensors

Sensors are a class of devices that have found widespread use. A sensor comprises an active sensing element and a signal transducer, and produces an electrical, optical, thermal or magnetic output signal. A biosensor can be described as a device which has a biological sensing element connected to (or integrated with) a transducer, thus transforming a biological event into a signal which can then be interpreted [80]. The first biosensors were reported in the early 1960s [81].

Its differ from classical chemical sensors in the following two ways:

1) The sensing element consists of a biological material such as proteins (e.g., cell receptors, enzymes, antibodies), oligo- or polynucleotides, microorganisms, or even whole biological tissues [82, 83]
2) The sensor is used to monitor biological processes or for the recognition of biomolecules.

For *in vitro* biosensing, the sample solution (such as blood serum, urine, milk products etc.) is dropped atop the biosensor, and the output signal gives information on the composition of the solution. By contrast, *in vivo* biosensing addresses dynamic systems, aiming for instance to measure the rate of uptake or efflux of relevant species or to estimate the spatial distribution of the concentration of an analyte in a living organism [82].

Because of unique physical properties including high surface area, semiconducting behavior, band gap fluorescence and strong Raman scattering spectra, carbon nanotubes allow subsequent applications in biosensing. In general, there are two types of biosensors that prepared with used from CNTs.

1) CNT-based paste electrodes
2) Electrodes modified by CNTs

3.3.1. CNT-Based Paste Electrodes

CNT paste electrodes (CNTPE) have been obtained by mixing CNT powder with deionized water, bromoform or mineral oil. For biosensing purposes, an enzyme is added to the mixture to obtain a CNTPE with incorporated enzymes. For biosensing purposes, an enzyme is added to the mixture to obtain a CNTPE with incorporated enzymes [80, 84].

3.3.2. Electrodes Modified by CNTs

Conventional electrochemical biosensors are based on either glassy carbon electrodes (GCE) or metal electrodes (Au, Pt or Cu for example) for amperometric or voltammetric analyte detection. Such electrodes have a series of disadvantages, including poor sensitivity and stability, low reproducibility, large response times and a high overpotential for electron transfer reactions. CNTs can overcome most of these disadvantages due to their ability to undergo fast electron transfer and the resistance of CNT-modified electrodes to surface fouling [85]. The simplest route to CNT-modified electrodes is to cast a solution of CNTs on to a glassy carbon electrodes (GCE). Since CNTs are insoluble in most solvents, ultrasonication is required during preparation in order to effectively disperse the tubes. Electrodes have been fabricated by dispersing CNTs in a phosphate buffer or concentrated sulfuric acid, and subsequent spin-casting onto a polished GCE [86, 87]. The dispersion of CNTs in aqueous solution can be facilitated by an appropriate surfactant.

3.3.3. Electrochemical Biosensors

Electrochemical biosensors are the oldest and most commonly used transducers in biosensors. Electrical detection methods are appealing because of their low cost, low power consumption, ease of miniaturisation, and potential multiplexing capability [81]. They are currently among the most popular of the various types of biosensors. Carbon materials have been used as components in electrochemical biosensors for over a decade. Biosensing can be performed using a broad spectrum of techniques. Many classical approaches like mass spectrometry and biolabeled fluorescence usually require a number of steps before the biomolecule are detected [88]. Such methods are highly sensitive, but are difficult to miniaturize. Electronic and electrochemical detection techniques, in comparison, are advantageous in this aspect. Carbon nanotubes are promising materials for sensing applications due to several unique properties. In particular, their large length to diameter aspect ratios provide for high surface to volume ratios. Also CNTs are attractive materials for application to biosensors due to the low-potential detection of hydrogen peroxide and NADH and the minimal surface passivation during the electrochemical oxidation of NADH. The major barrier for fabricating well-defined CNT-modified electrode is the low solubility of CNTs in most common solvents.

There are several ways for confining CNTs on to electrochemical transducers [89]. In addition, CNT chemical functionalization can be used to attach almost any favorite chemical species to them, which allows us for instance to enhance the solubility and biocompatibility of the tubes. This has permitted the realization of composite electrodes comprising CNTs well-dispersed in an appropriate polymer matrix [90]. Pristine or specifically functionalized CNTs have been shown to be capable of detecting biomolecules.

There several approaches to the development of electrochemical biosensors using CNTs. i) In the simplest method, CNTs are randomly deposited onto conductive surfaces in a mat configuration (CNT mats) or packed into a micropipette for use as electrodes. This method results in an unknown configuration of CNTs which, although easy to achieve, may not offer optimal signals. Alternatively, the CNTs can be coated with the biomolecule of interest after electrode fabrication. ii) The second approach involves vertically aligned CNT forests, with one end in contact with the underlying electrode and the other end exposed in the electrolyte solution. This configuration may be achieved by growing the CNTs directly from the surface or by self-assembly of shortened CNTs. CNTs are typically functionalized after this electrode type has been assembled. iii) A third type of nanoelectrode uses just a single CNT. If the type of CNT used could be controlled precisely (SWNT versus MWNT, metallic versus semiconducting), this would ultimately give the best performance. However, the fabrication and manipulation challenges involved will limit its practical use. Electrochemical methods for detecting biomolecules in solution are highly attractive due to their simplicity and the relative ease of calibration [91]. Electrochemical sensors can be based on potentiometry, amperometry, voltammetry, coulometry, AC conductivity or capacitance measurements. Most of the CNT-based electrochemical biosensors perform the detection of biomolecules amperometrically. CNT-based biosensors incorporating enzymes are then presented, starting with the glucose biosensors by Leland and Champ in 1962 [81].

There are enormous amount of literature exists on glucose biosensors[92, 93,94] Enzyme-free electrochemical biosensors have been successfully applied to the detection of various molecules such as Dopamine (Dopamine is a neurotransmitter and a neurohormone belonging to the catecholamine family of phenolic compounds.), NAD^+ (Nicotinamide adenine dinucleotide is an important cofactor of redox reactions inside living cells), Organophosphorus compounds [95], Cholesterol [96], nitric oxide [97], Morphine (Morphine the principal active agent in opium is a powerful analgesic drug) [98], Cysteine (Cysteine is a sulfur-containing amino acid commonly used in the food and pharmaceutical industry) [99], indole acetic acid (IAA) (a plant hormone) [100], Cytochrome c (Cytochrome c is a highly conserved protein present in a wide spectrum of plant and animal species) [101], and arsenite [102].

3.3.4. SWCNT-Based Field-Effect Transistors (Fets) and Chemiresistors

In addition to electrochemical sensors using CNTs as an electrode substrate, sensors based on transistor arrangements using CNTs have been developed [103]. SWCNTs are the most likely candidate for miniaturizing electronics beyond the microelectromechanical scale currently used in electronics. They exhibit electrical properties not shared by their multiwalled counterparts, and certain sizes of SWCNTs act as semiconductors. [104].

Since FET-based biomolecular detection does not employ fluorescence, electrochemical or magnetic tags, it has been termed a "label-free" methodology [105- 107]. FETs generally consist of a substrate (gate), two microelectrodes (source and drain) and a SWCNT or SWCNT network that bridges the electrodes SWCNTs are prospective candidates for molecular scale electronic devices [108,109].

The sensitivity of such devices towards specific gases could be further improved by chemically modifying the tubes in a covalent or noncovalent manner [110]. Sensors based upon SWCNT-FETs can be operated in two different ways. One possibility is to monitor the conductance of an individual SWCNT or a network of SWCNTs during the introduction of the analyte solution. In this chemiresistor configuration, the resistance of the device is directly or inversely proportional to the concentration of the analyte. A second method is to measure the complete field-effect modulation of conductance after introduction of the test solution. This latter methodology is referred to as chemFET, where the threshold voltage shift provides information about the analyte concentration [80].

In general, it could said due to their small size and excellent electrochemical properties, CNTs continue to attract enormous interest as components in biosensors. Meanwhile, it is now well established that CNT-based electrodes have electrochemical properties that are equal or superior to most other electrodes [111].

Further improvements may be expected from extending the range of modifying molecules that can be attached to the tubes; enzymes, nucleic acids and metal nanocrystals have been mostly employed for this purpose so far [112].

4. Toxicity

Although considerable research works has performed to evaluate the toxicity of nanomaterials and their effect on body and biological systems, this research filed is still in fancy and much more significant efforts is required in order to completely discern the effects of nanoscale materials on humans and the environment [113,114]. Toxicology studies of CNTs have been performed since 2003 [115]. As it mentioned the results are relatively few and it is not possible to make full conclusions and accurate human assessments. In a research work, SWNTs were injected to mice organs but no special toxic side effect was observed after two months [116], while other reports have suggested that nanotubes cause pulmonary damage to the lungs of mice and alter protein expression [117]. Toxicity of CNTs depend on their structural factors such as number of walls (SWNT or MWNT), length and aspect ratio, surface area, degree of aggregation, extent of oxidation, surface topology, bound functional group(s), and method of manufacturing (which can leave catalyst residues and produce impurities) strongly. Toxicity of CNTs is also depend on their concentration and dose to which cells or organisms are exposed [118]. Exposure of the human epidermal keratinocytes (HaCaT) to SWNTs [119] causes an accelerated oxidative stress which is due to the formation of free radicals and accumulation of peroxidative products. Source of free radicals is assigned to the metal catalysts remained in the structure of SWNTs. Effect of CNTs on rat macrophages (NR8383) and human A549 lung cell lines is studied [120]. It has been found that pristine CNTs show a toxicity on cell lines and causes necrosis and apoptosis deaths even after purification [121-124]. Carbon based materials such as carbon nanoparticles, carbon nanofibers, carbon black and active carbon seem to be more toxic than MWNTs. Interestingly SWNTs seem to be typically more toxic than MWNTs [124,125]. Functionalization of CNTs reduces their toxicity compared with pristine CNTs, due to their increased water solubility and diminished non-specific interactions with the biological molecules [126,127]. Toxicity of the pristine CNTs has been compared with those functionalized by different process and it has been found that pristine CNTs show higher toxicity than surfactant-aided dispersed CNTs. Toxicity of functionalized CNTs with positive surface charge is a function of their charge density and much lower than nonfunctionalized CNTs in vitro [128]. Toxicity of CNTs depends on their diameter reversely and aspect ratio directly [129]. The toxicity of CNTs is time and concentration dependent, so that 0.1 mg/mL of nonfunctionalized CNT and 5×10^{-5} μg/mL of functionalized CNTs can cause cell death. It seems that the biocompatibility of CNTs depends on controllable factors such as structural properties including size, morphology and surface charge of CNTs as well as the additives and impurities. If so, it may be possible to establish safe concentration ranges for different types of nanotubes.

5. Uptake

As it was explained in chapter one, the drug delivery systems are directed to the targeted cells via passive targeting (a methodology to increase the amounts of delivered drugs by minimizing non-specific interactions with non-target biological systems) or active targeting (that in which the therapeutic agent is delivered to tumors by attaching the drug delivery system with a ligand that binds to specific receptors that are over-expressed on target cells)

[130]. There are tow fates for the carrier systems after crossing different biological barriers and reaching the targeted sites (organs, tissues or cells): (i) the therapeutic agent cross the barrier of the targeted site (i.e., enters the cells) without internalization of the carrier system, (ii) both the therapeutic agent and the carrier system cross the barrier of the targeted site and enter the cells. The latter internalization method has greater delivery efficacy so that after entering cells, the intracellular environment will degrade the drug-carrier systems to the small molecules and release drug molecules inside the cells [72]. There are several factors and properties that dominate the cellular uptake of CNTs crucially. The first factor which is the surface properties of CNTs, greatly influence their interaction with the cells and biological macromolecules and therefore their internalization into the cells. For example, hydrophobicity and hydrophilicity (in modified CNTs) of CNTs surface influence their interactions with the cell surface, due to the presence of the hydrophobic and hydrophilic regions on the cell surface. Second factor that influence uptake of CNTs by cells is their size and shapes [131]. CNTs with a better water solubility and shorter lengths can be internalized by the cells than bundled CNTs or CNTs that have longer lengths. It seems CNTs are taken up by cells through clathrin-dependent endocytosis [131]. Different mechanisms for the cell uptake of CNTs have been reported [132]. For example, SWNTs functionalized by proteins or DNA were shown to enter cells in an energy-dependent manner [133]. This difference is assigned to the different surface characteristics and subcellular locations of CNTs. There are some evidences that SWNTs entered the cell nucleus [132- 135] and this entrance might be reversible [135], but there is no finding about nucleus cell entrance of MWNTs. Human embryonic kidney epithelial cells (HEK293) uptake single MWNTs and their bundles through direct penetration and endocytosis respectively. Single nanotubes penetrate from endosome membrane to the cytoplasm and MWCNT bundles then transport into lysosomes.

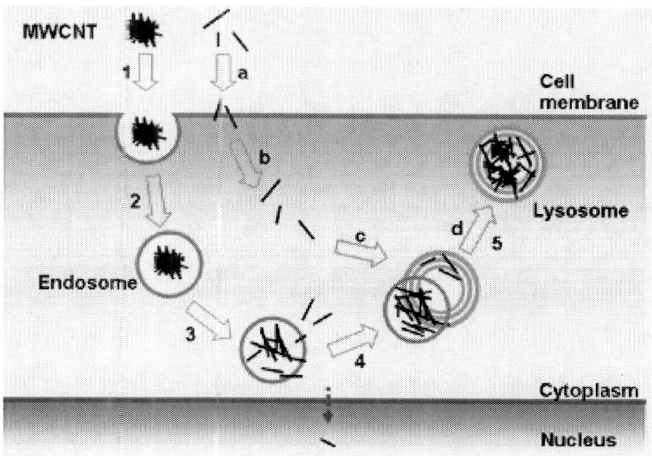

Figure 19. A mechanism for the cell uptake of MWNTs. Numbers (1-5) and letters (a-d) indicate different steps in two possible cellular translocation pathways of MWNTs. The bundled MWNTs bind to cell membranes (1) and are subsequently internalized into cells (2) inside endosomes. In the endosomes, bundles release single MWNTs that penetrate endosomal membranes and enter cytoplasm (3). Both residual bundled MWNTs in endosomes and free MWNTs in the cytoplasm are recruited into lysosomes for excretion (4, 5). Single MWNTs enter cells through direct membrane penetration (a) to enter cytoplasm (b). They are recruited into lysosomes for excretion (c, d). Short MWNTs are also able to enter the nucleus.

The accumulation of cytoplasmic MWNTs increased their chance to enter cell nucleus. Only short MWNTs can enter the cell nucleus. Other types of MWNTs and longer ones are recruited into lysosome for excretion. Although it has been reported that cell uptake of the CNTs don't depend on their surface charge, due to the protein absorption on their surface in biological mediums, but it seems in this stage more investigations is need to clear the effect of this parameter and it this factor could not be negligible in this case (figure 19)[136].

However more studies and investigations should be performed to fully understand interactions of CNTs with the cell membranes and especially their interactions with the biological macromolecules and objects in the cytoplasm, which is a very critical barrier for delivering and targeting the therapeutic agents.

Conclusion

Unique physical and chemical properties make carbon nanotubes (CNTs) as suitable candidates for biomedical applications but use of CNTs for biomedical applications is acquiring more and more obvious evidence for efficient development. It is clear that some important issues related to the health impact including the biodistribution, accumulation and elimination have to be addressed more thoroughly before CNTs can be proposed for clinical trials. However, CNTs show remarkable carrier properties, with a very strong tendency to cross cell membranes, and seem to perfectly fit in nanomedicine. Although, the toxicological studies on pristine CNTs are contradictory, showing a certain degree of danger, it is becoming evident that functionalised CNTs have reduced toxic effects. Therefore, the combination of cell uptake capacity with high loading of cargo molecules achievable with CNTs makes this new carbon nanomaterial a promising candidate for innovative therapies.

References

[1] Boccaccini, A. R.; Cho, J.; Roether, J. A.; Thomas, B. J. C. E.; Minay, J.; Shaffer, M. S. P. *Carbon.* 2006, *44*, 3149.

[2] Kong ,J.; Franklin, N.R.; Zhou, C.; Chapline, M.G.; Peng S, Cho, K. et al. *Science.* 2000, *287*, 622.

[3] (a) Kwon, S-H.; Jeong, Y-K.; Kwon, S.; Kang, M-CH.; Lee, H-W. *Transactions of Nonferrous Metals Society of China.* 2011 *21,* 126. (b) Besteman, K.; Lee, J.; Wiertz, F.; Heering. H.; Dekker, C. *Nano Letters.* 2003, *3*, 727.

[4] Wang, C.; Guo, Z. X.; Fu, S.; Wu, W.; Zhu, D. *Prog. Polym. Sci.* 2004, *29*, 1079.

[5] Breuer, O.; Sundararaj, U. *Polym. Comp.* 2004, *25*, 630.

[6] Xiea, X. L.; Mai, Y. W.; Zhou, X. P. *Mater Sci. Eng R-Rep.* 2005, *49*, 89.

[7] (a) Nakashima, N. *Int J Nanosci.* 2005, *4*, 119. (b) Ji, S.; Liu, C.; Zhang, B.; Yang, F.; Xu, J.; Long, J.; Jin, C.; Fu, D.; Ni, Q.; Yu, X. *Biochimica et Biophysica Acta* 2010, *1806*, 29–35. (c) Liu, Z.; Tabakman, S.; Welsher, K.; Dai, H. *Nano Res.* 2009, *2*, 85-120. (d) Chen, X.; Schluesener, H. J. *Nanotechnology* 2010, *21*, 105104.

[8] O'Connell, M. J.; Boul, P.; Ericson, L. M.; Huffman, C.; Wang, Y.; Haroz, E.; Kuper, C.; Tour, J.; Ausman, K. D.; Smalley, R. E. *Chem. Phys. Lett.* 2001, *342*, 265.

[9] Star, A.; Stoddart, J. F.; Steuerman, D.; Diehl, M.; Boukai, A.; Wong, E. W.; Yang, X.; Chung, S. W.; Choi, H.; Heath, J. R. *Angew. Chem.-Int. Ed.* 2001, *40*, 1721.

[10] (a) Gao, J.; Loi, M. A.; Carvalho, E. J. F. D; Dos Santos, M. C. *ACS Nano*, 2011, *5* (5), 3993. (b) Star, A.; Steuerman, D. W.; Heath, J. R.; Stoddart, J. F. *Angew. Chem.-Int. Ed.* 2002, *41*, 2508.

[11] (a)Vijayakumar, C.; Balan, B.; Kim, M-J.; Takeuchi, M. *J. Phys. Chem. C.* 2011, *115* (11), 4533. (b) Chen, J.; Liu, H.; Weimer, W. A.; Halls, M. D.; Waldeck, D. H.; Walker, G. C. *J. Am. Chem. Soc.* 2002, *124*, 9034.

[12] (a) Lou, S.; Daussin, R.; Cuenot, S.; Duwez, A. S.; Pagnoulle, C.; Detrembleur, C. et al. *Chem Mater.* 2004, *16*, 4005. (b) Chaudhuri, P.; Soni, S.; Sengupta, S. *Nanotechnology* 2010, *21*, 025102. (c) . b) Lay, C. L.; Liu, H. Q.; Tan, H. R.; Liu, Y. *Nanotechnology* 2010, *21*, 065101.

[13] Yang, M.; Koutsos, V.; Zaiser, M. *J. Phys. Chem. B.* 2005, *109*, 10009.

[14] Nakashima, N.; Tomonari, Y.; Murakami, H. *Chem Lett.* 2002,*31*, 638.

[15] Petrov, P.; Stassin, F.; Pagnoulle, C.; Jérome, R. *Chem. Commun.* 2003, *23*, 2904.

[16] Kharisov, B. I.; Kharissova, O. V.; Gutierrez, H. L.; Me´ndez, U. O. *Ind. Eng. Chem. Res.* 2009, *48*, 572.

[17] Li, L.; Li, B.; Hood, M. A.; Li, C. Y. *Polymer.* 2009, *50*, 953.

[18] Meuer, S.; Braun, L.; Schilling, T.; Zentel, R. *Polymer.* 2009, *50*, 154.

[19] (a) Wu, Y.; Hudson, J. S.; Lu, Q.; Moore, J. M.; Mount, A. S.; Rao, A. M.; Alexov, E.; ChunKe, P. *American Chemical Society.* 2006, *110*, 2475. (b) Moghimi, S. M.; Andersen, A. J.; Hashemi, S. H.; Lettiero, B.; Ahmadvand, D.; Hunter, A. C.; Andresen, T. L. Hamad, I.; Szebeni, J. *Journal of Controlled Release* 2010, *146*, 175–181.

[20] (a) Detriche, S.; Devillers, S.; Seffer, J.-F.; Nagy, J.B.; Mekhalif, Z.; Delhalle, J. *Carbon. 49 (9)*, 2011, 2935. (b) Lou, X.; Daussin, R.; Cuenot, S.; Duwez, A. S.; Pagnoulle, C.; Detrembleur, C. et al. *Chem Mater.* 2004, *16*, 4005.

[21] Kam, N. W. S.; O'Connell, M.; Wisdom. J. A.; Dai, H. *Proc. Natl. Acad. Sci. U. S. A.* 2005, *102*, 11600.

[22] Rinaudo, M. *Prog. Polym. Sci.* 2006, *31*, 603.

[23] Adeli, M.; Hamid, M.; Beyranvand, S. *Carbon.* 2011, submitted.

[24] Wang, S. F.; Shen, L.; Zhang, W. D.; Tong, Y. J. *Biomacromolecules.* 2005, *6*, 3067.

[25] Wu, Z.; Feng, W.; Feng, Y.; Liu, Q.; Xu, X.; Sekino, T. et al. *Carbon.* 2007, *45*, 1212.

[26] Moulton, S. E.; Minett, A. I.; Murphy, R.; Ryan, K. P.; McCarthy, D.; Coleman, J. N. et al. *Carbon.* 2005, *43*, 1879.

[27] Yang, M. H.; Yang, Y.; Yang, H. F.; Shen, G. L.; Yu, R. Q. *Biomaterials.* 2006, *27*, 246.

[28] Yang, M. H.; Jiang, J. H.; Yang, X. H.; Chen, Y. H.; Shen, G. L.; Yu, R. Q. *Biosens Bioelectron.* 2006, *21*, 1791.

[29] Huang, W.; Fernando, S.; Lin, Y.; Zhou, B.; Allard, L. F.; Sun, Y. P. *Langmuir.* 2003, *19*, 7084.

[30] Chen, R. J.; Zhang, Y.; Wang, D.; Dai, H. *J Am Chem Soc.* 2001, *123*, 3838.

[31] Tang, B. Z.; Xu, H. *Macromolecules.* 1999, 32, 2569.

[32] Yuan, W. Z.; Sun, J. Z.; Dong, Y.; Haussler, M.; Yang, F.; Xu, H. P.; Qin, A.; Lam, J. W. Y.; Zheng, Q.; Tang, B. Z. *Macromolecule.* 2006, *39*, 8011.

[33] Dodziuk, H.; Anczewski, W.; Ejchart, A.; Ueda, H.; Krinichnaya, E.; Dolgonos, G.; Kutner, W. *Chem. Commun.* 2003, *8*, 986.
[34] Gao, H.; Kong, Y.; Cui, D.; Ozkan, C. S. *Nano Lett*, 2003, *3*, 471.
[35] Ito, T.; Sun, L.; Crooks, R. M. *Chem. Commun.* 2003,*19*, 1482.
[36] Pantarotto, D.; Singh, R.; McCarthy, D.; Erhardt, M.; Briand, J. P.; Prato, M.; Kostarelos, K.; Bianco, A. *Angew. Chem., Int. Ed.* 2004, *43*, 5242.
[37] Wang, S.; Humphreys, E. S.; Chung, S. Y.; Delduco, D. F.; Lustig, S. R.; Wang, H.; Parker, K. N.; Rizz, N. W. O.; Subramoney, S.; Chiang, Y.M.; Jagota, A. *Nat. Mater.* 2003, *2*, 196.
[38] Caravan, P.; Ellison, J. J.; McMurry, T. J.; Lauffer, R. B. *Chem. Re*V. 1999, *99*, 2293.
[39] Merbach, A. E.; Toth, E. *John Wiley and Sons, New York*. 2001, 5
[40] Terreno, E.; Castelli, D. D.; Viale, A.; Aime, S. *Chem. Rev.* 2010, *110*, 3019.
[41] Sitharaman, B.; Kissell, K. R.; Hartman, K. B.; Tran, L. A.; Baikalov, A.; Rusakova, I.; Sun, Y.; Khant, H. A.; Ludtke, S. J.; Chiu, W.; Laus, S.; Toth, E.; Helm, L.; Merbach, A. E.; Wilson, L. J. *Chem. Commun.* 2005, *31*, 3915.
[42] Richard, C.; Doan, B. T.; Beloeil, J. C.; Bessodes, M.; Toth EÄ va, Scherman, D. *Nano Lett.* 2008, *8*, 232.
[43] Nakayama-Ratchford, N.; Bangsaruntip, S.; Sun, X. M.; Welsher, K.; Dai, H. *J. J. Am. Chem. Soc.* 2007*, 129*, 2448.
[44] (a) Robinson, J. T.; Welsher, K.; Tabakman, S. M.; Sherlock, S. P.; Wang, H.; Luong, R.; Dai, H. *Nano Res.* 2010, *3*, 779. (b) Welsher, K.; Liu, Z.; Daranciang, D.; Dai, H. *Nano Lett.* 2008, *8*, 586.
[45] Keren, S.; Zavaleta, C.; Cheng, Z.; de la Zerda, A.; Gheysens, O.; Gambhir, S. S. *Proc. Nat. Acad. Sci. USA*. 2008, *105*, 5844.
[46] Zavaleta, C.; Zerda, A. D. L.; Liu, Z.; Keren, S.; Cheng, Z.; Schipper, M.; Chen, X.; Dai, H.; Gambhir, S. S. *Nano Lett.* 2008, *8*, 2800.
[47] Liu, Z.; Tabakman, S.; Welsher, K.; Dai, H. *Nano Res.* 2009, *2*, 85.
[48] Zerda, A. D. L.; Zavaleta, C.; Keren, S.; Vaithilingam, S.; Bodapati, S.; Liu, Z.; Levi, J.; Ma, T. J.; Oralkan, O.; Cheng, Z. et al. *Nat. Nanotech.* 2008, *3*, 557.
[49] (a) Cheng, J. P.; Fernando, K. A. S.; Veca, L. M.; Sun, Y. P.; Lamond, A. I.; Lam, Y. W.; Cheng, S. H. *ACS Nano.* 2008, *2*, 2085. (b) Liu, Z.; Fan, A. C.; Rakhra, K.; Sherlock, S.; Goodwin, A.; Chen, X.; Yang, Q.; Felsher, D. W.; Dai, H. *Angew. Chem. Int. Ed.* 2009, *48*, 7668. (c) Yang, K.; Wan, J.; Zhang, Sh.; Zhang, Y.; Lee, Sh-T.; Liu, Zh. *ACSNano.* 2011, *5(1)*, 516. (d) Berlin, J. M.; Leonard, A. D.; Pham, T. T.; Sano, D.; Marcano, D. C.; Yan, S.; Fiorentino, S.; Milas, Z.L.; Kosynkin, D. V.; Price, B. K.; Lucente-Schultz, R. M.; Wen, X.; Raso, M. G.; Craig, S. L.; Tran, H. T.; Myers, J. N.; Tour, J. M. *ACSNano.* 2010; *4(8)*, 4621.
[50] Yang, S. T.; Fernando, K. A.; Liu, J. H.; Wang, J.; Sun, H. F.; Liu, Y.; Chen, M.; Huang, Y.; Wang, X.; Wang, H. et al. *Small.* 2008, *4*, 940.
[51] Chen, J.; Chen, S.; Zhao, X.; Kuznetsova, L. V.; Wong, S. S.; Ojima I. *J. Am. Chem. Soc.* 2008, *130*, 16778.
[52] Liu, Z.; Chen, K.; Davis, C.; Sherlock, S.; Cao, Q.; Chen, X.; Dai, H. *Cancer Res.* 2008, *68*, 6552.
[53] (a) Liu, Z.; Sun, X.; Nakayama, N.; Dai, H. *ACS Nano.* 2007, 1, 50. (b) Lee, J. H.; Yigit, M. V.; Mazumdar, D.; Lu, Y. *Advanced Drug Delivery Reviews* 2010, *62*, 592–605. (c) Ruenraroengsak, P.; Cook, J. M.; Florence, A. T. *Journal of Controlled*

Release 2010, *141*, 265–276. (d) Yu, X.; Zhang, Y.; Chen, C.; Yao, Q.; Li, M. *Biochimica et Biophysica Acta* 2010, 1805, 97–104.

[54] (a) Mullen, D. G.; McNerny, D. Q.; Desai, A.; Cheng, X-M.; DiMaggio, S. C.; Kotlyar, A.; Zhong, Y.; Qin, S.; Kelly, C. V.; Thomas, T. P.; Majoros, I.; Orr, B. G.; Baker, J. R.; Banaszak Holl M. M. *Bioconjugate Chem.* 2011, *22 (4),* 679. (b) Kelly, Y.; Kim, M.A. *Nanomedicine: Nanotechnology, Biology, and Medicine*. 2007, 3, 103.

[55] Dhar, S.; Liu, Z.; Thomale, J.; Dai, H.; Lippard, S. J. *J. Am. Chem. Soc.* 2008, *130*, 11467.

[56] (a) Pantarotto, D.; Partidos, C. D.; Graff, R.; Hoebeke, J.; Briand, J.P.; Prato, M.; Bianco, A. *J. AM. CHEM. SOC.* 2003, *125*, 6160. (b) Pantarotto, D.; Briand, J.P.; Prato, M.; Bianco, A. *Chem.Commun.* 2004, *1*, 16.

[57] Liu, Z.; Cai, W. B.; He, L. N.; Nakayama, N.; Chen, K.; Sun, X. M.; Chen, X. Y.; Dai, H.; *J. Nat. Nanotech.* 2007, *2*, 47.

[58] (a) Li, R.;Wu, R.; Zhao, L.; Wu, M.; Yang, L.; Zou, H. *ACS Nano*. 2010, *4(3)*, 1399. [59] Liu, Z.; Li, X.; Tabakman, S. M.; Jiang, K.; Fan, S.; Dai, H. *J. Am. Chem. Soc.* 2008, *130*, 13540.

[59] Chakravarty, P.; Marches, R.; Zimmerman, N. S.; Swafford, A. D.; Bajaj, P.; Musselman, I. H.; Pantano, P.; Draper, R. K.; Vitetta, E. S. *Proc. Natl. Acad. Sci. USA*. 2008, *105*, 8697.

[60] McDevitt, M. R.; Chattopadhyay, D.; Kappel, B. J.; Jaggi, J. S.; Schiffman, S. R.; Antczak, C.; Njardarson, J. T.; Brentjens, R.; Scheinberg, D. A. *J. Nucl. Med.* 2007, *48*, 1180.

[61] Zhang, X.; Lingjie, M.; Lu, Q.; Fei, Z.; Dyson, P. J. *Biomaterials*. 2009, *30*, 6041.

[62] Feazell, R. P.; Nakayama-Ratchford, N.; Dai, H.; Lippard, S. J. *J. Am. Chem. Soc.* 2007, *129*, 8438.

[63] Adeli, M.; Hakimpoor, F.; Ashiri, M.; Kabiri, R.; Bavadi, M. *Soft Matter*. 2011, *7*, 4062.

[64] Adeli, M.; Mirab, N.; Alavidjeh, M. S.; Sobhani, Z.; Atyabi, F. *Polymer*. 2009, *50*, 3528.

[65] Adeli, M.; Mirab, N.; Zabihi, F. *Nanotechnology*. 2009, *20*, 485603.

[66] Tavakoli Naeini, A.; Adeli, M.; Vossoughi, M. *Nanomed.: Nanotechnol., Biol. Med.* 2010, *6*, 556.

[67] Levi-Polyachenko, N.; Merkel, E.; Jones, B. T.; Carroll, D. L.; Stewart, J. H. *Molecular Pharmaceutics*. 2009, *5*, 1092.

[68] Connell, M.J.; Bachilo, S.M.; Huffman, C.B.; Moore, V.C.; Strano, M.S.; Haroz, E.H.; Rialon, K.L.; Boul, P.J.; Noon, W.H.; Kittrell, C.; Ma, J.; Hauge, R.H.; Weisman, R.B.; Smalley, R.E. *Science*. 2002, *297*, 593.

[69] Weissleder, R. *Nat. Biotech.* 2001, *19*, 316.

[70] Konig, K. *J. Microsc.* 2000, *200*, 83.

[71] Tran, A. P.; Zhang, L.; Webster, J. T. *Advanced Drug Delivery Reviews*. 2009, *61*, 1097.

[72] Chen, C.; Hayek, S; Mohite, V.; Yuan, H.; Chatterjee, J.; Haik, Y. *Scientific Publishers, California*. 2007, 160.

[73] Mehdipour, E.; Bavadi, M.; Sasanpour, P.; Rashidian, B.; Adeli, M. *Journal of Materials Chemistry*. 2011, Submitted.

[74] Korneva, G.; Ye, H.; Gogotsi, Y.; Halverson, D.; Friedman, G.; Bradley, J. C.; Korne, K. G. *Nano Lett*. 2005, *5*, 879.
[75] Panchapakesan, B.; Cesarone, G.; Liu, Sh.; Teker, K.; Wickstrom, E. *NanoBiotechnology*. 2005, *1*, 359.
[76] Ghosh, S.; Dutta, S.; Gomes, E.; Carroll, C.; D'Agostino, Jr.; Olson, J.; Guthold, M.; Gmeiner, W.H. *Acs. nano*. 2009, *3*, 2667.
[77] Helen Cathcart, S. Q.; Valeria, N.; John, M. K.; Werner, J. B.; Jonathan, N. C. *J. Phys.Chem. C*. 2007, *111*, 66.
[78] Zheng, M.; Jagota, A.; Semke, E. D.; Diner, B. A.; McLean, R. S.; Lustig, S. R.; Richardson, R. E.; Tassi, N. G. *Nat. Mater*. 2003, *2*, 338.
[79] Balasubramanian, K.; Burghard, M. *Anal. Bioanal. Chem*. 2006, *385*, 452.
[80] Lahiff, E.; Lynam, C.; Gilmartin, N.; O'Kennedy, R.; Diamond, D. *Anal. Bioanal Chem*. 2010, *398*, 1575.
[81] Wilson, G. S.; Gifford, R. *Biosens. Bioelectron*.2005, *20*, 2388.
[82] Malhotra, B. D.; Singhal, R.; Chaubey, A.; Sharma, S. K.; Kumar, A. *Curr. Appl. Phys*. 2005, *5*, 92.
[83] Rubianes, M. D.; Rivas, G. A. *Electroanalysis*. 2005,*17*,73.
[84] (a) Salimi, A.; Hallaj, R.; Khayatian, G. R. *Electroanalysis*. 2005, *17*, 873. (b) Shahrokhiana, S.; Ghalkhania, M.; Adeli, M.; Aminic, M.K. *Biosensors and Bioelectronics* 2009, *24*, 3235. (c) Jain, R.; Rather, J. A. *Colloids and Surfaces B: Biointerfaces*. 2011, *83*(*2*), 340.
[85] Wang, J.; Deo, R.P.; Musameh, M. *Electroanalysis*. 2003, *15*, 1830.
[86] Musameh, M.; Wang, J.; Merkoci, A.; Lin, Y. *Electrochem. Comm*. 2002, *4*, 743.
[87] Star, A.; Gabriel, J. C. P.; Bradley, K.; Gruener, G. *Nano Lett*. 2003, *3*, 459.
[88] Tsai, Y. C.; Huang, J. D.; Chiu, C. C. *Biosensors and Bioelectronics*. 2007, *22*, 3051.
[89] Wang, J.; Musameh, M.; Lin, Y. *J. Am. Chem Soc*. 2003, *125*, 2408.
[90] Wang, J. *Analyst*. 2005, *130*, 421.
[91] Sotiropoulou, S.; Chaniotakis, N. A. *Anal. Bioanal. Chem*. 2003, *375*, 103.
[92] Claussen, J. C.; Franklin, A. D.; Haque, A.; Porterfield, D. M.; Fisher, T. S. *Acs. nano*. 2009, *1*, 37.
[93] Lin, Y.; Lu, F.; Tu, Y.; Ren, Z. *Nano Lett*. 2004, *4*, 37.
[94] (a) Valentini, F.; Amine, A.; Orlanducci, S.; Terranova, M. L.; Palleschi, G. *Anal. Chem*. 2003, *75*, 5413. (b) Yuan, J.; Chen, J.; Wu, X.; Fang, K.; Niu, L. *Journal of Electroanalytical Chemistry*. 2011, *656*, 120. (c) Alwarappan, S.; Liu, G.; Li, C-Z. *Nanomedicine: Nanotechnology, Biology and Medicine*. 2010, *6*(*1*), 52.
[95] (a) Guo, M.; Chen, J.; Li, J.; Nie, L.; Yao, S. *Electroanalysis*. 2004, *16*, 1992. (b) Pauliukaite, R.; Doherty, A. P.; Murnaghan, K. D.; Brett, C. M. A. *Journal of Electroanalytical Chemistry*. 2011, *656*, 96. (c) Safavi, A.; Farjami, F. *Biosensors and Bioelectronics*. 2011, *26* (*5*), 2547.
[96] (a)Wu, F. H.; Zhao, G. C.; Wei, X. W. *Electrochem Commun*. 2002 , *4*, 690. (b) Noah, N. M.; Alam, S.; Sadik, O. A. *Analytical Biochemistry*. 2011, *413*(*2*),157.
[97] Bonanno, L. M.; DeLouise, L. A. *Anal. Chem*. 2010, *82*, 714.
[98] Fei, S.; Chen, J.; Yao, S.; Deng, G.; He, D.; Kuang, Y. *Anal. Biochem*., 2005, *339*, 29.
[99] Wu, K.; Sun, Y.; Hu, S. *Sens. Actuators. B*. 2003, *96*, 658.

[100] (a)Wang, J.; Li, M.; Shi, Z.; Li, N.; Gu, Z. *Anal Chem.* 2002, *74*, 1993. (b) Eguílaz, M.; Agüí, L.; Yáñez-Sedeño, P. Pingarrón, J.M. *Journal of Electroanalytical Chemistry.* 2010, *644*(*1*), 30.

[101] Male, K. B.; Hrapovic, S.; Santini, J. M.; Luong, J. H. T. *Anal. Chem.* 2007, *79*, 7831.

[102] Lin, Y.; Wang, J.; Liu, G.; Wu, H.; Wai, C. M.; Lin, Y. *Biosens. Bioelectron.* 2008, *23*, 1659.

[103] (a) Kim, S. N.; Rusling, J. F.; Papadimitrakopoulos, F. *Adv. Mater.* 2007, *19*, 3214. (b) Jones, C. S.; Lu, X.; Renn, M.; Stroder, M.; Shih, W-S. *Microelectronic Engineering.* 2010, *87*(*3*), 434.

[104] Chen, R. J.; Bangsaruntip, S.; Drouvalakis, K. A.; Kam, N. W. S.; Shim, M.; Li, Y.; Kim, W.; Utz, P. J.; Dai, H. *Proc. Natl. Acad. Sci. USA.* 2003, *100*, 4984.

[105] Star, A.; Tu, E.; Niemann, J.; Gabriel, J. C. P.; Joiner, C. S.; Valcke, C. *Proc. Natl. Acad. Sci. USA.* 2006, *103*, 921.

[106] Zheng, G.; Patolsky, F., Cui, Y.; Wang, W. U.; Lieber, C. M. *Nat. Biotechnol.* 2005, *23*, 1294.

[107] Javey, A.; Guo, J.; Wang, Q.; Lundstrom, M.; Dai, H. *Nature.* 2003, *424*, 654.

[108] Stokes, P.; Khondaker, S. I. *Nanotechnology.* 2008, *19*, 175202.

[109] Star, A.; Han, T. R.; Joshi, V.; Stetter, J. R. *Electroanalysis.* 2004, *16*, 108.

[110] Gooding, J. J. *Electrochim. Acta.* 2005, *50*, 3049.

[111] Balasubramanian, K.; Friedrich, M.; Jiang, C.; Fan, Y.; Mews, A.; Burghard, M.; Kern, K. *Adv. Mat.* 2003, *15*, 1515.

[112] Genaidy, A. W. K. *Hum. Factors Ergon. Manuf.* 2006, *16*, 247.

[113] Service, R. F. *Science.* 2007, *315*, 926.

[114] Cveticanin, J.; Joksic, G.; Leskovac, A.; Petrovic, S.; Valenta, Sobot A.; Neskovic, O. *Nanotechnology.* 2010, *21*, 015102.

[115] Liu, Z.; Davis, C.; Cai, W.; He, L.; Chen, X.; Dai, H. *Proc. Natl. Acad. Sci. U.S.A.* 2008, *105*, 1410.

[116] (a) Monteiro-Riviere, N. A.; Nemanich, R. J.; Inman, A. O.; Wang, Y. Y.; Riviere, J. E. *Toxicol. Lett.* 2005, *155*, 377. (b) Witzmann, F. A.; Monteiro-Riviere, N. A. *Nanomedicine.* 2006, *2*, 158.

[117] Tummala, N. R.; Morrow, B. H.; Resasco, D. E.; Striolo, A. *ACS Nano.* 2010, *4* (*12*), 7193.

[118] Shvedova, A. A.; Castranova, V.; Kisin, E. R.; Schwegler-Berry, D.; Murray, A. R.; Gandelsman, V. Z.; Maynard, A.; Baron, P. *J. Toxicol. EnViron. Health, Part A.* 2003, *66*, 1909.

[119] Pulskamp, K.; Diabate. S.; Krug. H. F. *Toxicol. Lett.* 2007, *168*, 58.

[120] Ding, L.; Stilwell, J.; Zhang, T.; Elboudwarej, O.; Jiang, H.; Selegue, JP. et al. *Nano Lett.* 2005, *5*, 2448.

[121] Manna, S. K.; Sarkar, S.; Barr, J.; Wise, K.; Barrera, E. V.; Jejelowo, O. et al. *Nano Lett.* 2005, *5*, 1676.

[122] Bottini, M.; Bruckner, S.; Nika, K.; Bottini, N.; Bellucci, S.; Magrini, A. et al. *Toxicol. Lett.* 2006, *160*, 121-.

[123] Tian, F.; Cui, D.; Schwarz, H.; Estrada, G. G.; Kobayashi, H. *Toxicol. In Vitro*, 2006, *20*, 1202.

[124] Magrez, A.; Kasas ,S.; Salicio, V.; Pasquier, N.; Seo, J. W.; Celio, M. et al. *Nano Lett.* 2006, *6*, 1121.

[125] Sayes, C. M.; Liang, F.; Hudson, J. L.; Mendez, J.; Guo, W.; Beach, J. M.; Moore, V. C.; Doyle, C. D.; West, J. L.; Billups, W. E.; Ausmanb, K. D.; Colvin, V. L. *Toxicol. Lett.* 2006, *161*, 135.

[126] Zhang, L. W.; Zeng, L.; Barron, A. R.; Monteiro-Riviere, N. A. *Int. J. Toxicol.* 2007, *26*, 103.

[127] Cui, H. F.; Vashist, S. K.; Al-Rubeaan,Kh.; Luong, J. H. T.; Sheu, F.S. *Chem. Res. Toxicol.* 2010, *23*, 1131.

[128] Gao, C.; Li, W.; Morimoto, H.; Nagaoka, Y.; Maekawa, T. *J. Phys. Chem. B Condens. Matter Surf. Interfaces Biophys.* 2006, *110*, 7213.

[129] Torchilin, V.P. *Handb. Exp. Pharmacol.* 2010, *197*, 3.

[130] (a) Chaudhuri, P.; Harfouche, R.; Soni, S.; Hentschel, D. M.; Sengupta, S. *ACS Nano.* 2010, *4*, 574. (b) Kam, N. W. S.; Liu, Z. A.; Dai, H. J. *Angew. Chem., Int. Ed.* 2006, *45*, 577. (c) Donaldson, K.; Murphy, F. A.; Duffin, R.; Poland, C. A. *Particle and Fibre Toxicology* 2010, 7, 5.

[131] Pantarotto, D.; Briand, J. P.; Prato, M.; Bianco, A. *Chem. Commun.* 2004, 16.

[132] Kostarelos, K.; Lacerda, L.; Pastorin, G.; Wu, W.; Wieckowski, S.; Luangsivilay, J.; Godefroy, S.; Pantarotto, D.; Briand, J. P.; Muller, S.; Prato, M.; Bianco, A. *Nat. Nanotechno.* 2007, *2*, 108.

[133] Mooney, E.; Dockery, P.; Greiser, U.; Murphy, M.; Barron, V. *Nano Lett.* 2008, *8*, 2137.

[134] Porter, A. E.; Gass, M.; Bendall, J. S.; Muller, K.; Goode, A.; Skepper, J. N.; Midgley, P. A.; Welland, M. *ACS Nano.* 2009, *3*, 1485.

[135] Mu, Q.; Broughton, D. L.; Yan, B. *Nano Lett.* 2009, *9*, 4370.

In: Hybrid Nanostructures in Cancer Therapy
Editor: Mohsen Adeli

ISBN: 978-1-62100-517-9
© 2012 Nova Science Publishers, Inc.

Chapter V

Functionalized Carbon Nanotubes: New Tools in Nanomedicine

Mohsen Adeli[1,2] and Masoumeh Bavadi[1]

[1]Department of chemistry, Faculty of Science, Lorestan University, Khoramabad, Iran
[2]Department of chemistry, Sharif University of Technology, Tehran, Iran

Abstract

With the prospect of cancer therapies, gene therapy and innovative new answers for life-threatening diseases and life-science problems, nanomedicine has become a fast-growing field that has an incredible ability to bypass barriers. Due to their ability to cross biological barriers and translocation easily into the cytoplasm or nucleus of a cell through its membrane without generating an immunogenic response and toxic effects, carbon nanotubes (CNTs) have became significant tools in nanomedicine, especially in the cancer therapy branch, as therapeutic agents or carriers for therapeutic agents with a high loading capacity. Because functionalized CNTs display low toxicity and are not immunogenic, such systems hold great potential in the field of nanobiotechnology and nanomedicine. Therefore in this chapter, we will show overview on recent advances in functionalization of CNTs for biomedical applications specifically their covalent conjugations with a variety of biological and bioactive molecules and macromolecules.

1. Introduction

Nanotechnology is the design, construction and application of objects, structures, devices, and systems by controlled manipulation of size, topology and property at the atomic, molecular, and macromolecular scale that produces devices and systems with at least one novel/superior characteristic or property at the subcellular level (<100 nm) [1,2].

Application of nanotechnology in the medicine field, to achieve efficient therapy strategies and overcome problems that current medicine has failed to overcome them, has created a new field called nanomedicine. As a definition, nanomedicine is a branch of science and technology to early diagnosis and efficient therapy of disease and hurtful injury, reducing pain, and preserving and improving human health, using nano-objects [3, 4].

Among diverse classes of nanomaterials carbon nanotubes (CNTs) have attracted particular attention as carriers for biologically relevant molecules [5-8]. They have fundamental advantages over bioorganic nanomaterials such as liposome, dendrimer, and biodegradable polymer in the case of their size, shape control and surface functionalization [9].

2. Carbon Nanotubes (CNTs)

Carbon nanotubes, first discovered by Iijima in 1991[10], are pseudo-one-dimensional carbon allotropes of high aspect ratio, ultra light weight, and excellent material properties such as mechanical strength, electrical conductivity, and high thermal conductivity. Conceptually the carbon nanotubes are viewed as rolled-up structures of single or multiple sheets of graphene to give single walled carbon nanotubes (SWNTs) and multi walled carbon nanotubes (MWNTs), respectively [11,12].

CNTs have a wide range of potential applications including nanoelectronic, sensors, fillers in composites materials and others [13–15].

Due to their high ability to cross the cell membrane, their optical and thermal properties and high loading capacity, CNTs are promising materials for nanomedicine and variety of delivery systems based on carbon nanotubes have been prepared and examined *in vitro* and *in vivo* for transferring the therapeutic agents and biological active molecules [16-18].

They have potential applications as carriers for delivery of drugs, RNA, DNA, peptides and other biological active molecules into cells because of the ability to cross cell membranes [19-24].

Despite the widely demonstrated potentials of CNTs in nanomedicine, research indicates these materials can potentially cause adverse effects on environment and specially health systems [25]. Hence toxicity profile of CNTs is important in biological systems.

The most important factor related to the toxicity of these materials is their high hydrophobicity or poor solubility in biological mediums which increases their interactions with cells membranes and causes formation of aggregated particles and therefore heterogeneous interactions with cell components [26].

However chemical modification or functionalization of carbon nanotubes reduce their aggregations and size polydispersity and raise their solubility, leading to an increase in their biocompatibility [27–29].

Varieties of organic molecules such as polymers and dendrimers are conjugated onto the surface and tip of CNTs by chemical reactions [30–36]. Depending on the type of interactions; two methods are used to modify the CNTs by polymers. This methods are based on either physical interactions or chemical bonding and are so called ''noncovalent'' or ''covalent'' approaches respectively.

Noncovalent approach is based on noncovalent interactions between CNTs and polymers and includes dispersion with the low molar mass polymers, polymer wrapping and polymer adsorption [37].

2.1. Covalent Functionalization of CNTs for Biomedical Applications

The most common method for the covalent functionalization of CNTs involves reactions with carboxylic acid (–COOH) residues on carbon nanotubes. These carboxylic acid groups are usually introduced by oxidation using strong acids, and they occur predominantly at the more reactive (open) end or defect sides of SWNTs and MWNTs rather than their side walls [38]. However, oxidized CNTs cannot be directly used for biological applications, because their solubility in aqueous solutions is not so high to overcome the solubility problems in the mediums with the high salt content such as the most biological solutions. Therefore –COOH functional groups of CNTs usually are used to attach macromolecules on the surface or ends of carbon nanotubes yielding CNT-polymer conjugates stable in biological environments [39].

In the covalent approach, molecules or macromolecules are grafted onto the surface of CNTs through chemical linkages. This method is very effective because grafted macromolecules raise the solubility of CNTs even with a low degree of functionalization [40–44]. Covalent attachment of polymer chains to the surface of CNTs can be accomplished by either ''grafting to'' or ''grafting from'' methods. In the ''grafting to'' method, polymers are connected to the functionalized CNTs through chemical reaction between their functional groups. The ''grafting to'' method is characterized by low grafting density because of the hindrance of the polymer chains which have reacted with CNTs [45]. The ''grafting from'' method involves the growth of polymers from the surface of CNTs by first covalently attaching of polymerization initiators and then exposing the nanotube-based macroinitiators to monomers. This method leads to the higher grafting density and control over the polymer growth with the possibility of designable structure [46, 47]. On the other hand among polymeric materials, dendrimers and hyperbranched polymers have attracted more interest due to their unique molecular features and properties [48–52]. Recently some hybrid materials containing carbon nanotubes and grafted hyperbranched polymers are synthesized through ''grafting from'' approach [53, 54].

1, 3-dipolar cycloaddition is also a widely and versatile used approach to attach molecular moieties and functional groups onto the surface of CNTs covalently. Subsequent attachment of macromolecules to CNTs through these functional groups leads to functionalized CNTs, suitable for delivery of therapeutic molecules [55].

3. Nanomedicine Applications of CNTs

3.1. Drug Delivery by CNTs

Drug delivery is an emerging field focused on targeting drugs or genes to a desirable group of cells. Some obstacles including poor water solubility, short blood circulation, damage the healthy cells, toxicity, and lack of the ability to select a particular cell type for treatment should be overcome to cure diseases by drugs. In recent years, these problems are subject to intensive research worldwide.

Within variety of nanomaterials, due to their unique properties especially their ultrahigh surface area and ability to carry molecules of interest across the cytoplasmic membrane and nuclear membrane without producing an immunogenic response; CNTs and their hybrid materials are promising and effective systems to deliver drugs and genes to target sites [56-59]. These potential applications often limited by their insolubility in solvents due to strong intertube van der Waals interactions. Therefore, functionalization of carbon nanotubes is the prerequisite for their solubility profiles and their manipulation into biological systems.

Mechanism for the internalization of carbon nanotubes into cells has not been fully understood. It has been found that functionalized CNTs cross the cell membrane by two mechanisms: i) via the endocytosis pathway and ii) via the endocytosis-independent pathway.

Endocytosis is a process in which cells encapsulate a foreign material from the outside by enclosing it with a small area of the cell membrane to form a vesicle inside the cytoplasm. Since endocytosis is energy dependent, a low energy environment (such as at temperatures lower than 37 °C) inhibits the endocytosis process.

Endocytosis-independent pathway is an energy-independent passive process, where the nanotubes diffuse across the cellular membrane [60].

Several studies have proved an endocytosis pathway as the cellular uptake mechanism of CNTs.

New biocompatible and water soluble hybrid materials containing MWNTs and hyperbranched polyglycerol (PG) or polycitric acid (PCA) have been synthesized by "grafting from" method (Scheme 1) [61].

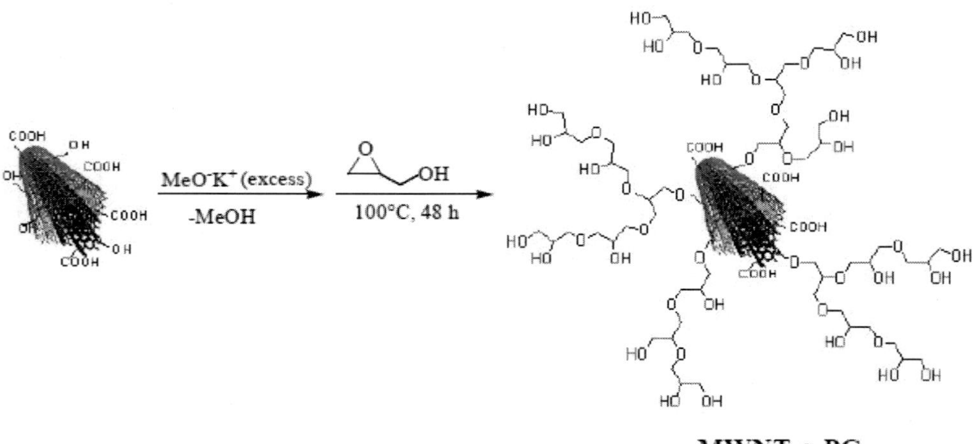

Scheme 1. Synthesis of hybrid nanomaterials consisting PG branches grafted onto the surface of MWNTs.

In order to investigate their potential application in nanomedicine and to understand the limitation and capability of these hybrid materials as nanoexcipients in biological systems, short-term *in vitro* cytotoxicity and hemocompatibility tests have been conducted on HT1080 cell line (human Fibrosarcoma). Because of this epithelial cell line is one of the first route of entry of the exogenous materials to the vascular system and therefore subsequent interactions with the whole body.

According to MTT assay results, a considerable toxicity up to concentration of 1mg/ml after 24 h and 48 h was not observed for MWNT-g-PG hybrid materials against HT1080 cell line. Crystal violet staining assay were also shown no sign of toxicity for these hybrid materials against above cell line up to concentration of 0.5 mg/ml. The results of LDH release from the treated cells (HT1080 cell line) were statistically equal to the negative controlled cells (%0.1 DMSO treated cells) up to concentration of 1 mg/ml after 24 h of incubation except for the concentration of 2 mg/ml which showed statistical significant difference (%150 increase against %0.1v/v DMSO as negative control, p<0.05). Annexinv-PI assay is a well-known method to differentiate early apoptosis and necrosis (secondary apoptotic cells) death of the cells. HT1080 cell line incubated with MWNT-g-PG hybrid materials showed a concentration-dependent behavior in the number of apoptotic cells, about 7-fold increase from higher (%3.5 against control) to lower (%0.56 against control) concentration. Also a concentration-dependent increase in the number of necrotic cells about 2-fold from the lower (%0.35 against control) to higher (%0.7 against control) concentration was observed. The data were also significant at each level (p<0.05) (Figure 1).

It can be found that at higher concentration (0.7 mg/ml) the ratio of apoptosis/necrosis is about 3.5/1 which is a good indicator; because the more the concentration increases, the much more apoptosis increases against necrosis, because materials can be liberated from the lysed cells instantly in necrosis process contrary to apoptosis which can induce instant unwanted inflammatory responses and subsequent harmful reactions which are not as good at all in particle designing and biocompatibility issues. These adverse reactions are not seen for apoptosis process, in that the living organism has time to identify (e.g., translocation of phosphatidyl serine to the outer membrane of the cell wall), treat and scavenge the cell debris before causing any harmful side effects in its natural.

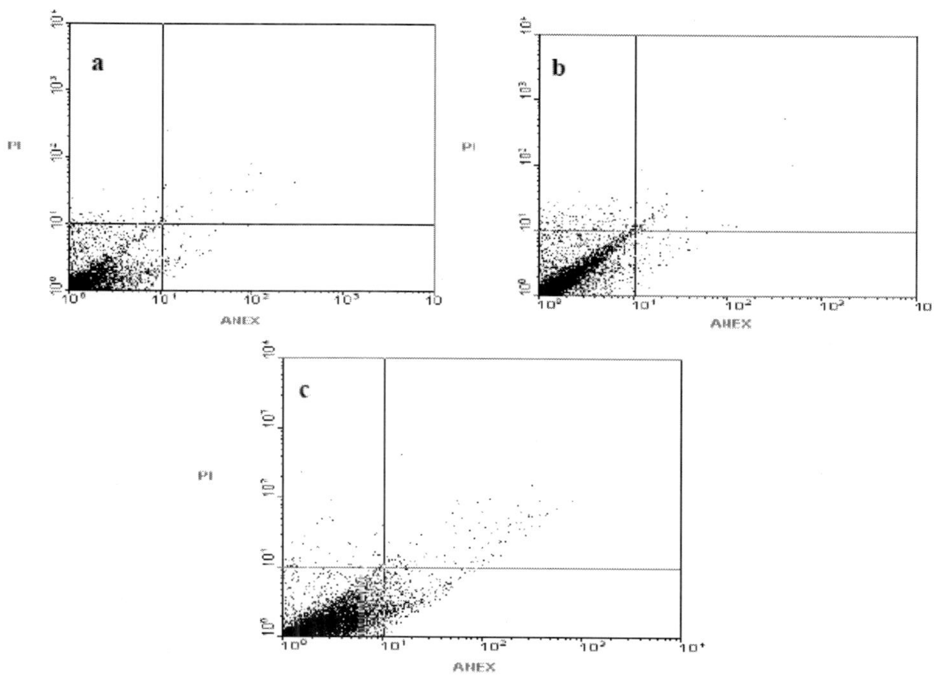

Figure 1. Dot plots of AnnexinV-FITC/PI staining of HT1080 cells. Three phenotype can be observed: viable (lower left quadrant); apoptotic (lower right quadrant), and necrotic or secondary apoptotic (upper right quadrant). a) untreated cells b) cells treated with 0.35mg/ml of MWCNT-*g*-PG, c) cells treated with 0.7 mg/ml of MWCNT-*g*-PG, after 24 h incubation time.

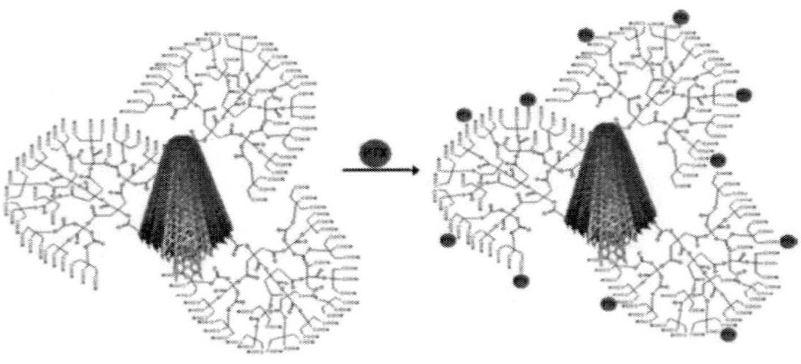

Figure 2. Attachment of PTX molecules to the end functional groups of MWNT-*g*-PCA hybrid materials to obtain MWNT-*g*-PCA-PTX drug delivery system.

In a research work, PCA branches as biocompatible segments were attached onto the surface of MWNTs to obtained MWNT-*g*-PCA hybrid materials. Then paclitaxel (PTX), a potent anticancer drug, was conjugated to the carboxyl functional groups of PCA branches via a cleavable ester bond to obtain a MWNT-*g*-PCA-PTX drug delivery system (Figure 2) [62].

To verify the pharmacological activity of paclitaxel-conjugated nanotubes, *in vitro* cytotoxicity tests were conducted on SKOV3 ovary and A549 lung cancer cell lines. Toxicity equal to PTX was observed for MWNT-*g*-PCA-PTX at shorter incubation times. For example at 40 nM concentration, the cytotoxicity of MWNT-*g*-PCA-PTX at 24 hours was equal to the effect of paclitaxel at 48 hours. In addition at a comparable incubation time, MWNT-*g*-PCA-PTX showed a higher cytotoxic effect than paclitaxel so that after 24 hours the cytotoxicity of this drug delivery system containing 40 nM of paclitaxel against A549 cells was approximately 20% greater than that for the same concentration of free paclitaxel. Therefore, MWNT-*g*-PCA-PTX drug delivery systems exhibited higher cytotoxicity at shorter incubation times than free PTX against cancer cells. The same results were obtained for MWNT-*g*-PCA-PTX drug delivery systems and free PTX against SKOV3 cell line. Higher toxicity for MWNT-*g*-PCA-PTX drug delivery systems against cancer cells could be assigned to the increased cell penetration of paclitaxel when conjugated to the MWNT-*g*-PCA. Due to the sufficient time for the penetration of the free PTX into the cells, at long range incubations a similar toxicity for free PTX and MWNT-*g*-PCA-PTX drug delivery systems against cancer cells was observed (Table 1).

Table 1. IC50s (nM) of paclitaxel and conjugated MWNT-*g*-PCA-PTX against A549 and SKOV3 cell lines at different incubation times

Incubation time (hours)	A549 PTX	A549 Conj	SKOV3 PTX	SKOV3 Conj
24	>2000*	>2000	>2000	>2000
48	>200	26.365±2.685	>2000	>2000
96	6.686±0.665	2.621±0.165	4.211±0.335	1.385±0.074
120	2.063±0.162	<I**	2.006±0.096	<I

Notes: Data are presented as means ± standard deviations (n = 3). *IC50s were obtained by extrapolation if the nonlinear regression was more than 2000 or 200 nM; **IC50s in this incubation time was smaller than the lowest concentration used (1 nM). Abbreviations: PTX, paclitaxel; Conj, conjugate; MWNT, multiwalled carbon nanotubes; PCA, poly citric acid.

Like all other drug delivery systems, those based on CNTs could be directed toward the targeted cancer cells by reorganization the receptors over expressed onto the surface of cancer cells with the help of specific ligands including folic acid, peptides and antibodies attached to CNTs [63]. This strategy leads to the accumulation of anticancer drugs in the target sites and therefore the serious and harmful side effects might be avoided [64].

Several tumor-targeting drug delivery systems based on carbon nanotubes have been synthesized and their efficiency to transport anticancer drugs to tumors is evaluated [65], for example biotin as a tumor-targeting modules and a second-generation taxoid as a cytotoxic drug warheads have been covalently connected to the side wall of SWNTs by different linkers to form a biotin-SWNT-linker-taxoid drug delivery system (Figure 3). This tumor-targeting drug delivery system has shown a high potency toward specific cancer cell lines. It has been found that the internalized drugs into the cytosol of the cancer cells using this drug delivery system is very high in compare to that for a simple extracellular exposure of the free drug to the same cancer cells [66].

Different analysis and imaging methods including confocal microscopy, single-photon emission computed tomography (SPECT) imaging, and gamma scintillation counting analyses revealed that the conjugates could be readily internalized by cells *in vitro* and exhibited relatively long blood circulation and high tumor accumulation *in vivo*.

Antitumor activity of drug delivery systems based on single walled carbon nanotubes having functional groups to coordinate with cisplatin (CDDP) as anticancer drug and epidermal growth factor (EGF) as a targeting agent has been evaluated *in vitro* and *in vivo* [67]. In other study, for preparing Pt(IV) complexes containing both a cell receptor targeting moiety and a delivery system, first a functionalized platinum (IV) complex (1) containing a folate derivative (FA) at an axial position, was prepared and then it was attached to the surface of an amine-functionalized SWNT and perfect drug delivery system (SWNT-PL-PEG-NH_2) was obtained (Figure 4).

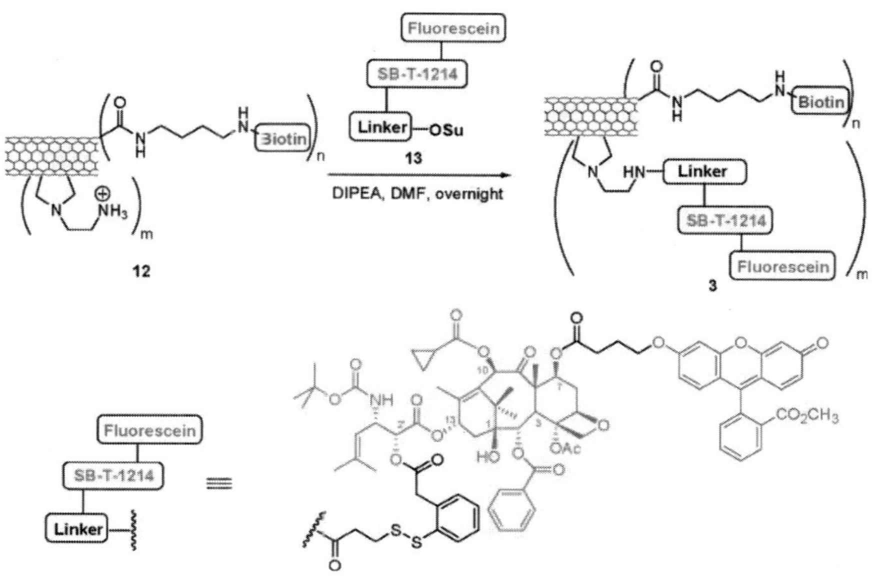

Figure 3. Synthesis of biotin-SWNT-linker-(Taxoid-Fluorescein) as a tumor-targeting drug delivery system. Reprinted with the permission of ref [66].

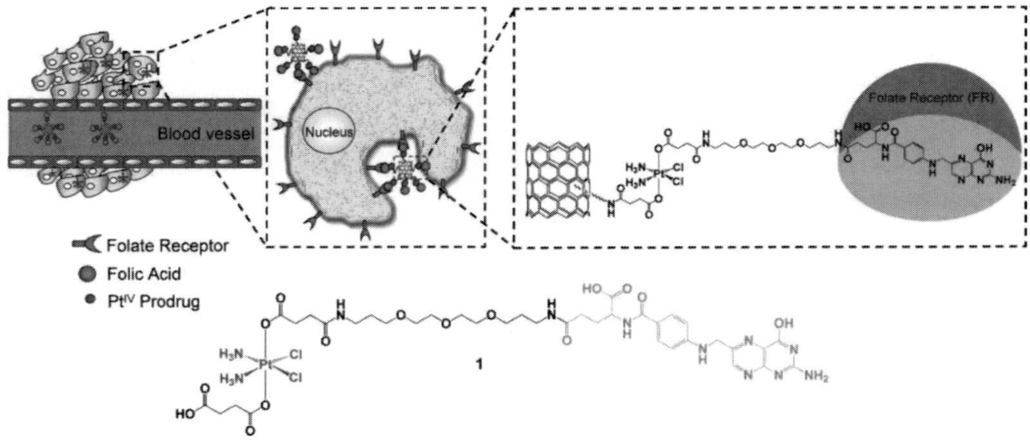

Figure 4. Folate receptor (FR)-mediated targeting and SWNT-mediated delivery of 1 by endocytosis and structure of 1. Reprinted with the permission of Ref [68].

The prepared drug delivery system was found more active by a factor of 8.6 compared to free CDDP. Intracellular reduction of a Pt (IV) prodrug was led to a form of this drug which is able to crosslink DNA of the cancer cell. The internalization studies showed high and specific binding of drug delivery system to the folic acid receptors over expressed onto the cancer cells [68].

It is highly probable that the type of molecules covalently or noncovalently attached to the external walls of the tubes play a key role in the process of transport into the cells.

For this purpose, CNT have been functionalized with amphotericin B, one of the most effective antibiotic molecules for the treatment of chronic fungal infections, and fluorescein. The antibiotic linked to the nanotubes was rapidly internalized into mammalian cells without toxic effects in comparison to the drug incubated alone [69].

In an alternative approach by a different group, SWNT have been functionalized with substituted carborane cages to develop a new delivery system for an efficient boron neutron capture therapy, these studies showed that some specific tissues contained carborane following intravenous administration of the CNT conjugate and, more interestingly, that carborane was concentrated mainly at the tumor site [70]. Overall, these results clearly indicate the potential applications of CNTs in tumor-targeted drug delivery in the near future.

3.2. Gene Delivery by CNTs

Gene therapy is a method in which genes are used to help cells to recover and produce their own therapeutic proteins. Two main methods are used to deliver genes into the cells: viral gene delivery or viral vector and non-viral gene delivery or non-viral vector including cationic lipids, liposomes, polyethylenimine (PEI), polyamidoamine, nanoparticles and other cationic polymers.

Viral vectors are more simple pathways and they are very efficient in gene expression but a big drawback for viral vectors concerns about their safety. Due to the variety of alternatives regarding the size, charge and type of vectors, non-viral vectors are chemically more controllable and display a reduced immunogenicity [71-75]. Affective non-viral vector should cross different biological barriers successfully, protect DNA from degradation and interaction with other biological molecules and create low immunogenicity. Since carbon nanotubes are able to cross the cell membrane easily, which is one of the most important steps among biological barriers; they are promising candidates to deliver genes into the cells safely [76].

DNAs and RNAs could be transferred by CNTs covalently [77, 78] and non-covalently [79] or through a bifunctional linker. In covalent approach CNTs are functionalized, for example by acid treatment, and then RNA and DNA attached to its carboxyl functional groups through a carbodiimide-activated coupling reaction either directly or through a bifunctional linker [80]. 50-thiol-modified single strands DNA (ssDNA) are attached to the surface of CNTs through a bifunctional linker to form CNTs-DNA gene delivery systems. It has been found that these systems are able to recognize their appropriate complementary sequence with a high degree of selectivity [81]. In addition, Thiol-modified short interfering RNA (siRNA) molecules similar to DNA are linked to aqueous solubilized SWNTs (functionalized with an amine-terminated surfactant) through cleavable disulfide linkages. According to results from in vitro delivery experiments, these delivery systems could effectively silence (50–60% knockdown) both CD4 receptor and CXCR4 co-receptor which are required for HIV to entry into human T cells and infection [82].

Macromolecules with a positive charge such as polyamidoamine (PAMAM) dendrimers are widely used for *in vitro* transfection of genes owing to their so-called proton sponge effect. Attachment of PAMAM dendrimers or other biocompatible macromolecules with positive charge to the surface of CNTs leads to new hybrid nanomaterials with a collection of desirable properties coffered from both macromolecules and CNTs. Antisense oligonucleotide is able to attach to the surface of CNTs through electrostatic interactions with PAMAMs attached to it surface [83]. In noncovalent method RNA and DNA macromolecules attached to CNTs by noncovalent interactions. It has been found that not only can DNA molecules be attached to the tips and walls of a CNT; it can also be encapsulated inside of the structure [84]. pDNA molecules have been immobilized onto the surface of a type of CNTs containing Ni particles enclosed in their tips to obtain gene delivery systems that are sensitive to a magnetic field. Then using a creative magnetic 'spearing' technique (exposure to an external magnetic field followed by centrifugation), the CNT–pDNA gene delivery systems have entered into the mammalian cells and a gene expression in 80–100% of the cell population has been achieved [85]. Release of DNA molecules from CNTs based delivery systems using thermal properties of CNTs has been investigated and it has been found that DNAs release from CNT transporters to the nucleus after the laser pulses [86].

3.3. Vaccine Delivery by CNTs

The ability to transport biomacromolecules including proteins and peptides of interest into living cells is another important application of CNTs in tissue engineering. The basic idea of using CNTs in vaccine delivery entails linking an antigene to CNTs, without losing its conformation, thereby inducing an antibody response with the right specificity [87, 88]. In general, Proteins such as lysozyme, histone, hemoglobin, myoglobin, ovalbumin, bovine serum albumin, trypsin, and glucose oxidase could be conjugated with carbon nanotubes via either spontaneous adsorption onto the carbon nanotubes surface or the immobilization more controllably in functionalization reactions. However, it is of particular importance that the

CNT-bound protein remains biologically active during its conjugation with carbon nanotubes [89, 90]. For this purpose, a B-cell epitope from VP1 protein of the foot-and mouth disease virus (FMDV) was covalently attached to the amine groups present on CNT, using a bifunctional linker. The peptides around the CNT adopt the appropriate secondary structure for recognition by specific monoclonal and polyclonal antibodies. The immunogenic features of peptide–CNT conjugates were subsequently assessed *in vivo*. Immunisation of mice with FMDV peptide–nanotube conjugates elicited high antibody responses as compared with the free peptide. These antibodies were peptide-specific since antibodies against CNT were not detected. In addition, the antibodies displayed virus-neutralizing ability [91].

3.4. Cnts in Lymphatic Targeting

The lymphatic system plays an important part in the defense of a subject against infectious diseases and cancer and is one of the main pathways for the metastasis of tumors. Lymphatic metastasis occurs extensively in cancers, resulting in frequent tumor relapse, even after extended lymph node dissection. Nonetheless, novel targeting delivery system may grant an opportunity to treat malignant tumors with lymph node metastasis locoregionally without systemic toxicity [92]. According to previous studies *in vivo* lymphatic targeting systems using liposomes and polymer particles demonstrated that smaller particles had better lymphatic uptake than larger particles. Furthermore, CNTs due to unique properties can be effectively taken up into lymphatic vessels and retained in the draining targeted lymph nodes for several days [93]. The lymphatic targeting drug delivery system using magnetic CNTs have been synthesized, which successfully delivered gemcitabine to lymph nodes with high efficiency under a magnetic field. According to results from delivery experiments, these delivery systems could confer an advantage over the way chemotherapeutic agents are currently delivered to lymph nodes [94, 95].

In another approach, CNTs can be successfully functionalized with poly (acrylic acid) (PAA) via *in situ* precipitation polymerization of acrylic acid and utilized for lymph node tracing. The results show that the PAA-*g*-CNTs have the potential to be used as a vital staining dye, which may simplify lymph node identification during surgery even when they are very small [96].

3.5. Thermal Therapy Applications

Hyperthermia therapy is a unique way to heat the tumor site and cancer cells and subsequently destroying them without creating significance side effects for the other parts of the body. One of the most important ways to dissipate heat of the cells and tissues is through blood fluid which is flowing inside their vessels. Fortunately cancer cells are surrounded with blood vessels that have an abnormal flow and therefore dissipate heat less efficiently than blood around healthy cells and this is way they are more susceptible to heat increases than healthy cells. CNTs are able to absorb light in the near-infrared (NIR) region (700-1100 nm), which is a harmless region of the light for body, and therefore increase heat of a site which are accumulated there. Internalization of CNTs into the cancer cells or accumulation those in the tumor sites and consequently exposing to the near-infrared radiation lead to increased heat in these sites and finally killing the cancer cells [97, 98]. Like cancer therapy by drug- or gene delivery systems, the major challenge for hyperthermia therapy is its selectivity, i.e selective photothermal ablation of tumor tissues to avoid damage the normal tissues [99-101].

In order to increase the selectivity of treatment and decrease undesirable effects to normal cells, CNTs are covalently functionalized by specific ligands including peptides or monoclonal antibodies (MAbs) and then subject to selective internalization into the cells via receptor-mediated endocytosis. However a drawback of this method is that covalent functionalization of CNTs damage their structure and interfere with their electronic and optical properties. Carboxylated CNTs keep their optical and thermal properties and hence retain significant background absorption in the NIR region that supports NIR-mediated photothermal therapy [102].

4. Are CNTs Safe?

Although CNTs have promised new and innovative tools in nanomedicine, their toxicity is still under question and their potential side effects have become an issue of strong concern for the environment and biological systems, which might cancel or delay the translation of appealing bench science data to relevant biomedical applications and to clinical stages [103]. Hence, safety of CNTs should be completely proved and questions concerning the toxicity of CNTs should be answered.

Due to the difficultness of the purification of pristine CNTs, impurities such as remained catalysts used for preparation of CNTs and amorphous carbon are one of the major sources of the toxicity of CNTs [104-106]. Structural factors and characterizes including long length of CNTs, size distribution, large surface area, diameter, hydrophobicity, aggregation status are other reasons for toxicity and immunogenicity of CNTs [107]. Pristine CNTs has been found to be toxic and unsafe to various mammalian cell lines *in vitro* and to the skin and lungs *in vivo* because they tend to accumulate due to their insolubility. Toxicity of pristine SWNTs (0.06–0.24 mg/mL) against human epidermal keratinocytes (HaCaT) has been investigated and it has been found that exposure to SWNTs resulted in accelerated oxidative stress, indicated by the formation of free radicals and accumulation of peroxidative products, depletion of total antioxidant reserves, and a loss of cell viability [108]. Fortunately functionalization of CNTs could change the undesirable structural characterizes and improve the desirable ones [109-116]. *In vitro* investigations had showed that SWNTs functionalized by phenyl-SO_3H or phenyl-$(COOH)_2$ groups, covalently, causes less cytotoxicity than pristine SWNT, stabilized with a surfactant-1% of Pluronic F108 in aqueous solutions [117].

Functionalization of CNTs, especially by hybdrophilic macromolecules or biomacromolecules, improves their water solubility and dispersion in biological fluids and therefore decreases the effect of some sources of their toxicity such as poor water solubility, hydrophobicity, assembly and long length. In a study amino-functionalized CNTs have been labeled with radioactive metal Indium-111 (^{111}In) through diethylene triamine pentaacetic acid (DTPA) as chelating agent and then they were administered to the mice intravenously and biodistribution of CNTs in different biological mediums (organs/tissues) was determined by measuring the radioactivity of the ^{111}In in these mediums. A rapid first order clearance from the blood fluid through renal excretion route was observed for both SWNTs and

MWNTs without any toxicity and side effects or mortality against biological systems. Although short circulation time was a disadvantage for these systems and very low toxicity of the functionalized CNTs may be was the result of the fast clearance and very limited interactions with the biological systems but this research work suggested that functionalized and water soluble CNTs are more safe and promising systems for use *in vivo* [118,119]. For example carbon nanotubes functionalized by 1, 3-dipolar cycloaddition reaction or oxidation by acid and then amidation could be taken up rapidly by B and T lymphocytes as well as macrophages without affecting the overall cell viability while highly water-soluble carbon nanotubes did not affect the functional activity of different types of immunoregulatory cells [120].

Inhalation is a major route to introduce CNTs into the body and a serious risk for persons who are working with CNTs for a long time. Histopathological studies on lungs for 7 and 90 days and after a single intratracheal instillation of an SWNT dispersion have showed that CNTs induced epithelial granulomas and interstitial inflammation at day 7, which persist and develop to peribronchial inflammation and necrosis around day 90 [121].

Conclusion

Although a large number of research works have proved the high potential of CNTs to accumulate in the tumor sites and promise them as effective agents for killing the cancer cells but the exact fate of these systems in body and long range toxicity and side effects as well as molecular and cellular mechanisms for cytotoxicity of this class of nanomaterial are not yet fully apparent. Therefore more results are needed to answer questions and introduce CNTs in the clinical phases.

References

[1] Kate, B.; Chiu, K.; Yamamoto, V.; Khalsa, B.; Black, K.; Ljubimova, J.; Ding, H, Patil, R.; Portilla-Arias, J.; Modo, M.; Moore, D.; Farahani, K.; Prakash, N.; Neman, J.; Ahdoot, D.; Grundfest, W.; Nikzad, Sh.; Heiss, J. *NeuroImage*. 2011, *54*, S106–S124 .

[2] Chang, C. *Journal of Autoimmunity*. 2010, *34*, J234– J246.

[3] Faraji, A. H.; Wipf, P. *Bioorganic and Medicinal Chemistry*. 2009, *17*, 2950– 2962.

[4] Kagan, V.; Bayir, H.; Shvedova, A. *Nanomedicine: Nanotechnology, Biology, and Medicine*. 2005, *1*, 313– 316.

[5] (a) Haniu, H.; Matsuda, Y.; Takeuchi, K.; Kim, Y.; Hayashi, T.; Endo, M. *Toxicology and Applied Pharmacology*. 2010, *242*, 256-262. (b) Thakare, V. S.; Das, M.; Jain, A. K.; Patil, *S.;* Jain, S. *Nanomedicine: Nanotechnology, Biology, and Medicine*. 2010, *5*, 1277-1301.

[6] Yarotski, D.A.; Kilina, S.V.; Talin, A.A.; Tretiak, S.; Prezhdo, O.V.; Balatsky, A.V, Taylor, A. J. *Nano Letters*. 2009, *9*, 12–7.

[7] Yang, X.; Zhang, Z.; Liu, Z.; Ma, Y.; Yang, R.; Chen, Y. *Journal of Nanoparticle Research*. 2008, *10*, 815–22.

[8] (a) Bianco, A.; Kostarelos, K.; Prato, M. *Expert Opinion Drug Delivery*. 2008, *5*, 331. (b) Adeli, M.; Mirab, N. Alavidjeh, M. S.; Sobhani, Z.; Atyabi, F. *Polymer*. 2009, *50*, 3528.
[9] Ferrari, M. *Nat. Rev. Cancer*. 2005, *5*, 161–171.
[10] Iijima, S. *Nature*. 1991,*354*, 56–58.
[11] Liu, Zh.; Sun, X.; Nakayama-Ratchford, N.; Dai, H. *ACS Nano*. 2007, *1*, 50–6.
[12] Singh, P. *Chalcogenide Letters*. 2010, *7*, 389-396.
[13] Jacobs, C.B.; Peairs, M. J.; Venton, B.J. *Analytica Chimica Acta*. 2010, *662*, 105–127.
[14] Wu, Y.; Phillips, J. A.; Liu, H. *ACS Nano*. 2008, *2*, 2023–8.
[15] Qiu, J.D.; Zhou, W.M.; Guo, J.; Wang, R.; Liang, R.P. *Analytical Biochemistry*. 2009, *385*, 264–9.
[16] Liu, Z.; Tabakman, S.; Welsher, K.; Dai, H. *Nano Res*. 2009, *2*, 85-120.
[17] (a) Veetil, J.; Ye, K. *Biotechnol. Prog*. 2009, *25*, 709-721. (b) Chen, X.; Schluesener, H. J. *Nanotechnology* 2010, *21*, 105104 (10pp).
[18] Liu, Z.; Chen, K.; Davis, C.; Sherlock, S.; Cao, Q.; Chen, X.; Dai, H. *Cancer Res*. 2008, *68*, 6652-6660.
[19] Tripisciano, C.; Kraemer, K.; Taylor, A.; Borowiak-Palen, E. *Chemical Physics Letters*. 2009, *478*, 200-205.
[20] McCarroll, J.; Baigude, H.; Yang, S-C.; Rana, T.M. *Bioconjugate Chem*. 2010, *21*, 56-63.
[21] Müller, K.; Malik, S.; Richert, C. *Acs NANO*. 2010, *4*, 649–656.
[22] Riggio, C.; Ciofani, G.; Raffa, V.; Cuschieri, A.; Micera, S. *Nanoscale Res Lett*. 2009, *4*, 668–673.
[23] Levi-Polyachenko, N.; Merkel, E.; Jones, B.; Carroll, D.; Stewart, J. *Molecular Pharmaceutics*. 2009, *6*, 1092–1099.
[24] Guo, Y.; Shi, D.; Cho, H.; Dong, Z.; Kulkarni, A.; Pauletti, G.M.; et al. *Advanced Functional Materials*. 2008, *18*, 1–9.
[25] Maynard, A.D.; Baron, P.A.; Foley, M.; Shvedova, A.A.; Kisin, E.R.; Castranova, V. *Journal of Toxicology Environmental Health, Part A*. 2004,*67*,87–107.
[26] Ding, L.; Stilwell, J.; Zhang, T.; Elboudwarej, O.; Jiang, H.; Selegue., J.P.; Cooke, P.A.; Gray, J.W.; Chen, F.F. *Nano Letters*. 2005, *12*, 2448–64.
[27] Wu, W.; Li, R.; Bian, X.; Zhu, Z.; Ding, D.; Li, X.; Jia, Z.; Jiang, X.; Hu, Y. *Acs NANO*. 2009, *3*, 2740-2750.
[28] Zhang, L.W.; Zeng, L.; Barron, A.R.; Monterio-Riviere, N.A. *International Journal of Toxicology*. 2007, *161*, 135–42.
[29] Zeineldin, R.; Al-Haik, M.; Hudson, L.G. *Nano Letters*. 2009, *9*, 751–7.
[30] Feng, Q.; Xie, X.; Liu, Y.; Zhao, W.; Gao, Y. *Journal of Applied Polymer Science*. 2007, *106*, 2413–21.
[31] Campidelli, S.; Sooambar, C.; Diz, E.L.; Ehli, C.; Guldi, D.M.; Prato, M. *Journal of American Chemical Society*. 2006, *128*, 12544–52.
[32] Yingkui, Y.; Xiaolin, X.; Zhifang, Y.; Xiaotao, W.; Wei, C.; Yiu-Wing, M. *Macromolecules*. 2007, *40*, 5858–67.
[33] Hahn, U.; Engmann, S.; Oelsner, C.; Ehli, C.; Guldi, D.M.; Torres, T. J. *Am. Chem. Soc*. 2010, *132*, 6329–6401.
[34] Qiao, R.; Ke, P.C. *Journal of American Chemical Society*. 2006, *128*, 13656–7.

[35] You, Y.Z.; Hong, C.Y.; Pan, C.Y. *Journal of Physical Chemistry C*. 2007, *111*, 16161–6.

[36] Shen, J.; Hu, Y.; Qin, C.; Li, C.; Ye, M. *Composites: Part A*. 2008, *39*, 1679-1683.

[37] (a) Meo, E.; Crescenzo, A.; Velluto, D.; O'Neil, C.; Demurtas, D.; Hubbell, A.; Fontana, A. *Macromolecules*. 2010, *43*, 3429–3437. (b) Madni, I.; Hwang, C-Y.; Park, S-D.; Choa, Y-H.; Kim, H-T. *Colloids and Surfaces A: Physicochem. Eng. Aspects*. 2010, *358*, 101 –107. (c) Moghimi, S. M.; Andersen, A. J.; Hashemi, S. H.; Lettiero, B.; Ahmadvand, D.; Hunter, A. C.; Andresen, T. L. Hamad, I.; Szebeni, J. *Journal of Controlled Release* 2010, *146*, 175–181.

[38] (a) Lacerda, L.; Raffa, S.; Prato, M.; Bianco, A.; Kostarelos. *Nano Today*. 2007, *2*, 38–43. (b) Lay, C. L.; Liu, H. Q.; Tan, H. R.; Liu, Y. *Nanotechnology* 2010, *21*, 065101 (10pp).

[39] Prato, M.; Kostarelos, K.; Bianco, A. *Accounts of Chemical Research*. 2008, *41*, 60-68.

[40] Chaudhuri, P.; Soni, S.; Sengupta, S. *Nanotechnology* 2010, *21*, 025102 (11pp).

[41] Spitalsky, Z.; Tasis, D.; Papagelis, K.; Galiotis, C. *Progress in Polymer Science*. 2010, *35*, 357–401.

[42] Capek, I. *Advances in Colloid and Interface Science*. 2009, *150*, 63-89.

[43] Chen, J.; Liu, H.; Weimer, W.A.; Halls, M.D.; Waldeck, D.H.; Walker, G.C. *Journal of American Chemical Society*. 2002, *124*, 9034–5.

[44] Narizzano, R.; Nicolini, C. *Macromolecular Rapid Communications*. 2005, *26*, 381–5.

[45] Sepahvand, R.; Adeli, M.; Astinchap, B. *Journal of Nanoparticle Research*. 2008, *10*, 1309–18.

[46] Adeli, M.; Bahari, A.; Hekmatara, H. *Nano: Brief Reports and Reviews*. 2008, *3*, 37–44.

[47] Adeli, M.; Mehdipour, E.; Bavadi, M. *Journal of Applied Polymer Science*. 2010, *116*, 2188–2196.

[48] Namazi, H.; Adeli, M.; Zarnegar, Z.; Jafari, S.; Dadkhah, A.; Shukla, A. *Colloid and Polymer Science*. 2007, *285*, 1527–33.

[49] Adeli, M.; Zarnegar, Z.; Kabiri, R. *European Polymer Journal*. 2008, *44*, 1921–30.

[50] Namazi, H.; Adeli, M. *Journal of Polymer Science, Part A: Polymer Chemistry*. 2005, *43*, 28–41.

[51] Adeli, M.; Zarnegar, Z.; Dadkhah, A.; Hossieni, R.; Salimi, F.; Kanani, A. *Journal of Applied Polymer Science*. 2007, *104*, 267–72.

[52] Namazi, H.; Adeli, M. *Polymer*. 2005, *46*, 10788–99.

[53] Xu, Y.; Gao, Ch.; Kong, H.; Yan, D.; Zhang Jin, Y.; Watts. *Macromolecules*. 2004,*37*,8846–53.

[54] Gao, Ch.; Muthukrishnan, Sh.; Li, W.; Yuan, J.; Xu, Y.; Müller, A. Macromolecules, 2007, *40*, 1803–15.

[55] Foldvari, M.; Bagonluri, M. *Nanomedicine: Nanotechnology, Biology, and Medicine*. 2008, *4*, 183–200.

[56] Martin, B. *Basic Biotechnology e Journal*. 2006, *2*, 26-30.

[57] Veetil, J. V; Ye, K. *Biotechnol. Prog*. 2009, *25*, 709-21.

[58] Bhirde, A. A.; Patel, V.; Gavard, J. *Asc Nano*. 2009, *435*, 307–316.

[59] Tran, Ph. J.; Zhang, l.; Webster, Th. J. *Advanced Drug Delivery Reviews*. 2009, *61*, 1097-1114.

[60] Firme, C. P.; Bandaru, P. R. *Nanomedicine: Nanotechnology, Biology, and Medicine*. 2010, *6*, 245-256.

[61] Adeli, M.; Mirab, N.; Alavidjeh, M. S.; Sobhani, Z.; Atyabi, F. *Polymer*. 2009, *50*, 3528–3536.

[62] Sobhani, Z.; Dinarvand, R.; Atyabi, F.; Ghahremani, M.; Adeli, M. *International Journal of Nanomedicine*. 2011, *6*, 705–719.

[63] (a) Li, R.; Wu, R.; Zhao, L.; Wu, M.; Yang, L.; Zou, H. *ACS Nano*. 2010, *4* , 1399–1408. (b) Lee, J. H.; Yigit, M. V.; Mazumdar, D.; Lu, Y. *Advanced Drug Delivery Reviews*. 2010, *62*, 592–605. (c) Ruenraroengsak, P.; Cook, J. M.; Florence, A. T. *Journal of Controlled Release*. 2010, *141*, 265–276. (d) Yu, X.; Zhang, Y.; Chen, C.; Yao, Q.; Li, M. *Biochimica et Biophysica Acta*. 2010, 1805, 97–104.

[64] Liu, Zh.; Tabakman, S.; Welsher, K.; Dai, H. *Nano Res*. 2009, *2*, 85-120.

[65] Wu, W.; Wieckowski, S.; Pastorin, G.; Klumpp, C.; Benincasa, M.; Briand, J-P.; Gennaro, R.; Prato, M.; Bianco, A. *Angewandte Chemie International Edition*. 2005, *39*, 6358-6362.

[66] Chen, J.; Chen, Sh.; Zhao, X.; Kuznetsova, L.; Wong, S.; Ojima, I. *J. Am. Chem. Soc.* 2008, *130*, 16778–16785.

[67] Bhirde, A.; Patel, V.; Gavard, J.; Zhang, G.; Sousa, A.; Andrius, M.; Leapman, R.; Weigert, R.; Gutkind, J. S.; Rusling, J. F. *Acs Nano*. 2009, *3* , 307–316.

[68] Dhar, Sh.; Liu, Zh.; Thomale, J.; Dai, H.; Lippard, S. J. *Am. Chem. Soc*. 2008, *130*, 11467–11476.

[69] Wu, W.; Wieckowski, S.; Pastorin, G.; Benincasa, M.; Klumpp, C.; Briand, J-P.; Gennaro, R.; Prato, M.; Bianco, A. *Angew. Chem., Int. Ed.* 2005, *44*, 6358– 6362.

[70] Yinghuai, Z.; Peng, A.T.; Carpenter, K.; Maguire, J.A.; Hosmane, N.S.; Takagaki, M. *J Am. Chem. Soc*. 2005, *127*:9875-9880.

[71] Tran, P. A.; Zhang, L.; Webster, T. *Advanced Drug Delivery Reviews*. 2009, *61*, 1097–1114.

[72] Klumpp, C.; Kostarelos, K.; Prato, M.; Bianco, A. *Biochimica et Biophysica Acta*. 2006, *1758*, 404 – 412.

[73] Mintzer, M. A.; Simanek, E.E. *Chemistry Review*.2009, *109*, 259–302.

[74] Kim, S.; Kim, W. *Pharm. Res*. 2009, *26*, 657–666.

[75] Zimmer, R. A. *Nanomed.: Nanotechnol. Biol. Med.* 2009, *5*, 8–20.

[76] Bianco, A.; Kostarelos, K.; Partidos, C.D.; Prato, M. *Chem Commun (Camb)*. 2005, 571–577.

[77] Li, S.; He, P.; Dong, J.; Guo, Z.; Dai, L. *J. Am. Chem. Soc*. 2005, *127*, 14-15.

[78] Wang, X.; Liu, F.; Andavan, G. T. S.; Jing, X.; Singh, K. V.; Yazdanpanah, R.; Bruque, N.; Pandey, R. R.; Lake, R.; Ozkan, M.; Wang, K. L.; Ozkan, C. S. *Small*. 2006, *2*, 1356-1365.

[79] Han, X.; Li, Y.; Deng, Z. *Adv. Mater*. 2007, *19*, 1518-1522.

[80] Lu, F.; Gu, L.; Meziani, M.; Wang, X.; Luo, P.; Veca, L.; Cao, L.; Sun, Y-P. *Adv. Mater*. 2009, *21*, 139–152.

[81] Lee, C.-S.; Baker, S. E.; Marcus, M. S.; Yang, W.; Eriksson, M. A.; Hamers, R. J. *Nano Lett*. 2004, *4*, 1713-1716.

[82] Liu, Z.; Winters, M.; Holodniy, M.; Dai, H. *Angew. Chem. Int. Ed.* 2007, *46*, 2023-2027.

[83] Bi-feng, P.; Da-xiang, C.; Ping, X.; Hao, C.; Feng-tao, L.; Qing, L.; Tuo, H .; Xiao-gang, Y.; Jun, S.; Chen-chen, B.; Feng, G.; Rong, H.; Meng-jun, S.H.U,; Yong-jie, M.A. *Journal of Cancer Research*. 2007, *19*, 1-6.

[84] Gao, H.; Kong, Y.; Cui, D. *Nano Letters*. 2003, *3*, 471-473.
[85] Cai, D.; Mataraza, J.M.; Qin, Z-H.; Huang. Z.; Huang, J.; Chiles, T.C.; Carnaham, D.; Kempa, K.; Ren, Z. *Nat. Methods*, 2005, *2*, 449–454.
[86] Kam, N.W.S.; O'Connell, M.; Wisdom, J. A.; Dai, H. *Proc. Natl. Acad. Sci. U. S. A.* 2005, *102*, 11600–11605.
[87] Pantarotto, D.; Partidos, C. D.; Graff, R.; Hoebeke, J.; Briand, J.P.; Prato, M.; Bianco, A. *J. Am. Chem. Soc.* 2003, *125*, 6160-6164.
[88] Bianco, A.; Hoebeke, J.; Godefroy, S.; Chaloin, O.; Pantarotto, D.; Briand, J.P.; Muller, S.; Prato, M.; Partidos, C.D. *J. Am. Chem. Soc*. 2005, *127*, 58-59.
[89] Ma, J.; Wang, J-N.; Tsai, C-J.; Nussinov, R.; Ma, B. *Front.Mater. Sci.China*. 2010, *4,* 17-28.
[90] Kam, N. W. S. Dai, H. *J. Am. Chem. Soc.* 2005, *127,* 6021-6026.
[91] Pantarotto, D.; Partidos, C.D.; Hoebeke, J.; Brown, F.; Kramer, E.; Briand, J.P.; Muller, S.; Prato, M.; Bianco, A. *Chem Biol*. 2003, *10*, 961-966.
[92] Yang, F.; Fu, D. L. P.; Long, J.; Ni, Q. X. *Medical Hypotheses*. 2008, *70*, 765–767.
[93] Reddy, S.T.; Rehor, A.; Schmoekel, H.G.; Hubbell, J. A.; Swartz, M.A. *J Control Release*. 2006, *112*, 26–34.
[94] Yang, F.; Hu, J. H.; Yang, D.; Long, *J.;* Luo, *G.;* Jin, *Ch.;* Yu, X.; Xu, *J.;* Changchun Wang, *Ch.;* Ni,Q.; Fu, *D. Nanomedicine*. 2009, *4*, 317–330.
[95] Yang, F.; Hu, J.H.; Yang, D.; Long, J.; Wang, C.C.; Fu, D.L.; Ni, Q . *Chem. Commun.* 2009, *29*, 4447-4449.
[96] Li, J.; Yang, F.; Guo, G.; Yang, D.; Long, J.; Fu, D.; Luc, J.; and Wang, Ch. *Polym. Int.* 2010, *59*, 169–174.
[97] Marches, R.; Chakravarty, P.; Musselman, I. H.; Bajaj, P.; Azad, R. N.; Pantano, P.; Draper, R. K.; Vitetta, E. S. *Int. J. Cancer* 2009, *125*, 2970–2977.
[98] Moon, H.; Lee, S.; Choi, H. Acs *Nano*. 2009, *3*, 3707-3713.
[99] Welsher, K.; Liu, Zh.; Daranciang, D.; Dai, H. *Nano Lett*. 2008, *8*, 586-590.
[100] Park, H.; Yang, J.; Lee, J.; Haam, S.; Choi, I-H.; Yoo, K-H. *Acs NANO*. 2009, *3*, 2919-2926.
[101] Levi-Polyachenko, N.; Merkel, E.; Jones, B.; Carroll, D.; Stewart, J.H. *Molecular Pharmaceutics*.2009, *6*, 1092–1099.
[102] Ji, Sh-r.; Liu, Ch.; Zhang, B.; Yang, F.; Xu , J.; Long, J.; Jin, Ch.; Fu, D-l.; Ni, Q-x.; Yu, X-j. *Biochimica et Biophysica Acta*. 2010, *1*, 29-35.
[103] Yang, W.; Thordarson, P.; Gooding, J.; Ringer, S.; Braet, F. *Nanotechnology*. 2007, *18*, 412001.
[104] (a) Shvedova, A. A.; Kisin, E. R.; Porter, D.; Schulte, P.; Kagan, V. E.; Fadeel, B.; Castranova, V. *Pharmacology and Therapeutics*. 2009, *121*, 192–204. (b) Chaudhuri, P.; Harfouche, R.; Soni, S.; Hentschel, D. M.; Sengupta, S. *ACS Nano*. 2010, *4*, 574-582.
[105] Coccini, A.; Roda, E.; Sarigiannis, D.A.; Mustarelli, P.; Quartarone, E.; Profumo, A.; Manzo, L. *Toxicology*. 2010, *269*, 41-53.
[106] Hussain, M. A.; Kabir, M. A.; Sood, A. K. *Current Science*. 2009, *96*, 664-673.
[107] Kato, H.; Mizuno, K.; Shimada, M.; Nakamura, A.; Takahashi, K.; Hata, K.; Kinugasa, S. *Carbon*. 2009, *47*, 3434–3440.

[108] Shvedova, A.A.; Castranova, V.; Kisin, E.R.; Schwegler-Berry, D.; Murray, A.R.; Gandelsman, V. Z.; Maynard, A.; Baron, P. *J Toxicol. Environ. Health A*. 2003, *66*, 1909-26.

[109] Murakami, T.; Fan, J.; Yudasaka, M.; Iijima, S.; Shiba, K. *Mol. Pharm.* 2006, *3*, 407–414.

[110] Tomonari, Y.; Murakami, H.; Nakashima, N. *Chem. Eur. J.* 2006, *12*, 4027– 4034.

[111] Cheng, F.; Adronov, A. *Chem. Eur. J.* 2006, *12*, 5053–5059.

[112] Liang, Z.; Lao, R; Wang, J; Liu, Y; Wang, L; Huang, Q; Song, S; Li, G; Fan, C. *Int. J. Mol. Sci.* 2007, *8*, 705–713.

[113] Karajanagi, S. S.; Yang, H.; Asuri, P.; Sellitto, E.; Dordick, J. S.; Kane, R. S. *Langmuir*. 2006, *22*, 1392–1395.

[114] Fei, B.; Lu, H.; Hu, Z.; Xin, J. H. *Nanotechnology*. 2006, *17*, 1589–1593.

[115] Ikeda, A.; Tanaka, Y.; Nobusawa, K.; Kikuchi, J. *Langmuir*, 2007, *23*, 10913–10915.

[116] Zou, J.; Liu, L.; Chen, H.; Khondaker, S.; McCullough, R. D.; Huo, Q.; Zhai, L. *Adv. Mater*. 2008, *20*, 2055–2060.

[117] Sayes, C. M.; Liang, F.; Hudson, J. L.; Mendez, J.; Guo, W.; Beach, J. M.; Moore, V.C.; Doyle, C. D.; West, J. L.; Billups, W. E.; Ausman, K. D.; Colvin, V. L. *Toxicol. Lett*. 2006, *161*, 135–142.

[118] Shvedova, A. A.; Kisin, E.R.; Castronova, V. *Am. J. Physiol. Lung Cell. Mol. Physiol.* 2005, *289*, 698–708.

[119] Singh, R.; Pantarotto, D.; Lacerda, L.; Pastorin, G.; Klumpp, C,.; Prato, M.; Bianco, A.; Kostarelos, K. *Proc. Natl. Acad. Sci. USA*. 2006, *103*, 3357–3362.

[120] Dumortier, H.; Lacotte, S.; Pastorin, G.; Marega, R.; Wu , W.; Bonifazi, D.; Briand, J.-P.; Prato, M.; Muller, S.; Bianco, A. *Nano Lett*. 2006, *6*, 1522-8.

[121] Lam, C. W.; James, J. T.; McCluskey, R.; Hunter, R. L. *Toxicol. Sci.* 2004, *77*, 126–34.

In: Hybrid Nanostructures in Cancer Therapy
Editor: Mohsen Adeli
ISBN: 978-1-62100-517-9
© 2012 Nova Science Publishers, Inc.

Chapter VI

Quantum Dot-Polymer Hybrid Nanomaterials in Nanomedicine

***Mohsen Adeli*[1,2], *Masoumeh Parsamanesh*[1], *and Elham Sadeghi*[1]**
[1]Department of Chemistry, Faculty of Science, Lorestan University, Khoramabad, Iran
[2]Department of chemistry, Sharif University of Technology, Tehran, Iran

Abstract

Semiconductor quantum dots are a new class of nanomaterials which have unique optical and electronic properties. Their novel properties promise them as candidates to use in many area of science such as nanomedicine. In this chapter, properties of quantum dots, their synthetic procedures, modification of their surface especially by polymers will be reviewed briefly. Biomedical applications of polymer-quantum dots and their toxicity concerns in biology and also strategies to reduce their toxicity will be discussed.

1. Introduction

Quantum dots (QDs) are semiconductor nanocrystals with a somewhat spherical shape (2–8 nm) which restricted in three dimensions. These nanocrystals which are about 100—10,000 times smaller than human cells are neither atomic nor bulk semiconductors [1, 2]. These nanocrystals which are prepared using II-VI or III-V column elements of the periodic table have size-tunable and unique optical and electronic properties including bright fluorescence, board excitation spectrum, narrow/symmetric emission spectrum and superior photostability that are not available from bulk counterparts or individual molecules [3-6]. They are usually insoluble in water. This factor limits their processability and considers the major drawback to use them for biomedical applications. In order to improve their water solubility the surface of QDs should be modified by suitable modifiers such as polymers and biomacromolecules. In addition to improve their water dispersesability, modification of the surface of QDs decreases their toxicity against biological systems and facilitates their specific interactions with biomacromolecules. High luminescence yield of QDs which can be survived in biological mediums for a long time in comparison to that for fluorescent dyes allow observation of biological phenomena including cancer cells detection, tumor vessels imaging, and cell trafficking studies inside the body over a prolonged period of time [7-9].

2. Properties of Quantum Dots

QDs which have attracted intensive attention during the last two decades are fluorescent semiconductor nanocrystals having a core-shell structure which their inner Semiconductor core consists of combinations of elements from groups II–VI or III–V of the periodic table such as CdSe and shell is a layer of other elements or their combinations such as zinc sulfide (ZnS). They are spherical in shape, typically with a diameter of 2–10 nm (on the order of 200–10000 atoms) depending on their final size, and their radius is known to be smaller than the bulk Bohr excitation radius [10-14].

As the size of QDs decreased to the nano-scale (less than the Bohr radius of the material), a three dimensional confinement of the electrons and holes in the particle occurs which makes the band gap energy dependent on particle size. Therefore, optical properties of QDs such as fluorescence excitation and emission can be "tuned" by altering the size [15, 16]. Physical size of nanocrystals compared to other entities is shown in figure 1 [17].

As it was mentioned, QDs which are highly luminescence nano-objects and exhibit size- and composition-tunable emission spectra are resistant to photobleaching and show exceptional resistance to photo and chemical degradation. All these properties and advantages promise QDs as excellent contrast agents for imaging and labels for bioassays [18].

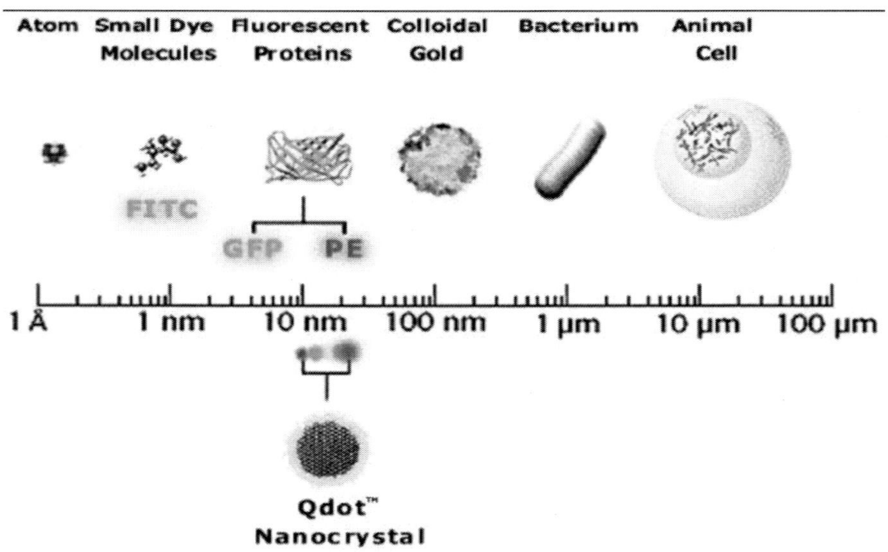

Figure 1. A comparison between the physical size of QDs and other biological entities. Reprinted with the permission of Ref [17].

3. Synthesis Procedures and Surface Chemistry of QDs

The emission wavelengths of QDs depend on their size; therefore it is important to obtain nanocrystals with a narrow size distribution. For this purposes several strategies for synthesis of II–VI semiconductor nanocrystals with various application has taken place during the last two decades [16]. These nanocrystals can be prepared either in nonpolar organic solvents, which yield nanoparticles non-soluble in water, or by water-based synthesis methods [19]. High quality QDs with a narrow polydispersity are typically prepared by the first method in which precursors of the used elements are injected to the organic solvents or oils at high temperatures. This strategy involves the introduction of the semiconductor precursors under conditions that thermodynamically favor crystal growth. Usually a capping agent such as trioctylphosphine oxide (TOPO) or hexadecylamine (HDA) which is able to interact with atoms onto the surface of a newly formed nanocrystal is added to the medium of reaction to kinetically control the crystal growth and to maintain its size within the nanoscale. Due to the coating of the surface of QDs by capping agents, their solubility is regular by these agents. Capping agents that used in the high temperature conditions, which provide high quality QDs, are usually hydrophobic molecules and therefore the obtained nanocrystals are only soluble in nonpolar hydrophobic solvents and are not soluble in water. However, high functionality and water solubility are two crucial characteristics that are necessary for QDs to be used in biomedical applications. Therefore, synthesis of QDs with hydrophilic surface or conversion of QDs with hydrophobic surface to those with hydrophilic surface and transfer them from organic phase into an aqueous phase has been extensively investigated [20-23]. Conversion of QDs with hydrophobic surface to those with hydrophilic surface can either be carried out by ligand exchange process or by encapsulation of QDs into the amphiphilic macromolecules such as performed polymers [24, 25]. In ligand exchange process hydrophobic surface capping agents such as TOPO are replaced with hydrophilic ones such as thiol-containing ligands and polymerized silica shells with polar groups [26-28]. Functionalization of QDs with carbohydrate molecules bearing reactive thiol functional groups at the end chains in aqueous solution is an example of ligand exchange process [29]. Chemical modification of the surface of QDs with small molecules or functional ligands even alters the characteristics of these particles. For instance, dopamine conjugation quenches the fluorescence of the QDs, which is a property that can be exploited for sensing applications if the conjugates are taken up into living cells [30].

Due to their larger size and longer chains, polymers are able to change the solubility and other properties of QDs more sufficiently than small molecules. Many strategies and methods including, introduction of the polymerizable ligands onto the surface of QDs, in situ polymerization, polymerizable surfactants and attachment of polymers to the capping agents of QDs by chemical linkages have been developed to produce QDs-polymer hybrid materials recently. Attachment of polymers and macromolecules onto the surface QDs by covalent linkages leads to hybrid materials with long-term stability [31, 32]. There are two different methods for attaching polymer chains onto the surface of QDs by a single-point chemical linkage strategy: the “grafting to” and the “grafting from” methods. In the “grafting to” technique the terminal end of a functionalized polymer chain react directly with the nanocrystal surface. In the “grafting from” method, polymers are growth from the surface of

QDs in a sufficient procedure with appropriate polymerization inhibitors to produce QD-polymer hybrid materials [16]. These methods which include the introduction of polymers directly onto the QDs surface require an intermediate ligand exchange step and usually lead to changes in the photophysical properties of QDs. Another strategy is including noncovalent interactions between polymers and surface of QDs. For example hydrophobic blocks of an amphiphilic macromolecule and hydrophobic surface of QDs leads to a thin polymeric coating on the QDs surface. Hydrophilic blocks of macromolecules attached onto the surface of QDs are responsible for its improved water solubility and functionality. Due to the absence of ligand exchange step in this method, it seems it do not change the photophysical properties of the QDs [33, 34, and 16]. Glycofunctionalized QDs with biotin end-terminated glycopolymers have been synthesized via a cyanoxyl-mediated free radical polymerization [31].

4. Quantum Dot-Polymer Systems and Nanomedicine

There have been numerous promises brought in with the appearance of nanomaterials in past few years. Use of nanodevices, nanomaterials and nanostructures for different biomedical applications constitutes a new field called "nanomedicine". Nanomedicine involves a regular and multi-step process from the design, synthesis, characterization, *in vitro* experiments and initial administration to cross different biological barriers including the tissue endothelium barrier and introduction into the interstitial space of tissues, through the cell membrane into organelles of cells and even through the perinuclear membrane into the nucleus of cells [35-41].

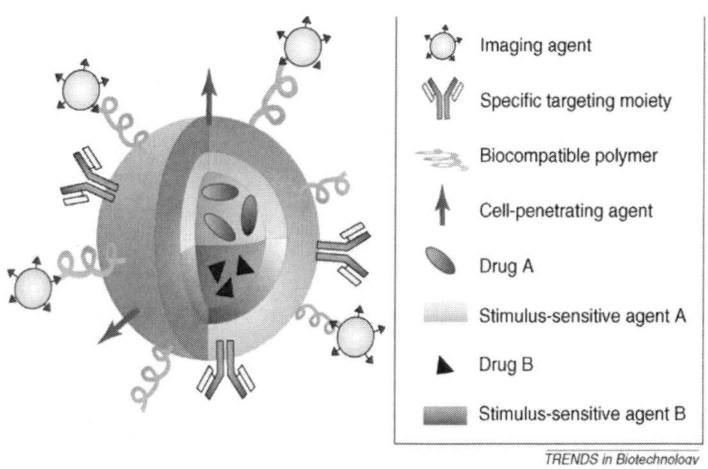

Figure 2. A perfect drug delivery system based on nanomaterials. It is consisting of a nanocapsule having different objects including imaging agent, specific targeting ligand, biocompatible polymer and cell-penetrating agents on its surface and encapsulated drugs inside. Reprinted with the permission of Ref [10].

The aim of the targeted cancer therapy is to improve the drug pharmacokinetics and pharmacodynamics and also diminish the non-specific interactions between the therapeutic systems and biological objects which lead to decrease the immunogenicity of these systems in the quest for developing the efficacy of anticancer drugs and killing the cancer cells. Drug delivery systems based on nanomaterials with an optimized size, between 10-200 nm, show above properties better than others. They can be tailored to cross the biological barriers actively or passively and to deliver therapeutic agents to the targeted sites and release them in a controlled manner. These characterizes for drug delivery systems based on nanomaterials lead to highest therapeutic efficacy and lowest side effects [42].

Blood-brain barrier (BBB) is the most difficult biological barrier to be crossed by delivery systems. Anticancer drugs such as doxorubicin (DOX) are loaded by nanomaterial-based delivery systems that can cross BBB to release DOX at therapeutic concentrations in the brain [10].

The most important advantage of QDs to be used in nanomedicine over current techniques is their ability to label cells and sub-cellular organelles *in vivo* easily and without needs to sacrificing tissues [43-45].

After administration and crossing the tissue endothelium barrier and introduction into the interstitial space of tissues, the most important barrier for drugs to reach their destinations is the cell membrane [46]. Cellular internalization process can be achieved by different mechanisms including non-specific entry by endocytosis, specific entry mediated by biomolecules attached to QD surface, micropipette injection, electroporation, and possibly by inducement of plasma membrane damage [19] (Figure 3).

Internalization of QDs into the cells through above routes usually leads to sequestration of aggregated QDs in different locations inside cells such as vesicles, showing strong colocalization with membrane dyes. Therefore labeling of the cells organelles by this method is difficult and in most cases is not possible [47-49].

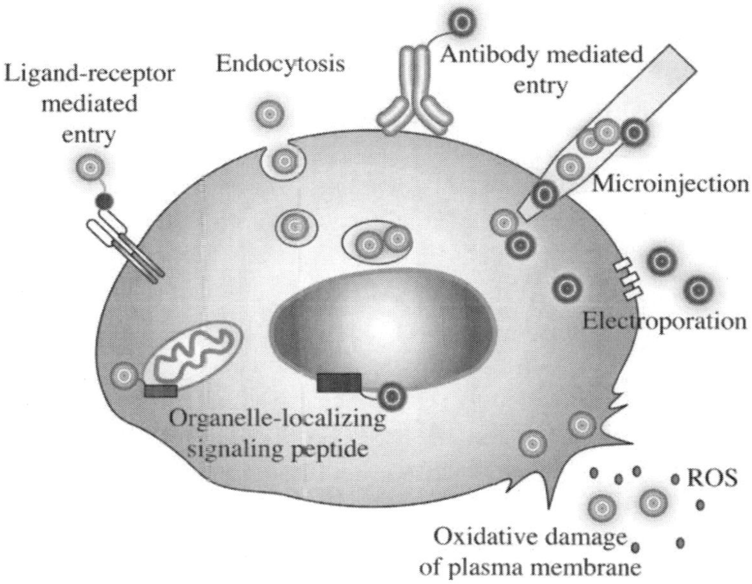

Figure 3. Different mechanisms by which QDs cross the cell membranes and internalize into the cells. Reprinted with the permission of Ref [19].

Despite the current technical challenges, due to the high quantum yield of QDs and their bright luminescent, they are garnering interest as intracellular probes after crossing the cell membrane and internalization into the cells. Some strategies to overcome mentioned challenges have been reported so that they can be tracked even in the cell organelles. Recently a size-dependence distribution of QDs in the sub-cellular organelles has been observed. It has been found that the non-functionalized CdTe QDs with 2.1 nm sizes are actively delivered into the nucleus of macrophages, while those with a size of 3.8 nm did not enter the nucleus and mainly end up in the cytoplasm [46].

Functionalization of the surface of QDs is a widely used method to confer them an ability to escape cytoplasm and label the intracellular organelles [50]. Because this process changes their interactions with the biological systems so that they can effectively internalize into the cells and ended up in endosomes/lysosomes [46]. Attachment of targeting ligands onto the surface of QDs dominates the route of their internalization into the cells and their localization into the organelles. Cell-penetrating peptides such as polyarginine and Tat are widely used to overcome the plasma membrane barrier and target QDs to cellular nuclei. This strategy have resulted in organelle-level resolution of intracellular targets for living cells, yielding fluorescent contrast of vesicles, mitochondria, and nuclei, but not the ability to visualize single molecules [51]. However the mechanism of delivery and the behavior and type of interactions of QDs in the cells are still a matter of debate.

Considerable research has been down for developing biodegradable polymeric nanoparticles for drug delivery and tissue engineering [52]. It has been found that the peptide-conjugated QDs are internalized to the cells by macropinocytosis and they are tethered to the inner surface of vesicles, and are trapped in intracellular organelles. Interestingly QD-loaded vesicles are actively transported by molecular machines (such as dyneins) along microtubule tracks to an asymmetric perinuclear region called the microtubule organizing center [53-60]

A comparison between the circulation lifetime of the PEG-functionalized QDs in the mouse blood stream and small organic dyes (which are eliminated from circulation within minutes after injection) has shown a longer blood circulation (half-life more than 3 hours) for PEG-functionalized QDs. This long blood circulation time is assigned to both PEG and suitable size of QDs. PEG is a well-known polymer which decreases the non-specific interactions between coated objects by this polymer and biological systems. On the other hand coating of the surface of QDs regulate their size to an intermediate state in which they are small and hydrophilic enough to slow down opsonization and reticuloendothelial uptake and also large enough to avoid renal filtration. Ampiphilic QDs (AMP-QDs) have been modified and functionalized by using PEG having a hydrophobic domain. Interactions between hydrophobic domains of PEG and AMP-QDs were lead to attachment of PEG onto the surface of QDs noncovalently. It has been found that functionalized QDs show improved passivation in biological environments and less susceptibility to nonspecific interactions with proteins [61,62]. Hyperbranched copolymers are also used to functionalize QDs. Multiarm star copolymers with a polyethylenimine core and PEG arms (PEI-g-PEG) are able to encapsulate and stabilize QDs in aqueous solution through direct ligand binding to the QD surface [63]. Due to the positive surface charge and a "proton sponge effect" associated with the large number of amino functional groups of PEI, these QDs could penetrate cell membranes and disrupt endosomal organelles in living cells. Amino functional groups of PEI give a buffering capability (pH 5–6) to QDs functionalized by PEI-g-PEG which lead to absorption of proton in acidic organelles and an increased osmotic pressure across the organelle membrane. This osmotic pressure causes transferring the water to organelle and swelling and finally rupturing of the acidic endosomes and a release of the trapped QDs or materials into the cytoplasm [64-66].

5. Cancer and Quantum Dots

5.1. Cancer Diagnosis

Control and cure of the cancer in the primary stages is much easier than progressed tumors. Tumors that their sizes exceed several millimeters are very difficult to eradicate and in the most cases they metastasis in the body and cure of patients having such tumors is impossible. Therefore the specific techniques to early diagnosis of cancer cells are important. Unfortunately the current treatment options are not effective, in most cases, and cancer patients are not satisfied with them. In the case of cancer therapy, the goal of nanomedicine is to develop safer and more effective delivery systems for therapeutic and diagnostic agents together with reducing the patient compliance, using nanomaterials and nanostructures [67, 68, 69, 3].

Several unique characteristics of these inorganic nanocrystals including, tunable to discreet narrow frequencies, broad band absorption spectra, narrow band emission, high photoluminescence, high resistance to photobleaching and high functionality promises them as efficient cancer diagnosis systems. Considerable success has been achieved in using QDs for *in vitro* bioassays, labeling fixed cells and tissue specimens, and for imaging membrane proteins on living cells. This has been demonstrated by following fluorescent QDs-injected Xenopus embryos through embryogenesis [70-78].

In this research work complete photobleaching was occurred for dextran-labeled controls after 80 minutes of constant illumination but any quenching or changes in the signal intensity of QDs fluorescent-labeled embryos was not observed. In addition to above advantages, synthesis of QDs is highly versatile so that they can be prepared that excite by a single light source but emit light or color at a wide range wavelengths. This property gives a possibility for independent labeling and identification of numerous biologic targets [79, 80].

In contrast to successful *in vitro* experiments and results, however, *in vivo* imaging of the biological systems inside cells has gotten limited progress.

A major problem is the lack of efficient methods for delivering individual QDs into the cytoplasms of living cells. Due to the non-specific interactions with the biological systems inside cells and also low pH QDs tend to assemble inside cells, and are often trapped in endocytotic vesicles such as endosomes and lysosomes [81].

One of the best methods to overcome problems of different barriers both *in vitro* and *in vivo* is the functionalization of QDs by polymers. Coating of the surface of QDs by hydrophilic macromolecules not only improved their water solubility and functionality but also minimizes their recognition by proteins and cells in the body, leading to a long circulation time in the blood and increased their efficiency [82, 83].

Polyethylene glycol (PEG) is the best polymer to modify QDs for biomedical applications [17 and 84] (Figure 4).

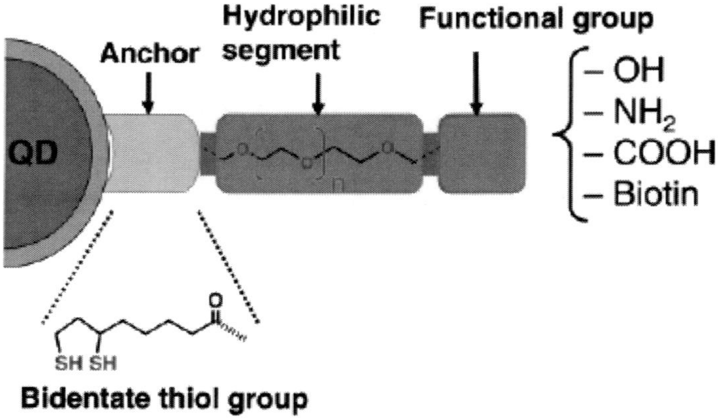

Figure 4. Schematic representation of the functionalization of QDs by PEG. Reprinted with the permission of Ref [84].

Thioglycolic-acid-stabilized CdTe QDs which have been synthesized directly in aqueous solution are successfully conjugated with biotin and polyethylene glycol. They are used for immunofluorescent labeling of cancer cells. Conjugated ligands onto the surface of QDs diminish the non-specific interactions with biological systems [85].

In order to improve the properties of QDs for biomedical applications, in addition to conjugation of polymer to their surfaces, their structures are modified by different modifier molecules such as antibodies and therapeutic agents [82]. Nanoparticles containing QDs entrapped in a lipid shell and post-loaded with a folate-lipid conjugate for targeting to mouse and human tumor cells expressing the folate receptor have been examined. Mixing of the hydrophobic QDs with 1,2 dipalmitoyl-sn-glycero-3 phosphocholine and methoxy-polyethylene glycol-distearoyl-phosphatidyl-ethanolamine (mPEGDSPE) generated a nanoparticle referred to as lipodot, with a mean diameter size of ~100 nm. Post-loading of folate-derivatized PEG-DSPE into the lipodots was led to nanoparticles having targeting ligands. It has been found that only folate-targeted lipodots were taken up by tumor cells [86].

Biodegradable and surfactant-free poly(lactide-*co*-glycolide) nanoparticles loaded with QDs has been synthesized through nanoprecipitation. Nanoparticles co-loaded with both QDs and hydrophobic drug (Coenzyme Q10) molecules are obtained using this strategy. Even though surfactants are not utilized during the nanoprecipitation procedure, these loaded nanoparticles have not aggregated [87]. CdTe-coated magnetic polystyrene nanospheres (MPN/CdTe) have been prepared via a stepwise electrostatic self-assembly. Conjugation of EGF to MPN/CdTe core-shell hybrid materials has been led to nanoobjects that not only emitted bright fluorescence and exhibited superparamagnetism but also could labeled human breast cancer MDA-MB-435S cells rapidly (Figure 5) [88]

Amphiphilic polymer consisting of a RAFT synthesized polyacrylic acid and octylamine are used to encapsulate hydrophobic CdSe/ ZnS NPs with a well-determined size [89].

Another problem for imaging by long-wavelengths light is autofluorescence of proteins and biological systems or tissues, like intestine and suboptimal tissue penetrance. This limitation could be overcome using QDs that fluoresce in the near infrared (NIR) spectra (700–1000 nm). Due to this property, QDs that emit in the NIR are attractive for in vivo tissue imaging [90-96]. Hybridization of QDs with other contrast agents develops their properties and diminishes above limitations for cancer diagnosis [97]. For example they can be embedded in the core of paramagnetic micelles to create bimodal nanoparticles visible by both MRI and fluorescence. These bimodal hybrid nanomaterials can be targeted to the specific epitopes by the incorporation of targeting ligands such as $\alpha_{\upsilon}\beta_3$-specific RGD peptides to their structures [98].

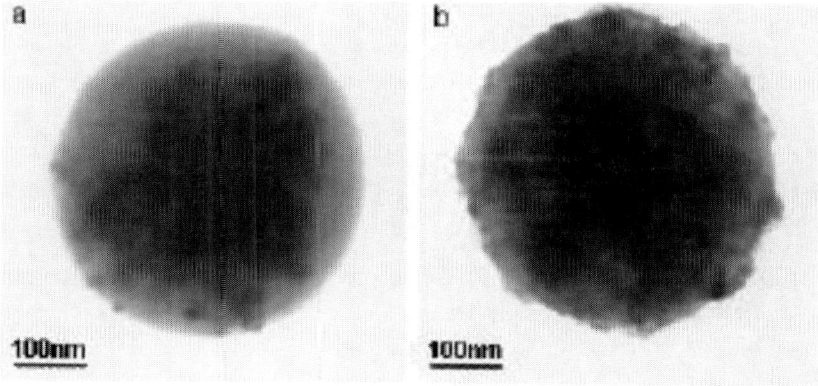

Figure 5. TEM images of (a) magnetic polystyrene nanospheres and (b) CdTe-coated magnetic polystyrene nanospheres. Reprinted with the permission of Ref [88].

5.2. Cancer Therapy

In addition to short circulation time, one of the main problems that limit the successes of the cancer therapy by anticancer drugs is the random distribution of anticancer drugs in the both normal tissues and tumor sites which result in a relatively low therapeutic index. Nanomaterials-based anticancer drug delivery systems not only increase the circulation time of loaded drugs but also target them to tumor sites passively or actively and therefore optimize their effects and also reduce their toxicity against normal cells [67-69]. CdS QDs are used as removable caps to controlled release of drugs encapsulated inside mesoporous silica nanospheres. The CdS cap ensures the drug is encapsulated inside the system until released by disulfide-bond reducing reagents.

The QDs avoid drugs of a defined size from leaking outside the spheres prematurely [99]. QDs having mercaptoacetic acid capping agent and grafted cyclodextrin molecules on their surface (QDs-CD-MAA) are synthesized and used to deliver paclitaxel (PTX) and folic acid (FA) by electrostatic interactions and inclusion complex formation (Sheme 1) [100].

Conjugation of the cyclodextrin molecules onto the surface of QDs decreased the viability of the L929 cell line. Decreasing of the viability of the cells upon conjugation of the cyclodextrin molecules onto the surface of QDs is assigned to the increasing of the transfer of QDs through cell membrane. However conjugation of a high number of cyclodextrin molecules onto the surface of QDs increased their biocompatibility interestingly. In this case, inherent biocompatibility of cyclodextrins dominates increasing of the toxicity of QDs caused by increasing their transfer to the cytoplasm.

A significance difference between cytotoxicity effects after 3 and 24 h incubation for these systems was not observed. This result confirmed that QDs pass through the cell membrane less than 3 hours extensively

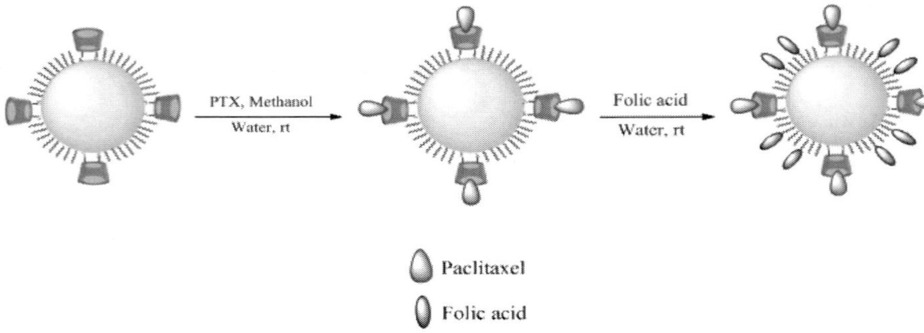

Scheme 1. Delivery of FA and PTX by QDs-CD-MAA through electrostatic interactions and inclusion complex formation.

Ability of QDs-CD-MAA and their host-guest systems (QDs-CD-MAA containing PTX and FA) as drug delivery systems for killing the tumor cell line c26 has shown that QDs-CD-MAA/PTX are able to kill cancer cells effectively. Table 1 shows the inhibitory concentration of PTX, QDs-MAA, QDs-CD-MAA, QDs-CD-MAA/PTX and QDs-CD-MAA/(PTX+FA) producing 50% cell growth inhibition or death, IC50. The IC50 for QDs-CD-MAA/PTX is much lower than that for QDs-MAA and QDs-CD-MAA. It is also small for QDs-CD-MAA in compared that for QDs-MAA. These results are in agree with the MTT results for the L929 cell line, because cyclodextrin molecules always increase the ability of the QDs and their host-guest systems to cross the cell membrane.

QDs are co-loaded with the blends of poly(lactide)-vitamin E TPGS (PLA-TPGS) and vitamin E TPGS-carboxyl (TPGS-COOH) copolymers and luminescent nanoparticles with a biocompatible shell and encapsulated QDs have been obtained. Absorption of folic acid onto the surface of these nanoparticles conferred them targeting capability (Figure 6) [101].

Functionalized-quantum-dot-liposome (f-QD-L) hybrid nanoparticles are prepared by encapsulating of PEG-coated QD in the internal aqueous phase of different lipid bilayer vesicles.

The cationic analogue of cholesterol was incorporated in the f-QD-L bilayers to enhance the interaction with the plasma membrane. f-QD alone at this concentration range has not shown any intracellular signal, indicating that no uptake by A549 cells taken place even after 3 h of incubation. This result has been attributed to the steric hindrance by the PEG molecules that reduce the nonspecific f-QD cell binding and the low concentration of f-QD used. In contrast, the cationic f-QD-L hybrids are internalized by A549 cells very efficiently [102].

Table 1. *In vitro* cytotoxicity of QDs-MAA, QDs-CD-MAA, QDs-CD-MAA/PTX, QDs-CD-MAA/(PTX+FA) and PTX on the tumor cell line (c26)

Sample	Tumor cell lines c26 (IC50 μg/ml)
QDs-MAA	0.63
QDs-CD-MAA	3.02
QDs-CD-MAA/PTX	0.05
QDs-CD-MAA/(PTX+FA)	0.36
PTX	0.029

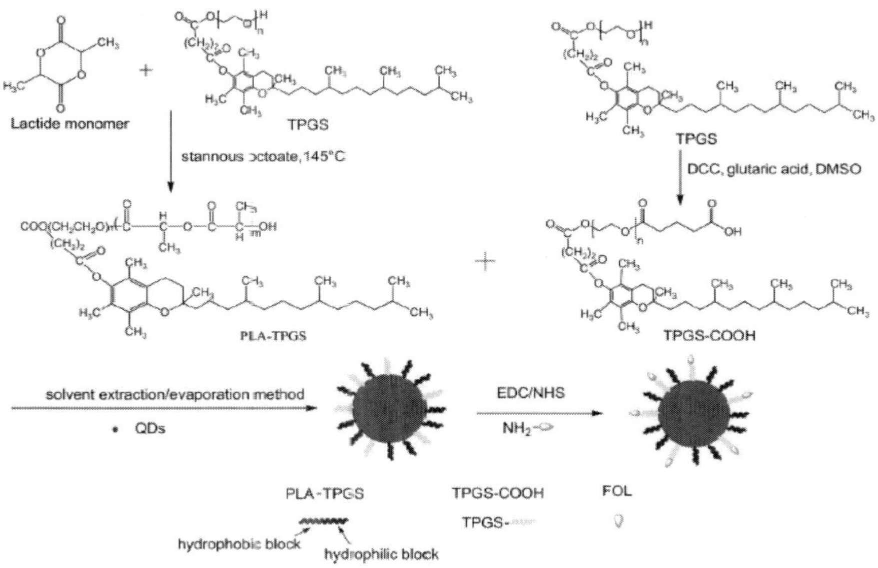

Figure 6. Preparation of QDs-loaded PLA-TPGS/TPGS-COOH NPs with folate molecules on their surface. Reprinted with the permission of Ref [101].

QDs-polyrotaxane supramolecules are also synthesized and used to deliver and controlled release of anticancer drugs [103].

β-CD-*graft*-QDs were first synthesized, then pseudopolyrotaxane (Ps-PR) consisting of α-CD rings and PEG axes were prepared and capped through host-guest relationship between their end hydrophobic groups as guest molecules and β-CD-*graft*-QDs as host molecules (Scheme 2a). Diagnosis and drug delivery systems were synthesized by conjugating of folic acid, as tumor-recognition module and cisplatin (CDDP), as an anticancer drug, to the functional groups of hybrid nanomaterials (Scheme 2b).

Molecular self-assemblies are products of what is so called the "bottom-up" approach in nanotechnology. Due to the noncovalent interactions between their building blocks, one of the potential applications of the molecular self-assemblies is recognized in drug delivery filed, because they will degrade back into individual monomers that can be broken down by the *in vivo* environment. MTT assay showed considerable toxicity for anticancer drug delivery systems so that IC50 for CDDP-QDs-polyrotaxane-FA and free CDDP were 35.2 and 40.12 ± 3.1% respectively, confirming that these systems are more efficient than free drug against C26 cell line.

Biocompatible nanomaterials have been utilized for delivery of chemotherapeutic drug docetaxel to localised tumours. Targeted delivery has been achieved using aptamers that recognized a prostate specific membrane antigen. Multifunctional nanoparticles consisting of nanocrystals, antibodies and the chemotherapeutic drug doxorubicin have been synthesized and used for cancer treatment [10].

Paclitaxel loaded nanoparticles with shells formed from a biodegradable polymer, poly (lactic-co-glycolic acid) (PLGA), are conjugated to transferrin via epoxy linkages. These nanoparticles have shown greater cellular uptake and reduced exocytosis, which yield greater antiproliferative activity and more sustained effects compared to the free drug or unconjugated nanoparticles [83].

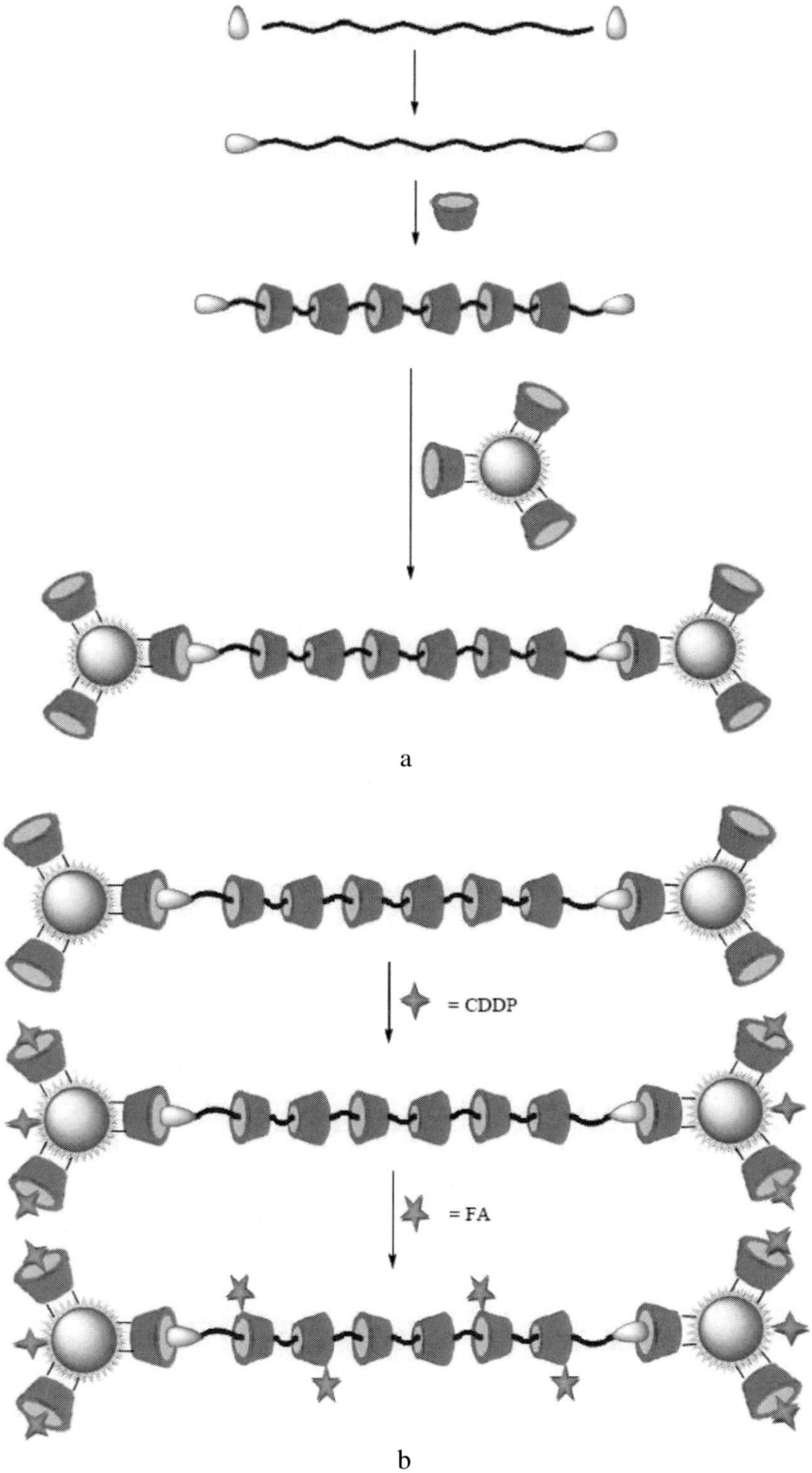

Scheme 2. (a) Synthesis of QDs-polyrotaxane supramolecules using an inclusion complex formation between functionalized pseudopolyrotaxane and CdSe QDs. (b) Preparation of CDDP-QDs-polyrotaxane and CDDP-QDs-polyrotaxane-FA conjugates.

6. Toxicity of QDs

In recent years, the toxicity of QDs has become a growing concern because of their increasing utilize in a wide range of biomedical applications, such as cancer therapy and diagnosis [104]. Hence the toxicity of QDs should be fully investigated and understand in all stages and conditions, and their safety should be proved before considering for any real biomedical application in clinical stages [105]. Like other nanomaterials the toxicity of QDs depends on structural and physicochemical parameters such as functional groups, surface charge, size, shape, and dosage [15].

Several mechanisms such as descrption and releasing of the free metal ions (Cd^{2+} in the case of cadmium-based QDs), free radical formation, and non-specific interaction with proteins and intracellular compartments have been proposed for toxicity of QDs [104]. Since UV radiation is used to excite QDs and energy of UV radiation is close to needed energy to break covalent chemical bonds, it usually dissolves the semiconductor nanomaterials in a process known as photolysis and metal ions as the products of this process leak from QDs into the culture medium and causes non-desirable toxicity and side effects [106-108].

Another source for toxicity of QDs is their ability to transfer the absorbed optical energy to other molecules in biological systems such as oxygen. This process leads to radicals and reactive oxygen species which can damage DNA strands and other cellular components that are in direct contact with them. The final result of this process is the apoptosis and necrosis deaths of the living cells [109].

In addition to their cytotoxicity, nonspecific interactions of QDs with the immune cells, biological molecules and proteins in blood lead to their fast clearance from the body or accumulation in kidney, liver and spleen for several months after systemic administration [22]. This behavior not only limits the biomedical applications of QDs but also open a big question concerning their fate in the body.

However there are some methods and strategies to reduce the short term cytotoxicity of QDs. A well-know method to decrease the cytotoxicity of QDs is to create a shell around them to keep their surface from the direct contact with the biological medium [111].

Core-shell quantum dots are prepared by coating an emissive semiconductor dot core with a thin shell of a second semiconductor of higher band gap, or other materials such as polymer or dendrimers (figure 8).

This procedure to avoid the direct contact of nanocrystal with surrounded medium is known as passivation [110]. The coating of QDs with the appropriate and biocompatible shells such as dendritic macromolecules, inorganic compounds and amphiphilic polymers repressed their surface oxidation and decreased their cytotoxicity [111].

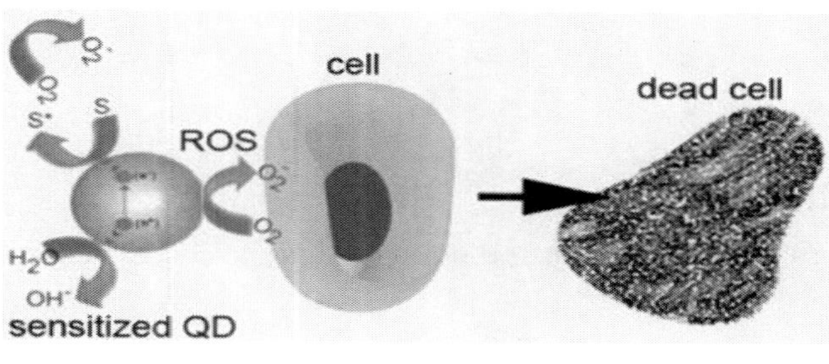

Figure 7. Toxicity and cellular death induced by QDs.

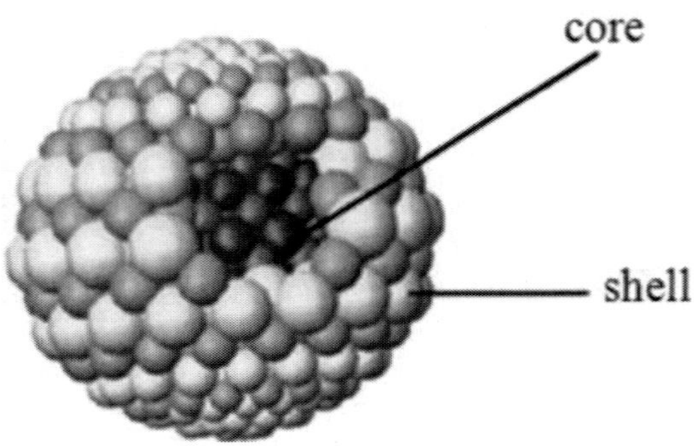

Figure 8. A nanocrystal is coated with a wider band gap semiconductor or another material in order to develop its optical and physiological properties.

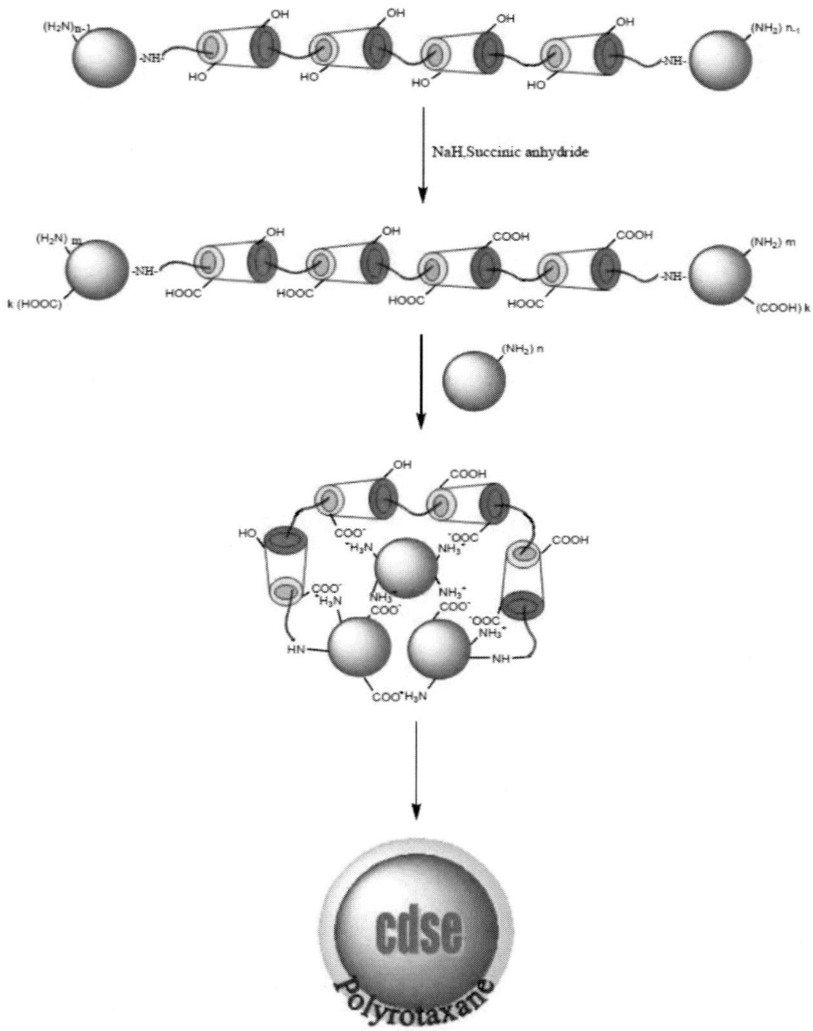

Figure 9. Preparation of PR@QDs using interaction between positively charged NH_2-CdSe QDs and negatively charged PR-CdSe QDs–COOH.

Polymer-encapsulated or polymer-co-loaded QDs have shown the lowest level toxicity for living cells [19, 108].

Molecular self-assembly of CdSe QDs-end-capped polyrotaxane hybrid nanostructures (PR-CdSe QDs) has been led to a new type of core-shell hybrid nanomaterials consisting of CdSe QDs core and polyrotaxane shell (PR@QDs) (Figure 9) [112].

Size of PR@QDs was between 20-25 nm and diameter of core and thickness of shell were between 15-20 and 2-3 nm, respectively. Short-term *in vitro* cytotoxicity tests were conducted on mouse tissue connective fibroblast adhesive cell line (L929) in order to investigate their potential application in nanomedicine and to understand the limitation and capability of these materials as nano-excipients in biological systems. Based on these experiments it has been found that polyrotaxane shell on the surface of QDs could increase the internalization rate of the QDs into the cells, more than two times, in compare to that without conjugated cyclodextrin.

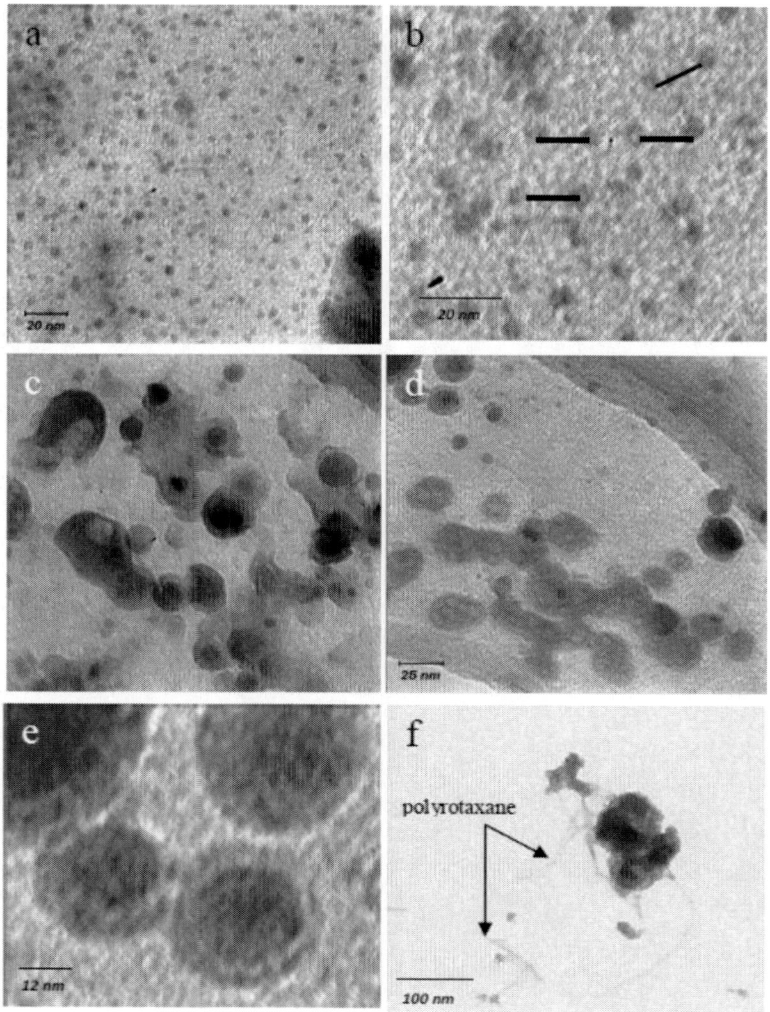

Figure 10. TEM images of NH_2-CdSe QDs(a), PR-CdSe QDs(b) and PR@QDs (c, d and e), a PR@QDs in which the axis of poltrotaxane is PEG 6000.

Figure 10 shows the TEM image of NH_2-CdSe QDs, PR-CdSe QDs and PR@QDs nanomaterials. TEM image of NH_2-CdSe QDs (Figures 10 a) shows QDs with an average size about 4 nm. In the figure 10 b, Ps-PR is not appeared because electron beam can transfer through its structure, but QDs are appeared in a necklace-like order and in most cases distance between QDs is around 10 nm where PEG axis and cyclodextrin rings are placed probably. TEM images of PR@QDs show that they are consisting of QDs cores and polyrotaxanes shells. Based on the TEM images of core-shell nanomaterials, diameter of the core and thickness of the shell are around 15 and 2 nm respectively. Figure 10 f shows the TEM image of a PR@QDs nanomaterial in which the axis of poltrotaxane is PEG 6000 molecular weight. In this figure polyrotaxanes, with a thickness around a 1 nm and a length around 100 nm, that are aggregating to create core-shell structures can be seen clearly.

The amino-functionalized QDs stoppers of polyrotaxanes are used as core to synthesize polyamidoamine, PAMAM, dendrons divergently and hybrid nanomaterials are obtained (Figure 11).

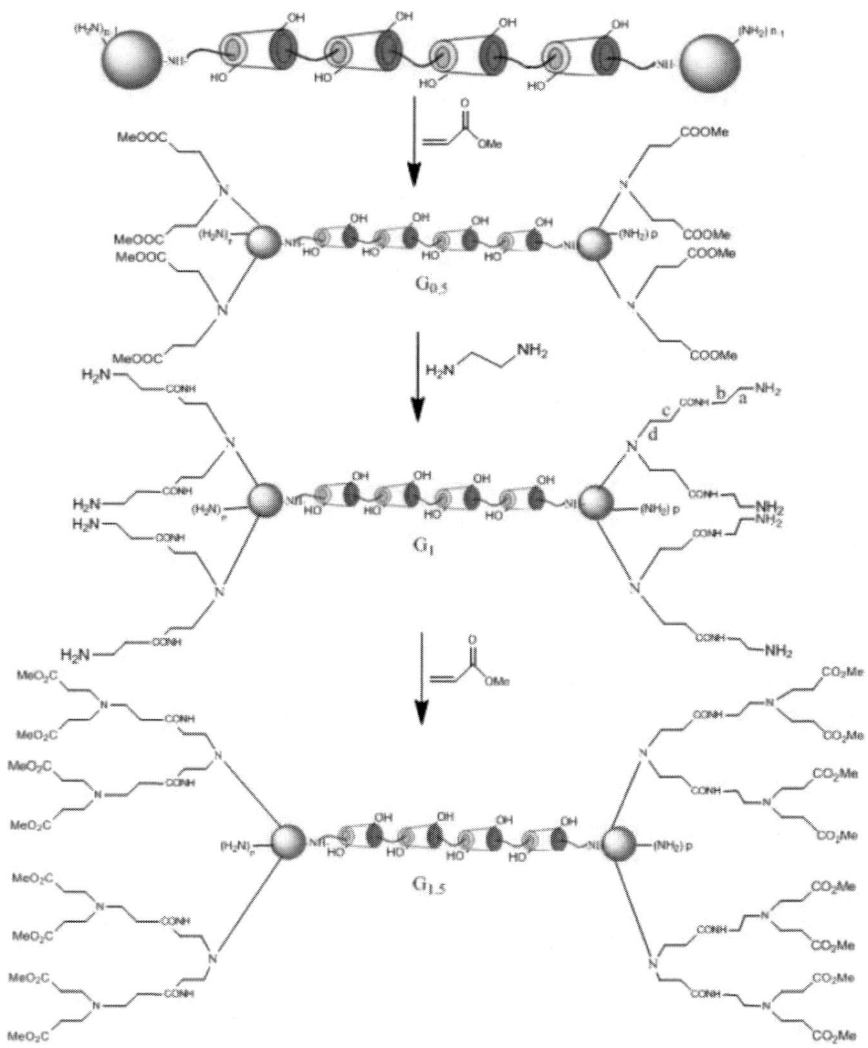

Figure 11. Representation of the synthesis route of hybrid nanomaterials.

Synthesized hybrid nanomaterials are freely soluble in water and their aqueous solutions are stable at room temperature over several months. Due to their biocompatible backbone, high functionality and water solubility synthesized hybrid nanomaterials are promising carriers and probes in order to use in cancer diagnosis and therapy [113].

Conclusion

Due to their unique optical properties, QDs are promising nanomaterials that could greatly improve biological imaging and detection of the cancer cells. It seems in the near future this area of research could lead to amazing results in the case of early diagnosis of cancer. However some of major challenges in this way are non-specific interactions of QDs with the biological systems, mechanisms to cross the biological barriers and their toxicity which should be improved and fully understand.

References

[1] Liang, J.; He, Z.; Zhang, S.; Huanga, S.; Ai, X.; Yang, H.; Hanb, H. *Talanta* 2007, 71, 1675–1678.

[2] Hong, H.; Zhang, Y.; Sun, J.; Cai, W. *Nano Today* 2009, 4, 399—41.

[3] Gao, J.; Chen, K.; Xie, R.; Xie, J.; Yan, Y.; Cheng, Z.; Xiaogang Peng, X.; Chen, X. *Bioconjugate Chem.* 2010, 21, 604–609.

[4] Zu, X.; Duan, D.; Madsen, S.; Publicover, N. G. *Anal. Bioanal. Chem.* 2010, 396, 1345-1353.

[5] Li, Z.; Huang, P.; He, R.; Lin, j.; Yang, S.; Zhang, X.; Ren, Q.; Cui, D. *Materials Letters* 2010, 64, 375–378.

[6] Choi, Y.; Kim, H. P.; Hong, S. M.; Ryu, J. Y.; Han, S. J.; Song, R. *small* 2009, 5, 2085–2091.

[7] Warnement, M.; Tomlinson, I.; Chang, J.; Schreuder, M.; Luckabaugh, C.; Rosenthal, S. *Bioconjugate Chem.* 2008, 19, 1404–1413.

[8] estephan, E.; Larroque, C.; Bec, N.; Martineau, P.; Cuisinier, F. J. G.; Cloitre, T.; Gergely, C. *Biotechnology and Bioengineering* 2009, 104, 1121-1131.

[9] Papagiannaros, A.; Levchenko, T.; Hartner, W.; Mongayt, D.; Torchilin, V. *Nanomedicine: Nanotechnology, Biology, and Medicine* 2009, 5, 216–224.

[10] Sanvicens, N.; Marco, M. P. *Trends in Biotechnology* 2008, 26,425-433.

[11] Yoffe, A.D. *Adv. In Phys.* 2001, 50, 1–208.

[12] Kim, Y.; Moon, S.; Kuritzkes, D. R.; Demirci, U. *Biosensors and Bioelectronics* 2009, 25, 253–258.

[13] Hu, M.; Yan, J.; He, Y.; Lu, H.; Weng, L.; Song, S.; Fan, F.; Wang, L. *American Chemical Society* 2010, 4, 488-494.

[14] Cheng, A. K. H.; Su, H.; Wang, Y, A.; Yu, H. *Anal. Chem.* 2009, 81, 6130–6139.

[15] Rzigalinski, B. A.; Strobl, J, S. *Toxicology and Applied Pharmacology* 2009, 238, 280–288.

[16] Tomczaka, N.; Jan czewski, D.; Hana, M.; Vancsoa, G. J. *Progress in Polymer Science* 2009, 34, 393–430.
[17] Hotz, C. Z.; *NanoBiotechnology Protocols,*2005, 303, 1-17.
[18] Medintz, I.L. et al. *Nat. Mater.* 2005, 4, 435–446.
[19] Maysinger, D.; Lovric, j.; Eisenberg, A.; Savic, R. *European Journal of Pharmaceutics and Biopharmaceutics* 2007, 65, 270–281.
[20] Smith, A. M.; Ruan, G.; Rhyner, M. N.; Nie, S. *Annals of Biomedical Engineering* 2006, 34, 3–14.
[21] Zhang, B.; Liang, X.; Hao, L.; Cheng, J.; Gong, X.; Liu, X.; Ma, G.; Chang, j. *Journal of Photochemistry and Photobiology B: Biology* 2009, 94, 45–50.
[22] Shi, C.; Zhu, Y.; Cerwinka, W. H.; Zhau, H. E.; Marshall, F. F.; Simons, J. W.; Nie, S.; Chung, L. W. K. *Urologic Oncology: Seminars and Original Investigations* 2008, 26, 86–92.
[23] Biju, V.; Mundayoor, S.; Omkumar, R.; Anas, A.; Ishikawa, M. *Biotechnology Advances* 2010, 28, 199–213.
[24] Shao, Q.; Yang, C.; Jiang, L.; He, J.; Li, S.; Jiang, B. *Journal of Polymer Science: Part A: Polymer Chemistry* 2010, 48, 751–755.
[25] Shen, H.; Chen, L.; Chen, S. *J. Inorg. Organomet. Polym.* 2009, 19, 374–381.
[26] Chan, W.C.; Nie, S. *Science* 1998, 281, 2016–2018.
[27] Pathak, S.; Choi, S.K.; Arnheim, N.; Thompson, M.E. *J. Am. Chem. Soc.* 2001, 123, 4103–4104.
[28] Bruchez Jr., M.; Moronne, M.; Gin, P.; Weiss, S.; Alivisatos, A.P. *Science* 1998, 281, 2013–2016.
[29] Jiang, X.; Ahmed, M.; Deng, Z.; Narain, R. *Bioconjugate Chem.* 2009, 20, 994–1001.
[30] Clarke, S.J.; Hollmann, C. A.; Aldaye, F. A.; Nadeau, J.L. *Bioconjugate Chem.* 2008, 19, 562–568.
[31] Shen, H.; Chen, L.; Chen, S. *J. Inorg. Organomet. Polym.* 2009, 19, 374–381.
[32] Wang, Q.; Seo, D. *J Mater Sci* 2009, 44,816–820.
[33] Idowu, M.; Lamprecht, E.; Nyokong, T. *Journal of Photochemistry and Photobiology A: Chemistry* 2008, 198, 7–12.
[34] Dubertret, B.; Skourides, P.; Norris, D.J.; Noireaux, V.; Brivanlou, A.H.; Libchaber, A. *Science* 2002, 298, 1759–1762.
[35] (a) Zhang, X.; Meng, L.; Lu, Q.; Fei, Z.; Dyson, P.J. *Biomaterials* 2009, 30, 6041. (b) Rannard, S.; Owen, A. *Nanotoday* 2009, 4, 382.
[36] (a) Wang, C.; Chen, J.; Talavage, T.; Irudayaraj, J. *Angew. Chem.* 2009, 121, 2797: *Angew. Chem. Int.* Ed. 2009, 48, 2759. (b) Liu, Z.; Tabakman, S.M.; Chen, Z.; Dai, H. *Nature Protocols* 2009, 4, 1372.
[37] Agrawal, A.; Deo, R.; Wang, G.D.; Wang, M.D.; Nie, S. *PNAS* 2008, 105, 3298.
[38] VanHandel, M.; Alizadeh, D.; Zhang, L.; Kateb, B.; Bronikowski, M.; Manohara, H. Badie, B. *Journal of Neuroimmunology* 2009, 208, 3.
[39] Choi, J.H.; Chen, K.H.; Han, J-H.; Chaffee, A.M.; Strano, M.S. *Small* 2009, 5, 672.
[40] Byrne, J.D.; Betancourt, T.; Brannon-Peppas, L. *Advanced Drug Delivery Reviews* 2008, 60, 1615.
[41] Zrazhevskiy, P.; Gao, X. *Nanotoday* 2009, 4, 414.
[42] Pison, U.; Welte, T.; Giersig, M.; Groneberg, D. A. *European Journal of Pharmacology* 2006, 533, 341–350.

[43] (a) Phan, J.H.; Moffitt, R.A.; Stokes, T.H.; Liu, J.; Young, A.N.; Nie, S.; Wang, M.D. *Trends in Biotechnology* 2009, 27, 350. (b) Jamieson, T.; Bakhshi, R.; Petrova, D.; Pococka, R.; Imani, M.; Seifalian, A.M. *Biomaterials* 2007, 28, 4717. (c) Bhang, S.H.; Won, N.; Lee, T-J.; Jin, H.; Nam, J.; Park, J.; Chung, H.; Park, H-S.; Sung, Y-E.; Hahn, S.K.; Kim, B-S.; Kim, S. *ACS Nano* 2009, *3*, 1389. (d) Chen, C.; Peng, J.; Xia, H-S.; Yang, G-F.; Wu, Q-S.; Chen, L-D.; Zeng, L-B.; Zhang, Z-L.; Pang, D-W.; Li, Y. *Biomaterials* 2009, 30, 2912.

[44] (a) Smith, B.R.; Cheng, Z.; De, A.; Koh, A.L.; Sinclair, R.; Gambhir, S-S. *Nano Lett* 2008, *8*, 2599. (b) Weng, K.C.; Noble, C.O.; Papahadjopoulos-Sternberg, B.; Chen, F.F.; Drummond, D.C.; Kirpotin, D.B.; Wang, D.; Hom, Y.K.; Hann, B.; Park, J.W. *Nano Lett* 2008, 8, 2851.

[45] Shi, C.; Zhu, Y.; Xie, Z.; Qian, W.; Hsieh, C-L.; Nie, S.; Su, Y.; Zhau, H.E.; Chung, L.W.K. *Urology* 2009, 74, 446.

[46] Zhang, Y.; Mi, L.; Xiong, R.; Wang, P.; Chen, J.; Yang, W.; Wang, C.; Peng, Q. *Nanoscale Res Lett* 2009, 4,606–612.

[47] Jaiswal, J.K.; Mattoussi, H.; Mauro, J.M.; Simon, S.M. *Nat. Biotechnol.* 2003, 21, 47-51.

[48] Parak, W.J.; Boudreau, R.; Le Gros, M,; Gerion, D.; Zanchet, D.; Micheel, C.M.; Williams, S.C.; Alivisatos, A.P.; Larabell, C. *Adv. Mater.* 2002, 14, 882-885.

[49] Bara, S.; Rege, k. *small* 2009, 5, 370–376.

[50] Derfus, A.M.; Chan, W.C.W.; Bhatia, S.N. *Adv. Mater.* 2004, 16, 961-966.

[51] Chen, F.; Gerion, D. *Nano Lett.* 2004, 4 1827-1832.

[52] Singh, R.; Lillard Jr, J. W. *Experimental and Molecular Pathology* 2009, 86, 215–223.

[53] Brooks, H.; Lebleu, B.; Vives, E. *Adv. Drug Deliv. Rev.*2005, 57, 559-577.

[54] Wadia, J.S.; Dowdy, S.F. *Adv. Drug Deliv. Rev.* 2005, 57, 579-596.

[55] Gupta, B.; Levchenko, T.S.; Torchilin, V.P. *Adv. Drug Deliv. Rev.* 2005,57, 637-651.

[56] Futaki, S. *Adv. Drug Deliv. Rev.* 2005, 57, 547-558.

[57] Zorko, M.; Langel, U. *Adv. Drug Deliv. Rev.* 2005, 57, 529-545.

[58] Medintz, I. L.; Pons, T ; Delehanty, J. B.; Susumu, K.; Brunel, F. M.; Dawson, P. E.; Mattoussi, H. *Bioconjugate Chem.* 2008, 19, 1785–1795.

[59] Ruan, G.; Agrawal, A.; Marcus, A.I.; Nie, S.M. *J. Am. Chem. Soc.* 2007, 129, 14759-14766.

[60] Lei, Y.; Tang, H.; Yao, L.; Yu, R.; Feng, M.; Zou, B. *Bioconjugate Chem.* 2008, 19, 421–427.

[61] Rhyner, M.N.; Smith, A. M.; Gao, X.; Mao, H.; Yang, L.; Nie, S. *Nanomedicine* 2006, 1, 209-217.

[62] Warnement, M.R.; Tomlinson, I.D.; Chang, J.C.; Schreuder, M.A.; Luckabaugh, C.M.; Rosenthal, S.J. *Bioconjugate Chem.* 2008, 19, 1404–1413.

[63] Duan, H.W.; Nie, S.M. *J. Am. Chem. Soc.* 2007, 129, 3333-3338.

[64] Neu, M.; Fischer, D.; Kissel, T. *J. Gene Med.* 2005, 7, 992–1009.

[65] Boussif, O.; Lezoualch, F.; Zanta, M.A.; Mergny, M.D.; Scherman, D.; Demeneix, B.; Behr, J.P. *Proc. Natl. Acad. Sci. U. S. A.* 1995, 92, 7297-7301.

[66] Pack, D.W.; Hoffman, A.S.; Pun, S.; Stayton, P.S. *Nat. Rev. Drug Discov.* 2005, 581-593.

[67] Sunderland, C.J.; Steiert, M.; Talmadge, J.E.; Derfus, A.M.; Barry, S.E. *Drug. Dev. Res.* 2006, 67, 70.

[68] Orive, G.; Gascon, A.R.; Hernandez, R.M.; Dominguez-Gil, A.; Pedraz, J.L. *Trends Pharm. Sci.* 2004, 25, 382.
[69] Tothill, I. E. *Seminars in Cell and Developmental Biology* 2009, 20, 55–62.
[70] Wang, H.; Yang, R.; Yang, L.; Tan, W. *American Chemical Society* 2009, 3,2451-2460.
[71] Setua, S.; Menon, D.; Asok, A.; Nair, S.; Koyakutty, M. *Biomaterials* 2010, 31, 714–729.
[72] Zrazhevskiy, P.; Gao, X. *Nano Today* 2009, 4, 414-428.
[73] Duconge, F.; Pons, T.; Pestourie, C.; Herin, L.; Theze, B.; Gombert, K.; Mahler, B.; Hinnen, F.; Kuhnast, B.; Dolle, F.; Dubertret, B.; Tavitian, B. *Bioconjugate Chem.* 2008, 19, 1921–1926.
[74] Howes, P.; Green, M.; Levitt, J.; Suhling, K.; Hughes, M. *AM. CHEM. SOC.* 2010, 132, 3989–3996.
[75] Fountaine, T.J.; Wincovitch, S.M.; Geho, D.H.; Garfield, S.H.; Pittaluga, S. *Mod. Pathol.* 2006, 19, 1181–1191.
[76] Glaus, C.; Rossin, R.; Welch, M. J.; Bao, G. *Bioconjugate Chem.* 2010, 21, 715–722.
[77] Bernardin, A.; Cazet A.; Guyon, L.; Delannoy, P.; Vinet, F.; Bonnaffe, D.; Texier, I. *Bioconjugate Chem.* 2010, 21, 583–588.
[78] Lee, J.; Choi, Y.; Kim, K.; Hong, S.; Park, H.; Lee,T.; Cheon, G. J.; Song, R. *Bioconjugate Chem.* 2010, 21, 940–946.
[79] Voura, E.B.; Jaiswal. J.K.; Mattoussi, H.; Simon, S.M. *Nat Med.* 2004, 10, 993–998.
[80] Jamieson, T.; Bakhshi, R.; Petrova, D.; Pocock, R.; Imani, M.; Seifalian, A. M. *Biomaterials* 2007, 28, 4717-4732.
[81] Smith, A.M.; Duan, H.; Mohs, A.M.; Nie, S. *Advanced Drug Delivery Reviews* 2008, 60, 1226–1240.
[82] Hardman, R. *Environmental Health Perspectives* 2006, 114, 165 –72.
[83] Park, J.H.; Leeb, S.; Kimb, J.H.; Park, K.; Kimb, K.; Kwonb, I. C. *Prog. Polym. Sci.* 2008, 33, 113–137.
[84] Susumu, K.; Uyeda, H. T.; Medintz, I.L.; Pons, T.; Delehanty, J. B.; Mattoussi, H. *J. Am. Chem. Soc.*, 2007, 129 (45), 13987-13996.
[85] Li, Z.; Wang, K.; Tan, W.; Li, J.; Fu, Z.; Ma, C.; Li, H.; He, X.; Liu, J. *Analytical Biochemistry* 2006, 354, 169–174.
[86] Schroeder, J.E.; Shweky, I.; Shmeeda, H.; Banin, U.; Gabizon, A. *Journal of Controlled Release* 2007, 124, 28–34.
[87] Nehill, B.J.; Allen, P.G.; Desai, T.A. *ACS Nano*, 2008, 2, 538-544.
[88] Chu, m.; Song, X.; Cheng, D.; Liu, S.; Zhu, J. *Nanotechnology* 2006, 17, 3268–3273.
[89] Chen, Y.; Thakar, R.; Snee, P.T. *J. Am. Chem. Soc.* 2008, 130, 3744-3745.
[90] Yong, K.T. *Nanotechnology* 2009, 20, 015102 (10pp).
[91] Gao, J.; Gu, H.; Xu, B. *ACCOUNTS OF CHEMICAL RESEARCH* 2009, 42, 1097-1107.
[92] Algar, W. R.; Massey, M.; Krull, U. J. *Trends in Analytical Chemistry* 2009, 28, 292-306.
[93] Yong, K.; Ding, H.; Roy, I.; Law, W.; Bergey, E. J.; Maitra, A.; Prasad, P. N. *American Chemical Society* 2009, 3, 502-510.
[94] Parungo, C.P.; Ohnishi, S.; Kim, S.W. et al. *J. Thorac. Cardiovasc. Surg.* 2005, 129, 844–850.
[95] Stroh, M.; Zimmer, J.P.; Duda, D.G.; et al. *Nat. Med.* 2005, 11, 678–682.

[96] Morgan, N.Y.; English, S.; Chen, W. et al. *Acad. Radiol.* 2005, 12, 313–323.
[97] Yang, H.; Santra, S.; Walter, G.A.; Holloway, P.H. *Adv. Mater.* 2006, 18, 2890–2894.
[98] (a) Mulder, WJM.; Koole, R.; Brandwijk, RJ.; Storm, G.; Chin, PTK.; Strijkers, GJ.; Donega, CD.; Nicolay, K.; Griffioen, AW. *Nano Lett*, 2006, 6, 1–6. (b) Waters, E.A.; Wickline, S.A. *Basic Res. Cardiol.* 2008, 103, 114–121.
[99] Azzazy, H.; Mansour, M.; Kazmierczak, S.; *Clinical Biochemistry* 2007, 40, 917–927.
[100] Adeli, M.; Hakimpour, F.; Sagvand, M.; Jaafari, M.R.; Kabiri, R.; Moshari, Z. *Supramolecular Chemistry*, 2011, In press.
[101] Pan, J.; Feng, S-S. *Biomaterials* 2009, 30, 1176–1183.
[102] Al-Jamal, W.T.; Al-Jamal, K.T.; Bomans, P.H.; Frederik, P.M.; Kostarelos, K. *Small* 2008, 4, 1406–1415.
[103] Adeli, M.; Hakimpoor, F.; Parsamanesh, M.; Kalantari, M.; Sobhani, Z.; Attyabi. F. *Polymer* 2011, 52, 2401-2413.
[104] Wu, C.; Shi, L.; Li, Q.; Jiang, H.; Selke, M.; Ba, L.; Wang, X. *Chem. Res. Toxicol.* 2010, 23, 82–88.
[105] Zhang, L. W.; Yu, W. W.; Colvin, V.L.; Monteiro-Riviere, N. A. *Toxicology and Applied Pharmacology* 2008, 228, 200–211.
[106] Ipe, B.I.; Lehnig, M.; Niemeyer. C.M. *Small* 2005, 1,706 –9.
[107] Lovric, J.; Cho, S.J.; Winnik, F.M. et al. *Chem. Biol.* 2005, 12, 1227–34.
[108] Gao, X.; Yang, L.; Petros, J.A.; Marshall, F. F.; Simons, J. W.; Nie, S. *Current Opinion in Biotechnology* 2005, 16, 63–72.
[109] Hild, W.A.; Breunig, M.; Goepferich A. *European Journal of Pharmaceutics and Biopharmaceutics* 2008, 68, 153–168.
[110] (a) Santos, B.; de Farias, P.; Menezes, F.; Ferreira, R.; Júnior, S.; Figueiredo, R.; Carvalho Junior, L.; Beltrão E. *phys. stat. sol. (c) 3*, 2006, 11, 4017–4022. (b) Bailey, R.; Smith, A.; Nie, S. *Physica E.* 2004, 25,1–12. (c) Yordanov, G.; Yoshimura, H.; Dushkin, C. *Colloid Polym. Sci.* 2008, 286, 1097–1102. (d) Cao, S.; Liu, B.; Deng, X.; Li, S.; *Macromol. Biosci.* 2005, 5, 669–676.
[111] Pan, J.; Feng, S. *Biomaterials* 2009, 30, 1176–1183.
[112] Sadeghi Sarabi, R.; Adeli, M.; Sadeghi, E.; Mahmoudi, M.; Kalantari, M.; Hosseinkhani, H. *Journal of Nanostructured Polymers and Nanocomposites,* 2011, In press.
[113] Adeli, M.; Sadeghi Sarabi, R.; Sadeghi, E. *Nano*, 2011, In press.

In: Hybrid Nanostructures in Cancer Therapy
Editor: Mohsen Adeli
ISBN: 978-1-62100-517-9
© 2012 Nova Science Publishers, Inc.

Chapter VII

Gold Nanoparticle-Polymer Hybrid Nanomaterials and Biological Applications

Mohsen Adeli, Fahimeh Madani, and Raziyeh Yadollahi
Department of Chemistry, Faculty of Science, Lorestan University,
Khoramabad, Iran

1. Introduction

Due to their interesting size–dependent properties such as electrical and optical characterizes [1], high stability, low toxicity, easy surface modification and functionalization and good biocompatibility, gold nanoparticles (Au NPs) have received considerable attention during the past decade [2, 3]. Specifically Au NPs functionalized by organic molecules as capping agents have recently interested as attractive candidates for delivering variety of therapeutic agents such as proteins, nucleic acids, peptides and drugs into cells and their targets [4]. Synthetic methods for preparation of Au NPs are various and cover a broad range of reagents especially those used as capping agents. The preparation of gold nanoparticles in colloidal form was first reported by Michael Faraday in 1857 since he synthesized Au NPs through reaction of gold chloride with sodium citrate to produce multicolored solutions [5]. One of the most widely used procedures to obtain Au NPs with a size between 10-100 nm (ca 10-100 nm) is Turkevich method in which gold salt is reduced in aqueous sodium citrate solution, thereby making nearly monodisperse spherical Au NPs over a tuneable range of sizes depending on the gold/citrate ratio [6, 7]. Hydrophobic gold nanoparticles with diameters in 1-3 nm range are usually prepared by Brust method. In this method $NaBH_4$ is used to reduce gold salts in the presence of alkanethiols as capping agents through either two-phase or one phase synthesis. By varying the capping agent, in most cases thiol molecules, concentration the size of synthesized gold nanoparticles can be regulated between 2 and 5 nm [8]. The most of amine compounds that are used as capping agents in the synthesis process of Au NPs are only soluble in organic solvents, therefore the reduction step has to take place in these types of solvents without irreversible aggregation or decomposition, and consequently the prepared Au NPs with those methods are not easily dispersed in aqueous solutions. However to use Au NPs in biological systems, it is critically needed to functionalize them with capping agents with a good solubility in aqueous solutions to transfer them from organic solvents to aqueous medium [9].

Polymer-modified Au NPs have attracted additionally interest recently. Polymers confer several properties in Au NPs simultaneously. They stabilize Au NPs in different mediums depend on intrinsic properties of polymers, raise their biocompatibility and other biological activities and develop their functionality and other useful properties [10]. Polymer attached to the surface of Au NPs through different methods. They can be used as capping agents in the synthetic process of these nanoparticles. For example some functional groups such as amino (-NH2), cyano (-CN) and mercapto (-SH) are known to have high affinity for gold, hence polymers having such functional groups are expected to be used as capping agents to produce gold nanoparticles with a quit narrow size distribution [11].

Variety of water-soluble polymers including poly(methoxy-oligo(ethylene glycol) methacrylate) PMOEGMA [12] Poly(*N*-vinyl-2-pyrroridone) PNVP [13], Poly(4-vinylpyridine) PVP [14], Poly(*N*-isopropylacrylamide) PPA [15] and poly(ethylene glycol) PEG [16]. have been used for synthesis of Au NPs. Polymers are conjugated onto the surface of gold nanoparticles by either "grafting from" or "grafting to" methods as schematically illustrated in Scheme 1. [17-22 , 10]. In addition to above categories, another route for preparation of polymer-Au NPs hybrids is producing Au NPs using small ligands such as alkanethiols and citrate and then modification by polymers [10]. Prencipe and coworkers showed that Au NPs, and NPs functionalized by the polymers exhibit high stability in aqueous solutions at different pH values, at elevated temperatures, and in serum [23].

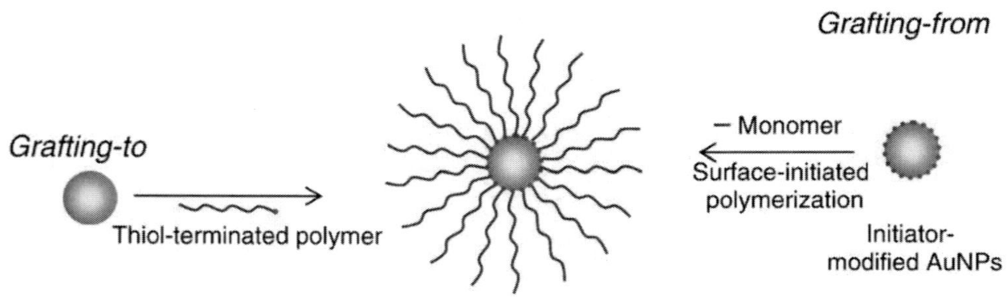

Scheme 1.The "grafting from" and "grafting to" approaches for preparation of polymer/gold nanoparticle hybrid materials. Reprinted with the permission from Ref [20].

2. Polymer Protected Au NPs: Preparation, Properties and Characterization

2.1. "Grafting from" Method

In the "grafting from" method, disulfide or thiol-terminated initiators are synthesized and linked onto the surface of Au NPs via the direct gold-sulfur covalent bond or the sulfurlingand exchange. Then functionalized Au NPS can be used as macroinitiators to polymerize monomers by usual polymerization methods.

Atom-transfer radical polymerization, ATRP, initiated by Au NPs macroinitiators is a "grafting from" technique in which controlled of the molecular weight and molecular weight distribution efficiently prevent the aggregation of nanoparticles and lead to a better uniformity and controlled on the thickness of the polymer shell on the surface of Au NPs. Higher surface graft density can be achieved by the "grafting from" technique but synthetic steps of this method are more tedious compared with those of "grafting to" technique [18-21, 24, 10].

Novel hybrid nanomaterials consist of Au NPs and poly(4-vinylpyridine) (Au@PVP) were fabricated through surface-initiated atom-transfer radical polymerization (SI-ATRP) at ambient conditions. For preparation of these hybrid nanomaterials, the citrate stabilized gold nanoparticles were first modified by a disulfide initiator, $[S\text{-}(CH_2)_{11}\text{-}OCOC(CH_3)_2Br]_2$ to confer the ability of initiating of polymerization to nanoparticles and then polymerization of 4-vinylpyridine (4VP) was occurred onto the surface of gold particles [14].

Stable thermosensitive gold nanosphere/poly(N-isopropylacrylamide) core/shell nanoparticles (Au@PNIPAAm) were prepared by SI-ATRP of monomer on to the surface of the initiator-modified gold nanoparticles [25]. Poly(*N*-isopropylacrylamide) (PNIPAAM) undergoes a thermosensitive conformation change at a lower critical solution temperature (LCST) near 32 °C in aqueous solution [12]. Applications involving NIPAM homopolymer hydrogels are somewhat limited. This limitation can be circumvented by incorporating acrylic acid (AAc) or acrylamide (AAm) moieties into the polymer backbone, which can shift the LCST of the copolymer hydrogels anywhere from 32 to 60°C depending on the ratio of components [26, 27]. Therefore, PNIPAAm is a promising material with many beneficial functions to develop a new concept in drug delivery systems (DDS) [28].

The fabrication of novel nanostructures of gold nanoparticles with a thermosensitive copolymer by SI-ATRP, as illustrated in Scheme 2, has been reported. A block copolymer of PNIPAAM and PMOEGMA were grafted onto the surface of initiator-functionalized Au NPs catalyzed by CuBr and *N,N,N',N',N''*-pentamethyldiethylenetriamine (PMDETA) in 2-propanol/water solvent [12]. Kim's group synthesized cross-linked Au NP/ PNIPAAm core/shell hybrid nanostructures as well as a brush type Au NP/PNIPAAm hybrid nanomaterials through SI-ATRP of NIPAAm, and studied the effect of the cross-linking on the thermoresponsiveness of hybrid nanomaterials [29].

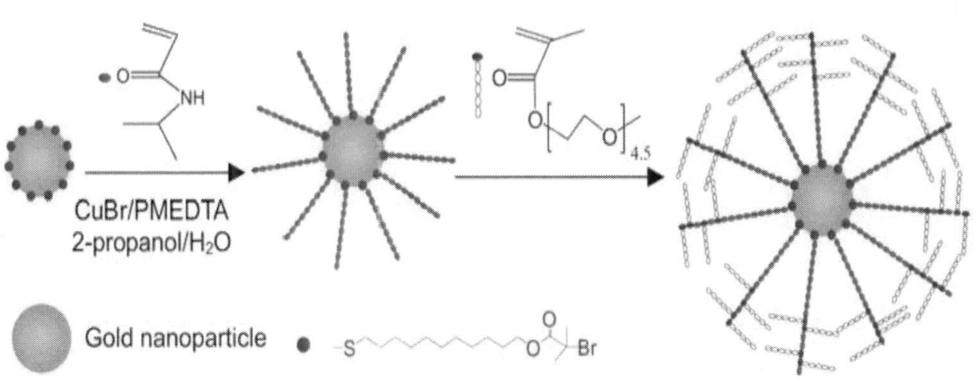

Scheme 2. Schematic representation of the synthesis of Au@PNIPAAm. Reprinted with permission from Ref [12].

Duan's et al. have used this method to prepare the polymeric nanocapsules. They fabricated cross-linkable copolymer brushes onto the surface of Au NPs by means of SI-ATRP, then the Au NPs cores were etched out and hydrophilic polymer capsules were formed [19]. The pH responsive nanoparticles consist of Au NPs cores and (PVP) have been synthesized and evaluated by different methods [30]. Robust Au NPs are prepared through a one-pot synthesis of a cross linked shell and linear tethered polymer brushes from the Au NP surface. The dual protecting polymer layers, i.e. an inner cross-linked shell and outer linear polymer brushes grafted to the inner shell, effectively stabilized the core/shell Au-NPs under harsh conditions such as elevated temperatures, because the cross-linked polymer shell prevented the dissociation of linear polymers from the nanoparticles [31].

2.2. "Grafting to" Method

The "grafting-to" method is a useful synthetic route to synthesize polymer protected gold nanoparticles. Polymers containing disulfide bonds or end thiol functional group are used as the stabilizer or capping agent during the preparation of gold nanoparticles. Polymers with these types of functional groups, sulfur-terminated polymers, also can directly bond to the surface of previously prepared gold nanoparticles through an approach called 'ligand exchange, procedure [17-21, 24, 10]. Au NPs containing copolymers of di(ethylene glycol) methyl ether methacrylate (MEO_2MA) and poly(ethylene glycol) methyl ether methacrylate (OEGMA) on their surface as stimuli-responsive shell has been synthesized and investigated. For preparation of these core/shell hybrid nanomaterials both above strategies in the "grafting to" method were used. Au@MEO_2MA-*co*-OEGMA NPs were formed by reducing $HAuCl_4$ in the presence of disulfide-functionalized poly (MEO_2MA-*co*-OEGMA) and Au@MEO_2MA-*co*-OEGMA NPs were generated by forming Au NPs with a citrate capping agent and then conjugation of a disulfide-functionalized poly (MEO_2MA*co*-OEGMA) through "ligand exchange" approach [32].

Thermosensitive diblock copolymers with a disulfide end moiety were prepared and used as capping agents to stabilize Au NPs/copolymer hybrid nanostructures. They were containing a gold nanoparticle core and a polymeric shell linked together by a polymeric intermediate [18]. In order to synthesized thermosensitive systems consist of Au NPs and PNIPAM shell, different types of this polymer with end thiol functional groups including PNIPAMs bearing dithiobenzoate end functional groups synthesized by reversible-addition fragmentation chain-transfer (RAFT) polymerizations, PNIPAM end-capped with a thiol functional groups obtained through hydrazinolysis of the former PNIPAM and thiol-functionalized PNIPAM prepared by conventional radical polymerization and following modification were prepared and conjugated onto the surface of Au NPs [24]. Poly(methyl methacrylate)-*b*-poly(*N*-isopropylacrylamide) (PMMA-*b*-PNIPAM)block copolymer having a dithiobenzoate chain end was synthesized by RAFT polymerization and used to protect gold nanoparticles in a one-pot synthesis where the polymer is bound to the gold surface by sulfur bonds [17, 22].

Au NPs with different sizes were prepared using thiol-terminated poly(ethylene glycol) (HS-PEG) with different molecular weights. PEG coated Au NPs were stable and soluble in phosphate buffered saline (PBS) solution and useful for biomedical applications [16, 33].

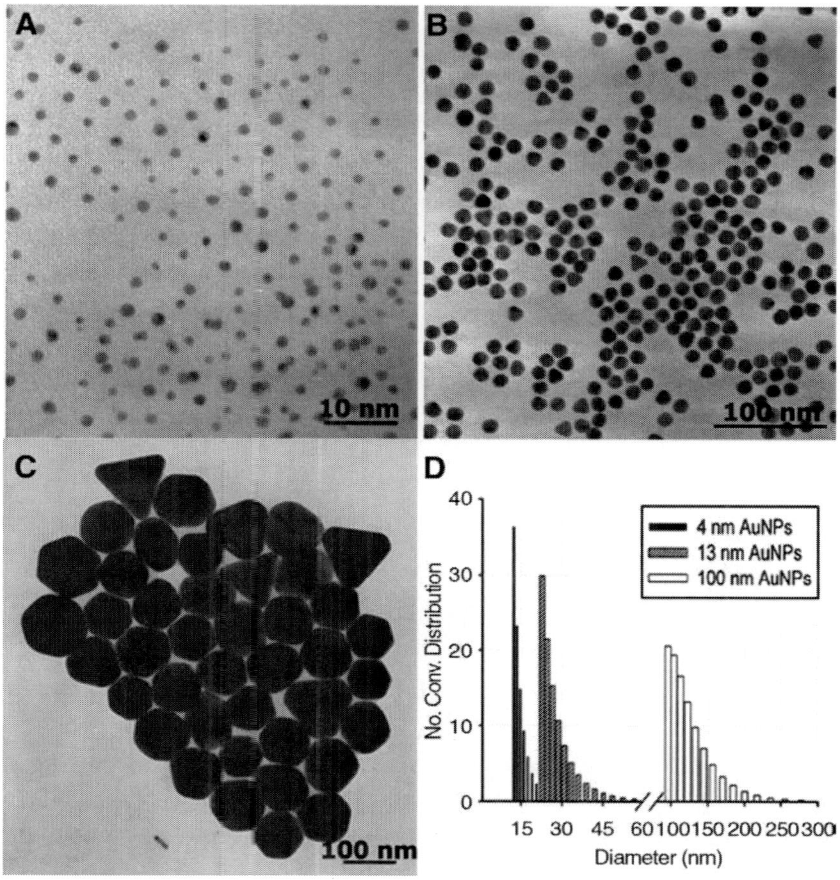

Figure 3.Transmission electron microscopy (TEM) images of (A) 4 nm, (B) 13 nm, and (C) 100 nm PEG protected Au NPs. (D) Diameter and size distribution of these Au NPs in the solution state. Reprinted with permission from Ref [33].

As it can be seen in figure 1 PEG protected Au NPs are well dispersed and especially in the case of small nanoparticles size distribution is narrow.

2.3. Characterization

It is important to know to how characterize metal nanoparticles and their structures and techniques to evaluate their behaviors in different mediums.

Here we have summarized the most common techniques and apparatus which have been used to characterized Au NPs. The morphology and size of Au NPs can be determined using microscopy observations. Scanning electron microscopy (SEM) is usually used for three-dimensional imaging and morphologies of nanoparticles [34], atomic force microscopy (AFM) is usually used to obtain topographical images and dimensions. Transmission electron microscopy (TEM) is used to record images with a high resolution, electron diffraction patterns and determination their sizes with high accuracy. UV-vis spectroscopy has been employed to characterize the optical properties of nanoparticles and determination of their surface plasmon resonance (SPR) bands and also evaluation the relation between the SPR of

Au NPs and their sizes [26, 35, 36]. The particle size distribution is measured by a quasi-elastic light scattering (QELS) [28]. Small angle X-ray scattering (SAXS) provided a wealth of information on the particle structure, especially polymer chain packing [22]. Fourier transform infrared spectrometer (FTIR) is used to evaluate the structure and determine functional groups of Au through their absorbance bands [36]. Field emission scanning electron microscopy (FE-SEM) and energy dispersive X-ray (EDX) analysis were used to characterize fully the morphology and elemental composition of the gold nanoparticle cores and hydrogel-coated gold nanoparticles [27]. Differential scanning calorimetry (DSC) and thermo gravimetric analysis (TGA) analysis are used to investigate the thermal behavior of the Au NPs and their capping agents and also the weight percent of conjugated polymers onto the surface of Au NPs [37]. Hydrodynamic particle size and solution properties of Au NPs coated by polymers are investigated by dynamic light scattering (DLS) experiments [22, 26, 37].

3. Biomedical Applications of Polymer Capped Au NPs

3.1. Drug Delivery

Drug delivery based on suitable and nontoxic cargos now is a wide range research field especially in the case of lethal daises such as cancer. Most anticancer drugs which are used for cancer therapy today are not targeted to tumors inherently. They are randomly distributed in the body and kill a large number of healthy cells upon administration. Delivered anticancer drugs by suitable cargos are targeted to tumors by two approaches so called "passive" and "active" targeting (Figure 4). In the "passive targeting" drug delivery systems (DDSs) based on nano-objects are transferred from different barriers such as endothelium barrier to tissues and targeted to tumors through physiochemical factors (e.g. size, molecular weight), extravasattion, or pharmacological factors [38, 39]. Basically tumors and normal tissues are different in their structures so that the barriers of tumor tissues are more susceptible to accept nanoparticles than normal tissues. The critical factor for this approach is the prolonged circulation in the blood for nanoparticles as drug delivery systems. Fortunately in the most cases conjugation of polymers to drug delivery systems or nanoparticles increases their circulation in the blood and therefore accumulates passively in tumors even in the absence of targeting ligands [40]. In the "active targeting" approach conjugated ligands onto the surface of carriers recognizes target cells by interactions with their surface receptors. Ligands could be small molecules, peptides or proteins that are conjugated onto the surface of DDSs directly or through a spacer. In some cases a combination of both approaches leads to targeted drug delivery systems with a high efficiency [41].

A comprehensive study was carried out to evaluate the physicochemical properties such as particle size, surface charge, surface hydrophilicity, PEGylation and galactose surface density on regulation of non-specific versus target-specific uptake by Pun and coworkers. In this research work unmodified and modified nanoparticles including negatively-charged NP, PEG-NP, and galactose-PEG-NP with different sizes in a range from 50 to 150 nm were administered systemically to mice.

In order to target PEG modified nanoparticles to liver, the galactose-PEG-thiols were conjugated onto the surface of PEG-NPs and they were administrated to mice. Blood and liver of mices were separated after 2 h post-injection in order to investigation the biodistribution of nanoparticles and hepatocytes and nonparenchymal cells (NPCs) of the liver were analyzed. These experimental works were led to important results which can be used in a wide range of biomedical applications of nanoparticles. They are summarized as follows: (i) PEGylation of nanoparticles increase the circulation half life of nanoparticles in the blood (ii) Galactose as a targeting ligand increases the filtration of nanoparticles by liver and (iii) The PEGylation of nanoparticles diminish their uptake by hepatocytes. The Size of nanoparticles is a critical factor in determination of the type of cells which nanoparticles will uptake by them [41, 42].

Tumor necrosis factors (TNF) and paclitaxel (PTX), were targeted to solid tumors by colloidal gold-based drug delivery systems. These systems are named CYT-6091 and are considered as an anticancer compounds which are constructed by attachment of TNF and thiol-terminated poly(ethylene glycol) (PEG-SH) onto the surface of the colloidal gold nanoparticles.TNF is a multidisciplinary molecules which not only has a strong anticancer effect but also target the gold nanoparticle specifically to tumors (Figure 5) [5].

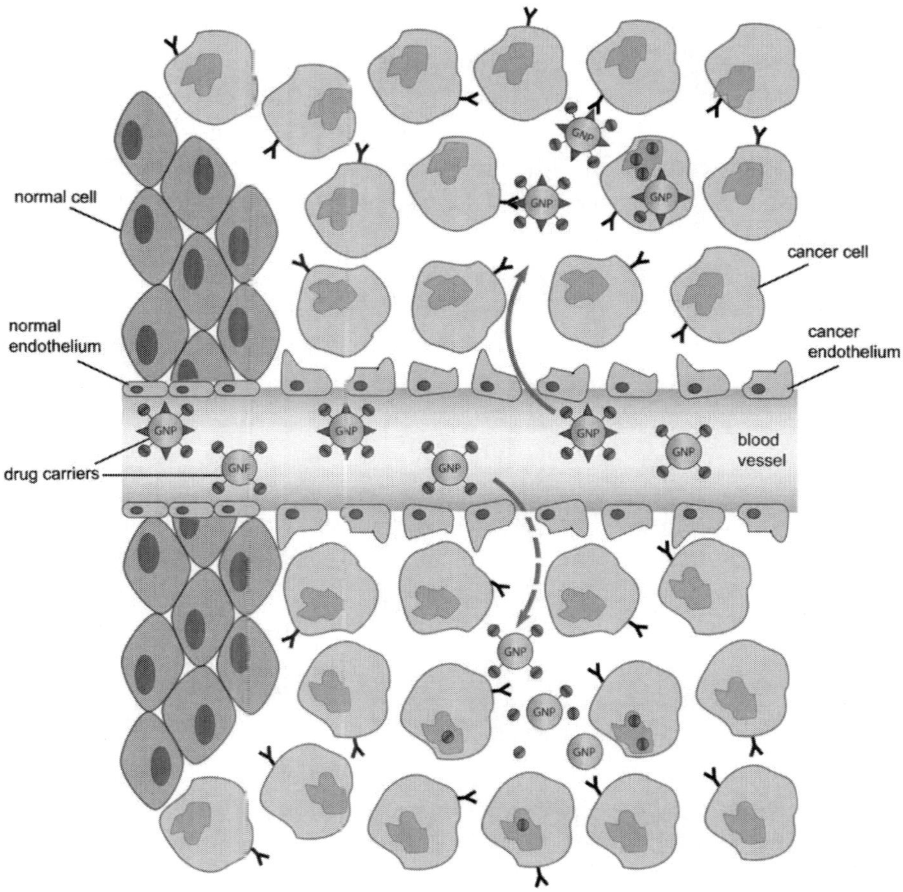

Figure 4. A schematic illustration of drug delivery via “active” and “passive” targeting, solid and dotted line respectively. Reprinted with permission from Ref [41].

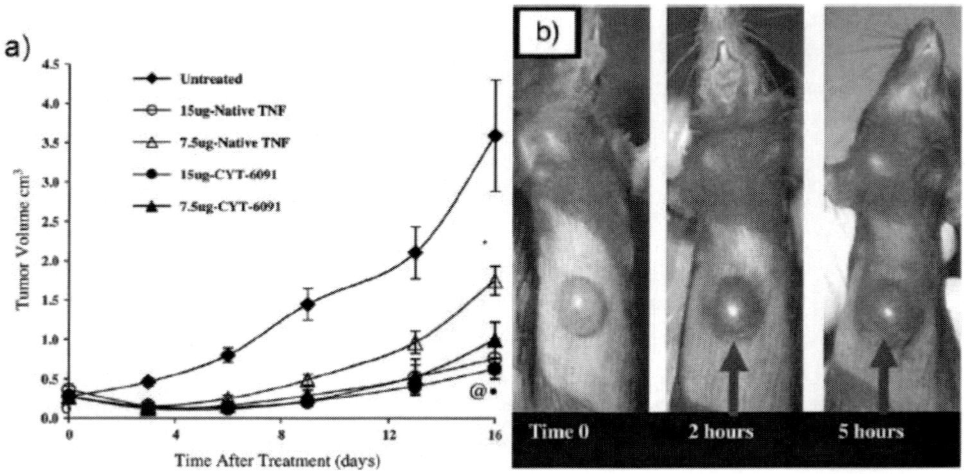

Figure 5. (a) Change in tumor volume over days after treatment with TNF and CYT-6091. (b) Visual documentation of the accumulation of CYT-6091 (red arrows indicate location of the particle drug) in MC-38 tumors. Reprinted with permission from Ref [5].

Another research work to investigate the effect of PEGylation on the biodistribution of Au NPs was carried out by Niidome and coworkers. One-third of gold nanorods without PEG capping agent, dispersed by CTAB, were found in the liver 0.5 h after the injection while PEG-protected gold nanoparticles were found in the blood 0.5 h after injection dominantly. However passing the time clearance was occurred so that after three days Au NPs were cleared from the blood completely [43]. PEGylated Au NPs with a long blood circulation were found in tissues having phagocytic cells such as liver and spleen for one week after administration [44].

Another research work focused on the role of PEG, as capping agent, and size of nanoparticles on their clearance from the blood upon administration was performed by Zhang el al. recently. They investigated effects of molar mass of PEG, used as capping agent, and size of Au NPs on the stability of Au NPs solutions. There was a direct relationship between stability of Au NPs coated by PEG so that PEG. Au NPs with three different 20, 40 and 80 nm sizes were capped by PEG5000 and subjected to the mice cells. Among three different nanoparticles, Au NPs with the 20 nm showed the longest blood circulation and lowest uptake by reticuloendothelial cells [45]. This research work clearly indicates that size and type of capping agent are two critical factors that dominate the circulation of Au NPs in blood [46].

Effect of Au NPs with 4 and 100 nm sizes and protected by PEG on DNA of cells was evaluated by intravenously administration to mice for 30 minutes. Only 0.38% (170 genes) and 0.50% (224 genes) of total genes (45000 genes) were significantly changed by the treatment of 4 or 100 nm PEG-coated Au NPs, respectively. These results indicate that 4 and 100 nm Au NPs induce similar host responses in the liver [47].

Based on *in vitro* and *in vivo* studies, it has been proved that PEG is the best capping agent in order to stabilize nanoparticles in biological systems. However, as above discussed different structural parameters affect the role of PEG in stabilizing nanoparticles. Au NPs modified by coumarin-PEG-thiol did not aggregate even in high ionic strength solution and they found to be quickly internalized into cells by non-specific endocytosis [48]. Recently the effect of the molecular weight and functionality of PEG on its key role in stabilizing and interaction with the cells has been investigated. PEG-diamine with molecular weights 2000

(PAM2-2K) and 10000 (PAM2- 10K), PEG-tetramine with molecular weight 20000 (PAM4-20K), and PEG-dithiol with molecular weight 2000 (PSH2-2K) were used not only as capping agents for stabilizing Au NPs but also as spacer to conjugate folic acid on their surface. It was found that conjugation of folic acid to the surface of gold nanoparticle have an important role for folate receptor-targeted drug delivery [49]. Folate-receptor is over expressed on the membrane of brain, kidney, breast, and lung cancer cells. Due to its high binding affinity for the folate receptors ($Kd{\sim}10^{-10}$ M), folic acid was conjugated to the PEG, then the folic acid-modified, activated-PEG functionalized Au NPs (FOL-aPEG-Au NPs) were conjugated to the anticancer drug DOX for targeted drug delivery applications [50]. A thiol-PEGylated tamoxifen derivative has selectively target and deliver plasmonic gold nanoparticles to estrogen receptor positive breast cancer cells with up to 2.7-fold enhanced drug potency in vitro [51]. Drug delivery systems consist of an Au core, a hydrophobic poly (L-aspartate-doxorubicin) (P(LA-DOX)) inner shell, and a hydrophilic PEG and folate-conjugated PEG outer shell (PEG-OH/FA) were synthesized and used in order to pH-triggered DOX release. The anticancer drug, doxorubicin (DOX), was covalently conjugated onto the hydrophobic inner shell by acid cleavable hydrazone linkage (Scheme 6) [52].

The thiolated analogue of silicon phthalocyanine has been attached to the surface of the PEGylated Au NPs through a covalent Au-S bond. This work highlights that varying the bond strength between the drug and Au NP surface can aid in timing and targeting the drug delivery as well as in optimizing the therapeutic agent [53]. Thiolated cyclodextrin (SH-CD) has also been used to modify the surface of Au NPs and increase their loading capacity to deliver anticancer drugs. It has been found that this systems as a drug carrier has the potential to prolong the blood circulation time of the drug, thereby increasing the accumulation of the drug in target tumors [54].

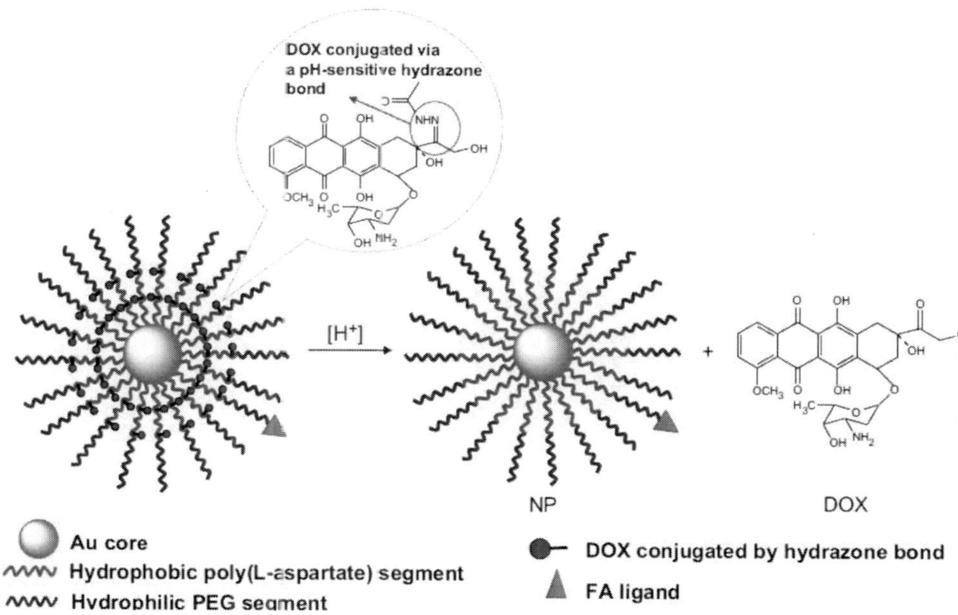

Scheme 6. Schematic representation of the Au-P(LA-DOX)-b-PEG-OH/FA NPs and its pH-triggered drug release. Reprinted with permission from Ref [52].

3.2. Gene Delivery

With the advent of nanotechnology, a number of metal nanoparticles, especially those of gold, have received widespread interest in the nonviral gene carriers owing to their unique optical properties, ease of bioconjugation and potential non-cytotoxicity. The pioneering work carried out by Mirkin and his co-workers on gold nanoparticle labeling of DNA molecules has attracted attention as an alternative to the various conventional labeling strategies for monitoring DNA hybridization as well as single base mismatch detection [55, 38, 56].

They have synthesized the composites including Au NPs that electrostatically bound to plasmid DNA via functionalization with cationic quaternary ammonium groups. This composite particle could protect the DNA from enzymatic degradation and could regulate DNA transcription of T7 RNA polymerase. Thereafter the investigations showed that the same groups caused releasing DNA from the modified Au NPs after treatment with glutathione (GSH), (Figure 7) [38].

In other example Niidome and co-workers, reported the conjugates based on nanorods that were attached to the gene of enhanced green fluorescence protein (EGFP) and used them for the remote control of gene expression in living cells.

The shapes and sizes of gold nanorods of EGFP-GNR conjugates changed after exposure to NIR irradiation for femto second. DNA was released after introducing the EGFP-GNR conjugates into HeLa cells and irradiating with the NIR source at the dose that did not cause significant lethality (Figure 8). GFP expression was specifically observed in areas locally exposed to laser irradiation. These results show that EGFP-GNR conjugates combined with NIR irradiation allow the induction of gene expression in specific cells [56].

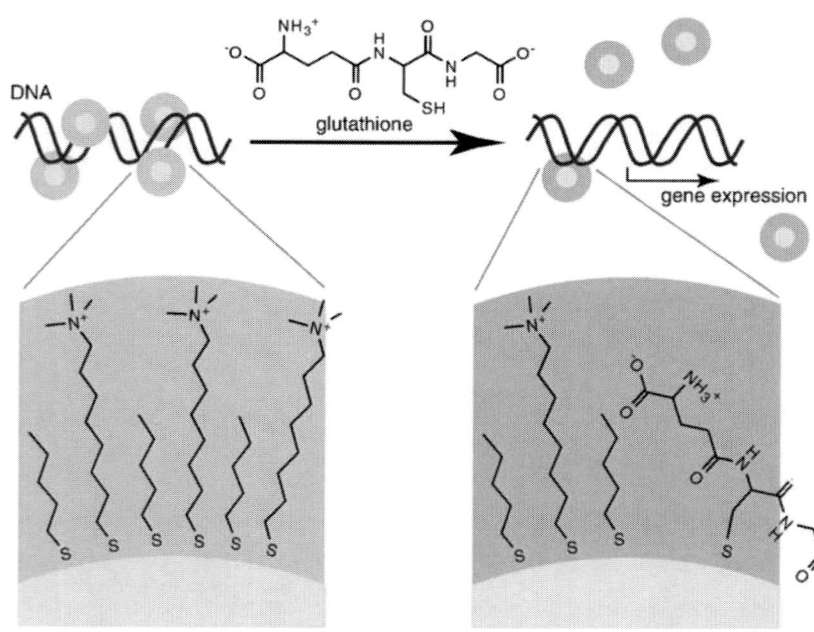

Figure 7. Au NPs functionalized with cationic quaternary ammonium–DNA complexes that were dissociated by GSH to release DNA after treatment with GSH. Reprinted with permission from Ref [38].

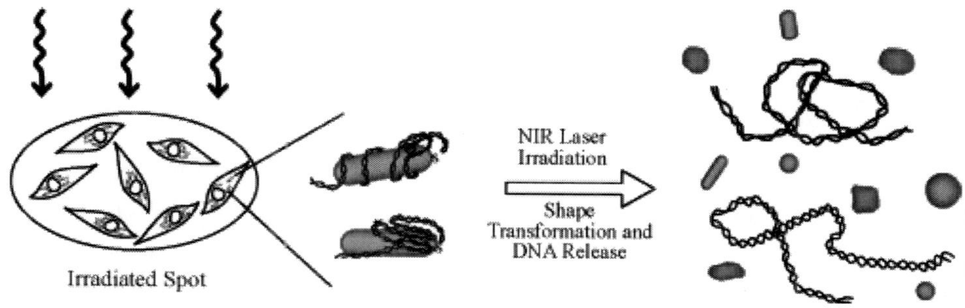

Figure 8. Cells containing EGFP-GNR conjugates are irradiated by NIR laser, leading to shape transformation and consequently release of EGFP DNA. Reprinted with permission from Ref [56].

3.3. Photothermal Therapy

Photothermal effects that induce increased temperature and thus leads to cell or tissue alterations through hyperthermia, coagulation or vaporization processes are now a promising strategy to cure cancer [57]. Usually in the photothermal therapy (PTT) both normal and tumor cells in the path of the laser light are destroyed. In addition, high power laser output up to tens to hundreds of watts should be used to efficiently induce the tumor ablation [58]. These disadvantages can be overcome by photothermal contrast agents that enable not only high efficiency by lowering the laser power but also selectivity by targeting only tumor cells. Plasmonic nanoparticles show strongly enhanced optical properties originating from the surface Plasmon resonance fields rendering them ideal in cancer diagnostics and therapy. The absorption property of Au NPs and their hybrids in the near infrared (NIR) region between 700 and 1100 nm is particularly important for application in photothermal treatment because biological chromospheres water molecules do not absorb significantly within this spectral region. Thus, the NIR photons can penetrate deep in to biological samples such as tissue or whole blood and then to be absorbed in the localized regions where the metallic nanoshells are present. The absorbed light energy by the gold nanoshells is released as heat and transferred to the surrounding biological tissues. Au NPs have been found to be non-toxic and highly biocompatible and the shell surface can readily be modified chemically for applications in the field of bioconjugation [59-67]. Compared to the above nanostructures, spherical gold nanoparticles are especially interesting because of their easy methods of synthesis and bioconjugation. Highly monodispersed gold nanospheres can be obtained within minuets by the citrate reduction method [68].

Nanoshells, new class of optically tunable nanoparticles, which are thin coatings deposited on dielectric core such as silica have gained considerable attention in this case [35]. Gold nanoshells with optical absorption in the NIR has been intravenously injected and allowed to circulate then it has been found that treated tumors displayed complete regression and mice remained healthy and tumor-free 90 days following treatment [69]. Gold nanoparticles, nanorods or their nanoshells used for PTT are usually stabilized and modified by PEG or its derivatives [70].

Gold nanoobjects modified by PEG inject directly into the tumor region or delivered intravenously. It was shown that NIR light of 820 nm at 4 W/cm^2 for 4 minutes caused irreversible tumor tissue damage [71, 72].

Selective PTT by targeting gold nanoobjects conjugated with antibodies to cells over expressed their receptors has been investigated [73, 74]. For example gold nanoshells conjugated with anti-HER2 via a bifunctional PEG linker are investigated for active targeting breast cancer cells. A diode laser at 820 nm is used for photothermal killing, 7 min, of the labeled cells (Figure 9). Two cell types including SK-BR-3 and HDF were also incubated with gold nanoshells conjugated with anti-HER2 and irradiated with NIR laser. It was found that only the HER2-overexpressing SK-BR-3 cells bound with anti-HER2 immunonanoshells died. Although the HDF cells were also exposed to the NIR light but they did not die (Figure 10) [75].

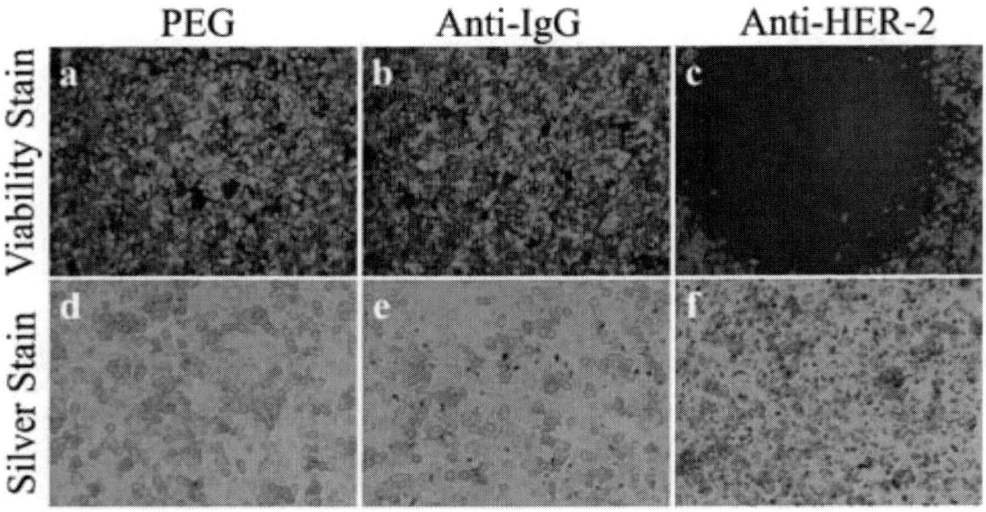

Figure 9. Selective PTT for cancer cells by using PEG-coated nanoshells (a, d), anti-IgG conjugated nanoshells (b, e), and anti-HER2 conjugated gold nanoshells (c, f) Only the cells incubated with anti-Her2 antibody conjugated gold nanoshells are damaged under NIR irradiation. Reprinted with permission from Ref [75].

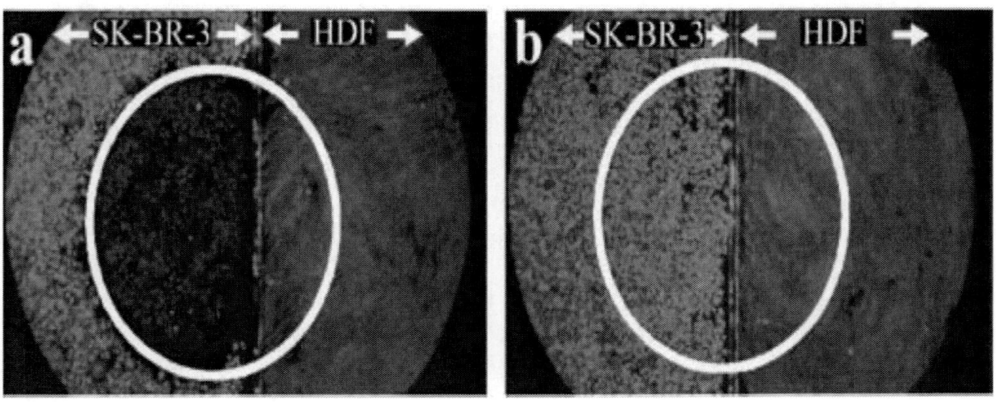

Figure 10. Two cell types, SK-BR-3 (left side of a and b) and HDF (right side of a and b) cells, Only the HER2-expressing SK-BR-3 cells bound with anti-HER2 immuno nanoshells and irradiated with NIR laser died. The HDFs, also exposed to the NIR light, did not die. Reprinted with permission from Ref [75].

Gold nanorods are also used for PTT of cancer cells, due to their absorption property in the long wavelengths of NIR region. PEG-protected gold nanorods GNR display superior spectral bandwidth, photothermal heat generation per gram of gold, and circulation half-life *in vivo* (t1/2,~17 hours). Gold nanorods coated and stabilized by PEG are injected into mice both intravenously and directly and they are studied using the transmission imaging of the NIR laser with a customized camera. The tumor was well identified after nanorod accumulation either via intravenous or subcutaneous injections (Figure 11a). NIR irradiation of the nanorod-treated tumors leads to significant inhibition of the tumor growth rate compared to control tumors [76]. The spectral profiling of the images clearly shows the difference in average tumor growth between the two administration methods (Figure 11b) [77, 78].

It has been found that conjugation of drugs onto the surface of Au NPs increase their efficiency for treatment of intracellular disease [79, 80].

Drugs can be conjugated onto the surface of Au NPs via noncovalent interactions such as electrostatic interactions or covalent bonding, or by physical absorption. For example, methotrexate, an antimetabolite and antifolate drug used in treatment of cancer, has been conjugated onto the surface of a 13 nm colloidal Au NP [81] (Figure 12). It can be physically absorbed onto the surface of Au NPS through its carboxylic groups after overnight incubation. Higher effective concentration and probably passive targeting leads to a cytotoxic effect for Au NPs-methotrexate conjugates about seven times higher than that of free methotrexate against Lewis lung carcinoma cells [81].

Photo-activated gene or drug release by plasmonically active particles reported for the first time 2000 [82, 83], followed by recorded patents and published articles [84, 78]. In these works a polymer-gel permeated with gold nanoshells was used to control drug release. Photo-activated release by spherical gold nanoparticles was also used to light-induced bursting of lysozyme containing packages in order to destroy Micrococcus lysodeikticus [85].

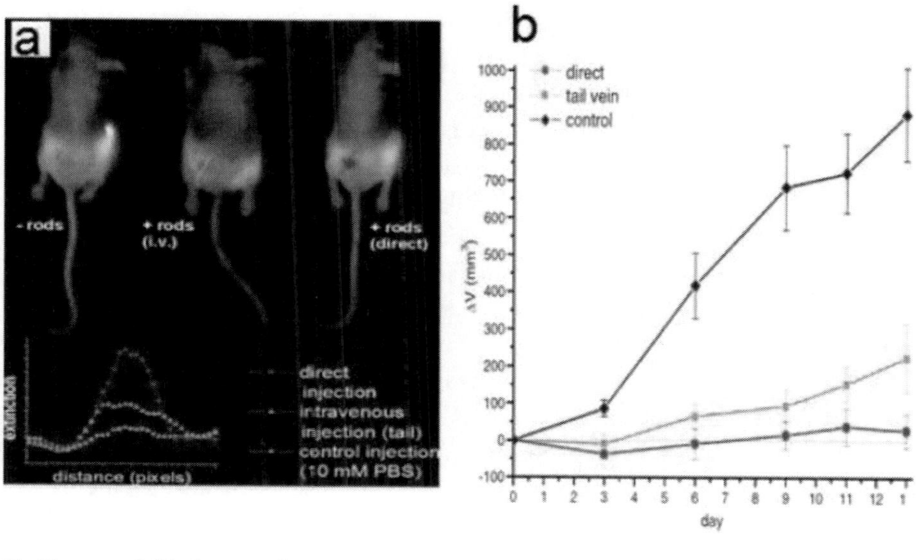

Figure11. Show a >96% decrease in average tumor growth for directly treated HSC-3 xeno grafts and a >74% decrease in average tumor growth for intravenously- treated HSC-3 xeno grafts at day 13 (relative to control tumor). Reprinted with permission from Ref [77].

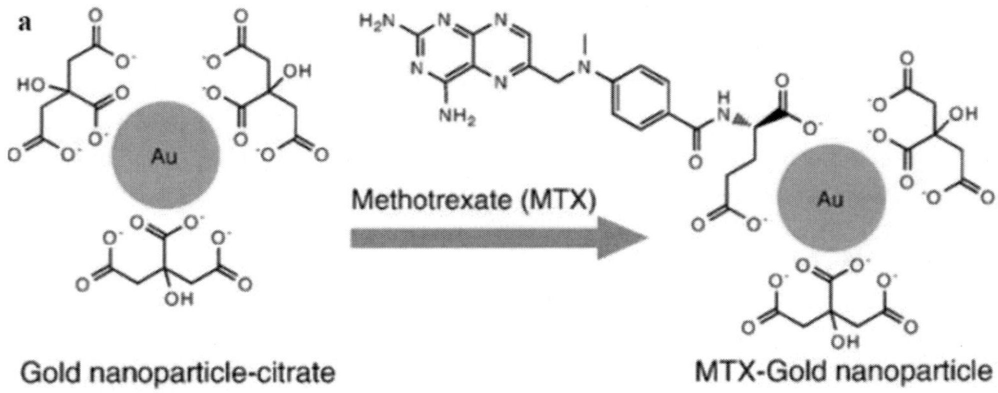

Reprinted with permission from Ref [81].

Figure 12. Schematic representation of methotrexate conjugated to the surface of spherical gold nanoparticles.

3.4. Photodynamic Therapy

Photodynamic therapy (PDT) is a promising strategy for killing the cancer cells and treatment other malignant diseases. Naturally photosensitizers used in PDT are nontoxic against cells in the absence of light. When exposed to an appreciated region of light, these sensitizers can induce apoptosis or necrosis to surrounding tissue or cells via generation the highly reactive oxygen species ROS (e.g., singlet oxygen, ($^1O_2$)). ROS produced by exciting and transferring energy from photosensitizers to oxygen of the surrounding tissue [86-89]. The ROS cause deactivation of biomolecules such as unsaturated lipids, amino acid residues in proteins, and nucleic acid bases in DNA through reaction with them. Cell membranes, which consist of the lipids, cholesterol, and proteins, are the potential targets of PDT [88].

An advantage of PDT is selective destruction of tumors using local illumination. Hydrophobicity of photosensitizers used in PDT allow them to transport through the lipophilic membranes in order to incorporate into the relevant sites (e.g., mitochondria, endoplasmic reticulum, and the Golgi apparatus), so that the initial oxidative damage can occur on proteins that exist in the membranes of those organelles. In spite of its benefit to cross the lipophilic membranes, poor water solubility of PDT agents is a significant problem for their intravenous delivery *in vivo*. Due to this limitation, a long time administration (1-3 days) of such photosensitizers to achieve the desirable concentration in a tumor for effective PDT treatment is needed [89]. This condition leads to non-specific interactions of PDT with the biological systems and ultimately toxicity and side effects for these objects. Therefore, one needs a delivery vector that can confer hydrophilicity and increase the water solubility of photosensitizers during the intravenous delivery without elimination their hydrophobicicity. Variety of nanomaterials such as liposomes, polymeric micelles, conjugated polymer nanoparticles, colloidal silica-based nanoparticles, magnetic nanoparticles, and gold nanoparticles (Au NPs) are used to stabilize PDT agents in aqueous systems [87-89].

Conjugation of PDT drugs or agents onto the surface of PEGylated Au NPs leads to hybrid amphiphilic nano-systems that are highly efficient for PDT. This strategy efficiently improves the accumulation of drugs into the tumor site relative to conventional drug administration. Because PEG arms conjugated onto the surface of Au NPs increase the solubility of the whole system in the biological media and also minimizes its non-specific interactions with the proteins and increase its blood circulation time. On the other hand hydrophobic drugs keep its fast transferring through the cell membrane. These advantages beside the intrinsic properties of Au NPs such as biocompatibility, conversion of the light to the desirable forms of energy, light scattering (imaging) and their suitable sizes (passive targeting) lead to perfect PDT systems. Attachment of receptor-specific targeting ligands onto the surface of Au NPs result in further specified for active targeting to tumor sites [87, 88].

Silicon phthalocyanine 4 (Pc 4) is a hydrophobic PDT drug currently under phase I clinical trials. Usually a time as long as 1 or 2 days is needed to accumulate Pc 4 in the tumor site sufficiently, which then can be irradiated with 672 nm light for PDT. However when Pc 4 is conjugated onto the surface of Au NPs (NP-Pc 4 conjugates), the time for the maximum drug accumulation in the tumor site is reduced to lower than 2 h (Figure 13) [88].

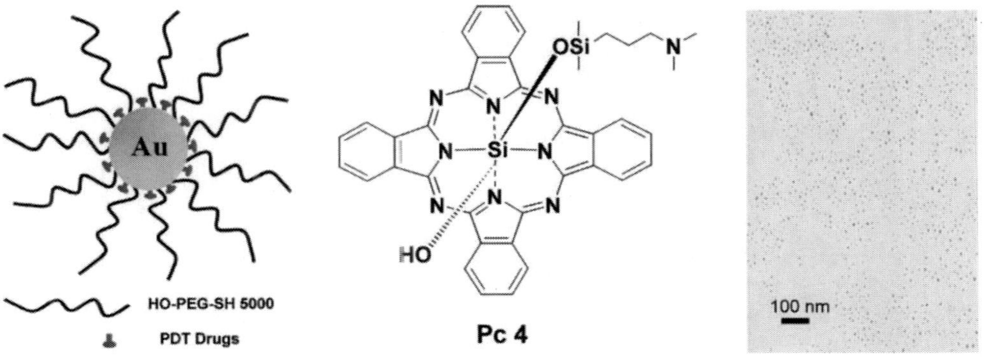

Figure13. Au NPs conjugates as PDT systems, Pc 4 structure, and transmission electron microscopy image of the conjugates. Reprinted with permission from Ref [88].

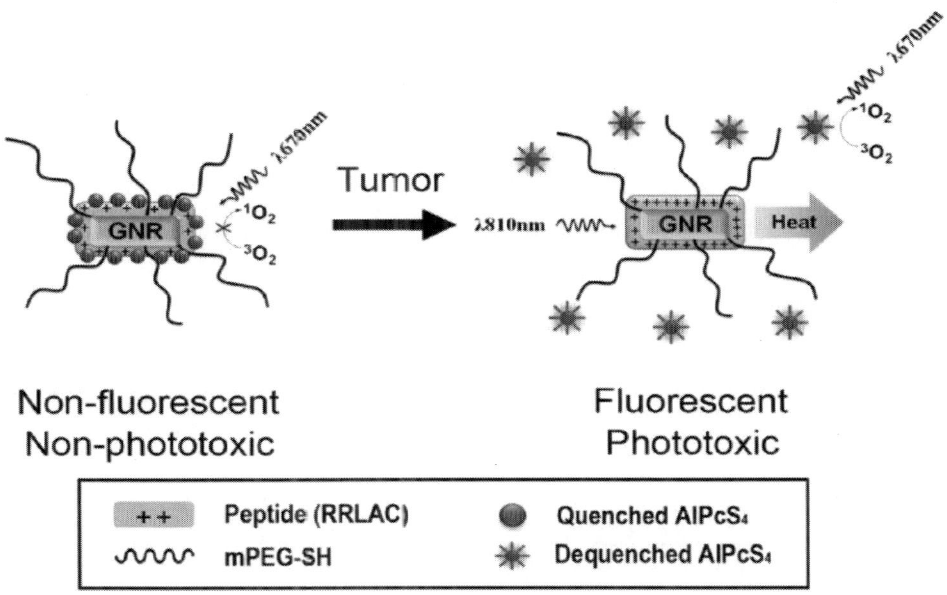

Figure 14. GNR-AlPcS4 hybrid therapy system for NIR fluorescence imaging and tumor phototherapy. Reprinted with permission from Ref [86].

A gold nanorod (GNR)-photosensitizer system has been developed for noninvasive near-infrared fluorescence imaging and cancer therapy. By combining Al(III) phthalocyanine chloride tetrasulfonic acid ($AlPcS_4$) with the GNR, highly effective photothermal therapy/photodynamic therapy (PTT/PDT) system as a hybrid therapy system with imaging capability has been produced (figure 14) [86].

In the mice receiving both free $AlPcS_4$ and the GNR-$AlPcS_4$ hybrid therapy system, tumor sites showed higher fluorescence intensities from the initial imaging time point, indicating higher accumulation of the injected photosensitizers in the tumor sites. In particular, tumor sites in the GNR-$AlPcS_4$ hybrid therapy system group were clearly discriminated from the surrounding normal tissues 1 h after injection (figure 15) [86].

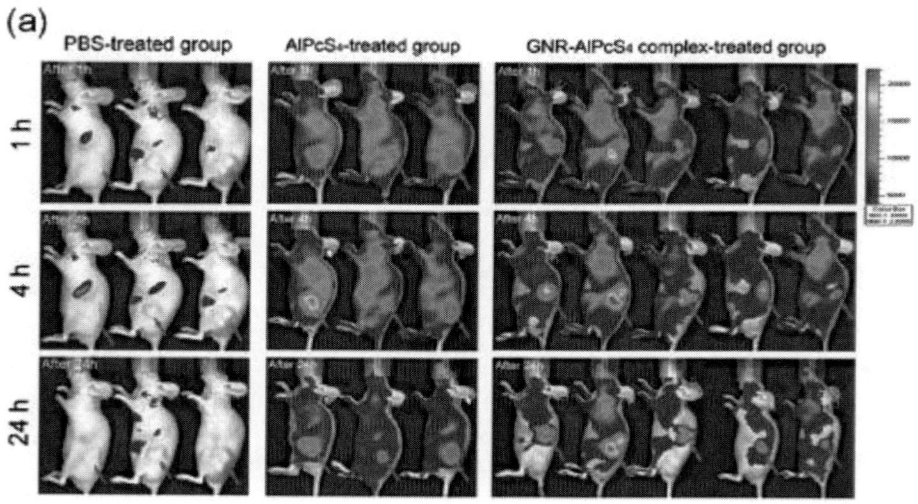

Figure 15. NIR fluorescence images *in vivo*. (a) Near-infrared (NIR) fluorescence images (Cy5.5 channel) of PBS(left), free AlPcS4-treated (middle), and GNR-$AlPcS_4$ hybrid therapy system -treated (right) mice were obtained 1, 4, and 24 h after injection. The arrows indicate tumor sites. Reprinted with permission from Ref [86].

3.5. Molecular Imaging

Computed tomography (CT) is one of the most useful diagnostic tools for various diseases in clinical applications. However other techniques such as magnetic resonance imaging (MRI) have been discovered that have advantages over CT including high spatial resolution. Recently researchers have used gold nanoparticles as contrast agents, due to their controllable size and shape, low level of toxicity and higher X-ray absorption coefficient compared with iodine-based compounds [37, 89-91].

Hybrid nanoparticles including an iron oxide core and a thin gold shell have been synthesized and modified using PEG and then they were used as a contrast agent for CT and MRI [37]. While detection of the hepatoma in the pre-enhanced CT image was difficult (Figure 16a), a good contrast enhancement (2-fold) between the hepatoma and the surrounding normal liver 5 minutes after intravenous injection of Au NPs was achieved. Difference between the contrast of the hepatoma and the surrounding normal tissue was detectable up to 24 h after injection [89].

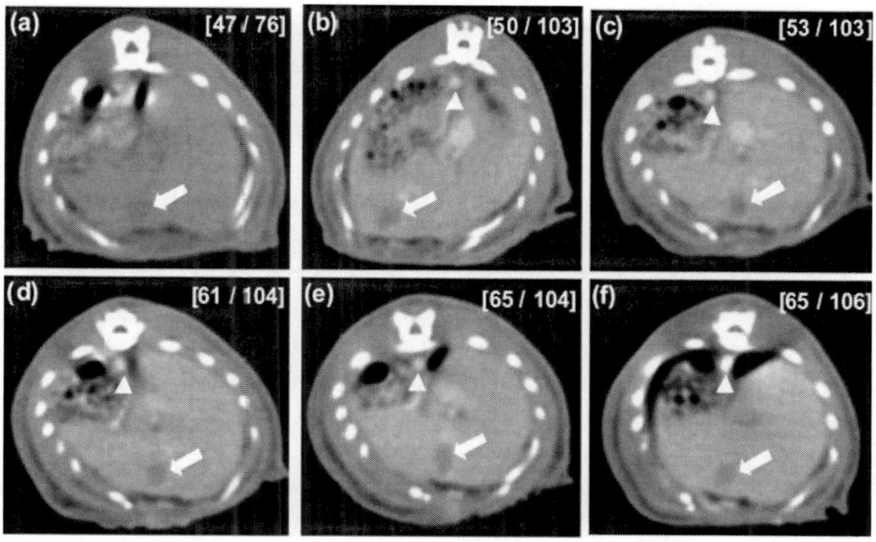

Figure 16. Serial CT images of a rat liver bearing a hepatoma. Arrows and arrowheads indicate the hepatoma region and aorta respectively. Images were obtained at (a) 0 h (before injection) and (b) 5 min, (c) 1 h, (d) 2 h, (e) 4 h, and (f) 12 h after injection. Reprinted with permission from Ref [89].

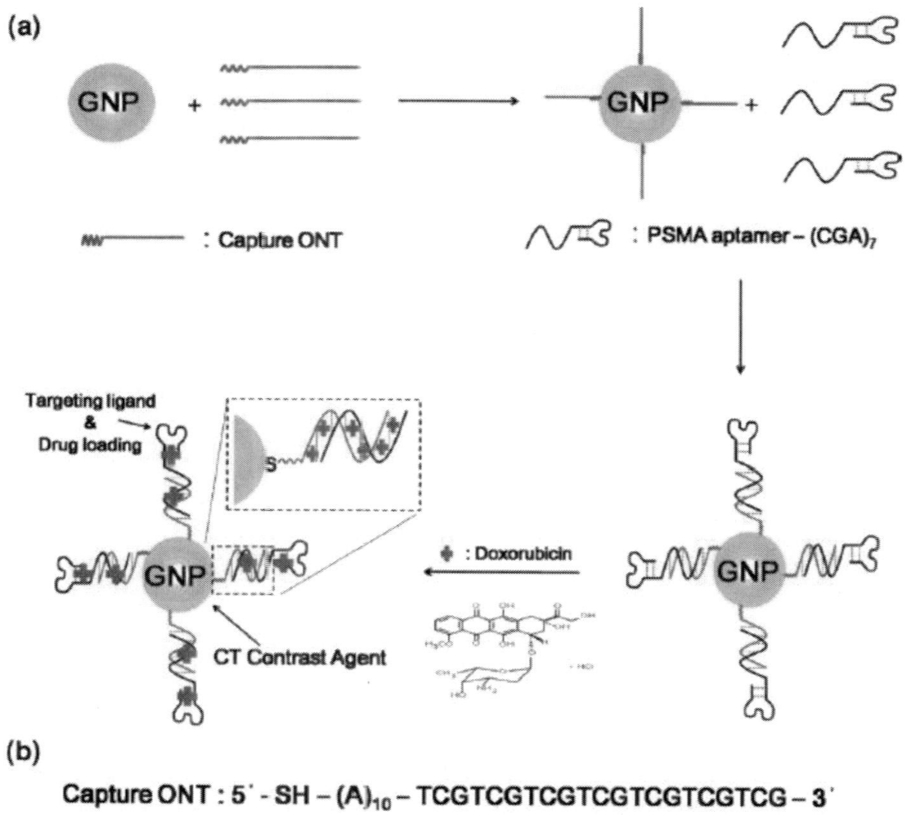

Figure 17. (a) Preparation of the Dox-loaded aptamer-conjugated Au NPs. (b) PSMA aptamer and oligonucleotide (ONT) sequences used to synthesize DOX-loaded aptamer-conjugated GNP. Reprinted with permission from Ref [90].

Mussel-inspired heparin–DOPA modified gold nanoparticles as a liver-specific CT imaging agent in vivo, eXIA 160, HEPA–Au NPs and saline as a control were injected into mice. Two hour post injection more than 50% of Au NPs accumulated in the liver and spleen while saline and eXIA 160 did not produce significant contrast. The excellent properties of this platform system highlight its potential as a novel liver-specific CT imaging agent and a molecular imaging probe [92]. Au NPs hybrids stabilized by diacid PEG and functionalized by an antibody, Erbitux (ERB), have been used as contrast agents for targeted cancer detection by MRI [90, 93].

Very recently, it has been reported that prostate specific membrane antigen PSMA-specific, aptamer-conjugated multifunctional Au NPs are able to act as both anticancer drug delivery vehicles and as CT nanocontrast agents simultaneously, because of the presence of gold. This strategy was led to combined prostate cancer imaging and anticancer therapy (Figure 17) [90].

The obtained PSMA aptamer-conjugated Au NPs showed more than 4-fold greater CT intensity for a targeted LNCaP cell than that of a nontargeted PC3 cell. Furthermore, the PSMA aptamer-conjugated Au NPs after loading of doxorubicin were significantly toxic against targeted LNCaP cells than nontargeted PC3 cells [90].

Conclusion

Typical properties of nanoparticles including size-dependent properties and unique properties such a slow toxicity, easy surface functionalization and especially photothermal properties promise Au NPs as multidisiplinary nanomaterials to be used for variety of biomedical applications.

References

[1] kisailus, D.; Najaria , M.; Weave, J.; Mors, D. *Adv. Mater.* 2005, *17*, 1234.
[2] Pal, A.; Srivastava, A; Bhattacharya, S. *Chem. Eur. J.* 2009, *15*, 9169.
[3] Zhang, H.;H, N. *Biosensors and Bioelectronics*. 2007, *23*, 393.
[4] Wang, Z.; Ma, L. *Coordination Chemistry Reviews*. 2009, *253*, 1607.
[5] Paciotti, G.; Kingston, D.; Tamarkin, L. *Drug Development Research*. 2006, *67*, 47.
[6] Pujals, S.; Bastús, N.; Pereiro, E.; Iglesias, C.; Puntes, V.; Kogan, R.; Giral, E. *Chem. Bio. Chem.*2009, *10*, 1025.
[7] Cao,Y.; Wang, Z.; Jin, X.; Hua, X.; Liu, M.; Zhao, Y. *Eur. Physicochem*. 2009, *33*, 453.
[8] Schmid, G.; Corain, B. *J. Inorg. Chem*. 2003, *17*, 3081.
[9] Tavakoli Naeini, A.; Adeli, M.; Vossoughi, M. *European PolymerJournal*. 2009, *46*, 165.
[10] Shan, J.; Tenhu, H. *Chem. Commun*. 2007, *72*, 4580.
[11] Aryal, S.; B.K.C, R.; Dharmaraj, N.; Bhattarai, N.; Kim, Ch.; Kim, H. *Spectrochimica Acta Part A*. 2006, *63*, 160.
[12] Li, D.; Cui, Y.; Wang, K.; He, Q.; Yan, X.; Li, J. *Adv. Funct. Mater.* 2007, *17*, 3134.

[13] Yusa, Sh.; Yamago, Sh.; Sugahara, M.; Morikawa, S.; Yamamoto, T.; Morishima, Y. *Macromolecule*. 2007, *40*, 5907.

[14] Li, D.; He, Q.; Cui, Y.; Li, J. *Chem. Mater*. 2007, *19*, 412.

[15] Zhu, M.; Wang, L.; Exarhos, G., D. Q. Li, A. *J. Am. Chem. Soc.* 2004, *126*, 2656.

[16] Cho, W., Kim, S.; Han, B.; Son, W.; Jeong, J. *Toxicology Letters*. 2009, *19*, 196.

[17] Nuopponen, M.; Tenhu, H. *Langmuir*. 2007, *23*, 5352.

[18] Yuan, Y.; Liu, X.; Wang, Y.; Wang, J. *Langmuir*. 2009, *25(17)*, 10298.

[19] Duan, H.; Kuang, M.; Zhang, G.; Wang, D.; Kurth, D.; Mohwald, H. *Langmuir*. 2005, *121*, 1495.

[20] Li, D.; He, Q.; Li, J. *Advances in Colloid and Interface Science*. 2009, *149*, 28.

[21] Tang, Q.; Cheng, F.; Lou, X.; Liu, H.; Chen, Y. *Journal of Colloid and Interface Scienc*. 2009, *337*, 485.

[22] Tang, T.; Krysmann, M.; Hamley, I. *Colloids and Surfaces A: Physicochem. Eng. Aspects*. 2008, *317*, 764.

[23] Prencipe, G.; Tabakman, S.; Welsher, K.; Liu, Z.; Goodwin, A .; Zhang, L; Henry, J.; Dai, H. *J. Am. Chem. Soc*. 2009, *131 (13)*, 4783.

[24] Shan, J.; Nuopponen, M.; Jiang, H.; Kauppinen, E.; Tenhu, H., *Macromolecul*. 2003, *36*, 4526.

[25] Wei, Q.; Ji, J.; Shen, J. *Macromol. Rapid Commun*. 2008, *29*, 645.

[26] Kim, J.; Lee, T. R. *Journal of Biomedical and Pharmaceutical Engineering*. 2008, *21*, 29.

[27] Kim, J.; Lee, T. R . *Drug Development Research*. 2006, *67*, 61.

[28] Jo, Y.; Kim, D.; Jeong, Y.; Kim, K.; Muhammed, M. *Macromol. Rapid Commun*. 2003, *24*, 957.

[29] Kim, D.; Kang, S.; Kong, B.; Kim, W.; Paik, H.; Choi, H.; Choi, I. *Macromol. Chem. Phys*. 2005, *206*, 1941.

[30] Li, D.; He, Q.; Yang, Y.; Möhwald, H.; Li, J. *Macromolecules*. 2008,*41* ,7254.

[31] Dong, H.; Zhu, M.; Yoon, J.; Gao, H.; Jin, R.; Matyjaszewski, K. *J. AM. Chem. Soc*. 2008, 130(39), 12582.

[32] Edwards, E.; Chanana, M.; Wang, D. *J. Phys. Chem*. 2008, *112*, 15207.

[33] Cho, W.; Cho, M.; Jeong, J.; Choi, M.; Han, B.; Shin, H.; Hong, J.; Chung, B.; Jeong, J.; Cho, M. *Toxicology and Applied Pharmacology*. 2010, *225*, 116.

[34] Feng, M.; Lee, D.; Li, P. *International Journal of Pharmaceutics*. 2006, *311*, 209.

[35] Kalele, S.; Gosavi, S.W.; Urban, J.; Kulkarni, S. K. *Current Science* . 2006, *91*, 25.

[36] Seoudi, R.; Fouda, A.A.; Elmenshawy, D.A. *Physica .,B*. 2010, *405*, 906.

[37] Kim, D.; Kim, J.; Jeong, Y.; Jon, S.; Korean, B. *J. Am. Chem. Soc*. 2009, *30*, 1855.

[38] Pissuwan, D.; Niidome, T.; Cortie, M. *Journal of Controlled Release*. 2011, *149*, 65.

[39] Niidome, T.; Ohga, A.; Akiyama, Y.; Watanabe, K.; Niidome, Y.; Mori, T.; Katayama, Y. *Bioorganic and Medicinal Chemistry*. 2010, *18*, 4453.

[40] Parka, J.; Leeb, S.; Kimb, J.; Parkb, K.; Kim, K.; Kwon, I. *Prog. Polym. Sci*. 2008, *33*, 113.

[41] Ghosh, P.; Han, G.; De, M.; Kim, Ch.; Rotello, V.M. *Advanced Drug Delivery Reviews*. 2008, *60*, 1307.

[42] Bergen, J.M.; Recum, H.; Goodman, T.; Massey, A.; Pun, S. *Macromol. Biosci*. 2006, *6*, 506.

[43] Niidome, T.; Yamagata, M.; Okamoto, Y.; Akiyama, Y.; Takahashi, H.; Kawano, T.; Katayama, Y.; Niidome, Y. *Journal of Controlled Release.* 2006, *114*, 343.
[44] Cho, W .; Cho, M.; Jeong, J.; Choi, M.; Cho, H.; Han, B.; Kim, Sh.; Kim, H.; Lim, Y.; Chung, B.; Jeong, J. *Toxicology and Applied Pharmacology*. 2009, *236*, 16.
[45] Zhang, G.; Yang, Z.; Lu.a, W.; Zhang, R.; Huang, Q.; Tian, M.; Liang, L.; Li, Ch. *Biomaterials*. 2009, *30*, 1928.
[46] Mu, C.; LaVan, D.; Langer, R.; Zetter, B. *ACSNano*. 2010, *4(3),* 1511.
[47] Choa, W.; Kimb, S.; Hanb, B.; Sonc, W.; Jeongd, J. *Toxicology Letters*. 2009, *191*, 96.
[48] Shenoy, D.; Fu, W.; Li, J.; Crasto, C.; Jones, G.; Dimarzio, Ch.; Sridhar, S.; Amiji, M. *Int. J. Nanomedicine.* 2006, *1(1)*, 51.
[49] Bhattacharya, R.; Patra, Ch.; Earl, A.; Wang, Sh.; Katarya, A.; Lu, L.N.; Kizhakkedathu, J. Yaszemski, M..; Greipp, Ph.; Mukhopadhyay, D.; Mukherjee, P. *Nanomedicine: Nanotechnology, Biology, and Medicine*. 2007, *3*, 224.
[50] Asadishad, B.; Vossoughi, M.; Alemzadeh, I. *Ind. Eng. Chem. Res*. 2010, *49*, 1958.
[51] Dreaden, E.; Mwakwari, S.; Sodji, Q.; Oyelere, A.; El-Sayed, M. *Bioconjugate Chem.* 2009, *20*, 2247.
[52] Prabaharan, M.; Grailer, J.; Pilla, S.; Steeber, D.; Gong, Sh. *Biomaterials.* 2009, *30*, 6065.
[53] Cheng, Y.; Samia, A.; Li, J.; Kenney, M.; Resnick, A.; Burda, C. *Lngmuir*. 2010, *26(4),* 2248.
[54] Park, Ch.; Youn, H.; Kim, H.; Noh, T.; Kook, Y.; Oh, E.; Park, H.; Kim, Ch. *J. Mater. Chem,* 2009, *19*, 2310.
[55] Parab, H.J.; and et al. *Biosensors and Bioelectronics*. 2010, *26*, 667.
[56] (a) Chen, Ch.; Lin, Y.; Wang, Ch.; Tzeng, H.; Wu, Ch.; Chen, Y.; Chen, Ch.; Chen, L.; Wu, Y. *J. Am. Chem. So.* 2006, *128*, 3709. (b) Guo, Sh.; Huang, Y.; Jiang, Q.; Sun, Y.; Deng, L.; Liang Z.; Du, Q.; Xing, J.; Zhao, Y.; Wang, P.C.; A Dong, n.; Liang, X.J. *ACS Nano*. 2010, *4* (9), 5505.
[57] (a) Brunetaud, JM.; Mordon, S.; Maunoury, V.; Beacco, C. *Lasers Med Sci*. 1995, *10*, 3. (b) Broek, B.V.; Devoogdt, N.; Hollander, A.D.; Gijs, H-L.; Jans, K.; Lagae, L.; Muyldermans, S.; Maes, G.; Borghs, G. *ACS Nano*. 2010, *4(10)*, 5887.
[58] (a) Sultan, RA, Tumour ablation by laser in general surgery. *Lasers Med. Sci.* 1990, 5, 185. (b) Tam, J.; Murthy, A.; Ingram, D.R.; Ma, L.L.; Kort, T.; Johnston, K.P.; Sokolov, K.V. *ACS Nano*. 2010, *4 (4)*, 2178.
[59] (a) Huang, X.; El-Sayed, I.H.; El-Sayed, M.A. *J Am.Chem Soc.* 2006, *128(6),* 2115. (b) Grabinski, C.; Schaeublin, N.; Wijaya, A.; Couto, H.; Baxamusa, S.H.; Hamad-Schifferli, K.; Hussain, S.M. *ACS Nano.* 2011, *5* (4), 2870.
[60] (a) Hirsch, L.R.; Stafford, R.J.; Bankson, .A.; Sershen, S.R.; Price, R.E.; Hazle, JD.; Halas, N.J.; West, J.L. *Proc Nat Acad Sci USA*. 2003, *100(23),* 13549.
[61] Loo, C.; Lowery, A.; Halas, N.J.; West, J.L.; Drezek, R. *Nano lett*. 2005, *5(4),* 709.
[62] Turkevich, J.;*Colloidal gold. Part II. Color, coagulation, adhesion, alloying and catalytic properties. Gold Bull.* 1985, *18(3)*, 125. (b) Shi, X.; Sun, K.; Baker, J.R.; Jr. *J. Phys. Chem. C*. 2008, *112* (22), 8251.
[63] Huang, X.; Qian, W.; El-Sayed, I.H.; El-Sayed, M.A. *Lasers in Surgery and Medicine.* 2007, 39, 747.
[64] Daniel, M.C.; Astruc, D. *Chem. Rev*. 2004, *104,* 293.

[65] Choi, W.I.; Kim, J.Y.; Kang, Ch.; Byeon, C.C.; Kim, Y.H.; Tae, G. *ACSNano*. 2011, *5,* 1995.

[66] Huang, Y.F.; Sefah, K.; Bamrungsap, S.; Chang, H.T.; Tan, W. *Langmuir*. 2008, *24* , 11860.

[67] Zhang, J.Z. *J. Phys. Chem. Lett.* 2010, *1(4)*, 686.

[68] (a) Turkevich, J.; Stverson, PC.; Hillier, J. *Disc Farad Soc*. 1951, *11,* 55. (b) Perraul, S.D.; Chan, W. *J. Am. Chem. Soc*. 2010, *132* (33), 11824.

[69] (a) Neal, D.P.; . Hirsch, L.R.; Halas, N.J.; Payne, J.D.; West, J.L. *Cancer Letters*. 2004, *209,* 171.(b) Huang, H.CH.; Rege, K.; HeysH, HeysH, J.J. *ACS Nano*. 2010, *4 (5)*, 2892.

[70] (a) Kasili, P.M.; Vo-Dinh, T. *NanoBiotechnology*. 2005 ,*1,* 245. (b) Huang, H-Ch.; Rege, K .; Heys, J.J. *Bioconjugate Chem*. 2010, *21 (8)*, 1559.

[71] Hirsch, L.R,.; R.J, Stafford.; J.A, Bankson.; R.E, Sershen Price.; J.D, Hazle.; N.J, Halas.; J.L, West. *Proc. Natl. Acad. Sc.* 2003, *100,* 13549.

[72] Huang, X.; K. Jain, P.; El-Sayed. I.H.; El-Sayed, M.A. *Lasers Med. S.* 2008, *23,* 217.

[73] Ding, A.A.; Ying-Yi. Chen, Ch-R.; Wang, Ch.; Li, P-Ch.; Bin.shieh, D. *Nanotechnology*. 2008, 882.

[74] Li, J L.; Day, D.; Gu, Min. *Adv. Mater.* 2008, *20,* 3866.

[75] Lowery, R.A.; Gobin, A.M.; Day, E.S.; Halas, N.J.; West, J.L. *International Journal of Nanomedicine,* 2006, *1(2)*, 149.

[76] Kawasaki, E.S.; Player, A. *Nanomedicine: Nanotechnology, Biology, and Medicine*. 2005, *1,* 101.

[77] Dickerson, E.B.; Dreaden, E.C.; Huang, X.; El-Sayed, I.H.; Chu, H.; Pushpanketh, S.; McDonald, J.F.; El-Sayed, M.A. *Cancer Letters*. 2008, *269,* 57.

[78] Huang, X.; Neretina, S.; El-Sayed, M.A. *Adv. Mater.* 2009, *21,* 1.

[79] (a) Saha, B.; Bhattacharya, J.; Mukherjee ,A.; Ghosh, A.K.; Santra, C.R.; Dasgupta, A.K.; Karmakar, P. *Nanoscale Res. Lett.* 2007, *2,* 614. (b) Cho, T.J.; Zangmeister, R.A.; MacCuspie, R.; P.A.; Hackley, V.A. *Chem. Mater.* 2011, *23* (10), 2665.

[80] (a) Gu, H.; Ho, P.L.; Tong, L.; Wang, L.; Xu, B. *Nano Lett*. 2003, *3,* 1261.(b) Abdullin, T.I.; Bondar, O.V.; Shtyrlin, Y.G.; Kahraman, M.; Culha, M. *Langmuir*. 2010, *26* (7), 5153.

[81] Chen, Y-H.; Tsai, C.-Y.; Huang, P.-Y.; Chang, M.-Y.; Cheng, P.-C.; Chou, C.-H.; Chen, D.-H.; Wang, C.-R.; Shiau, A-L.; Wu, C.-L. *Mol. Pharm.* 2007, *4 (5),* 713.

[82] Sershen, S.R.; Westcott, S.L.; Halas, N.J.; West, J.L. *J. Biomed. Mater. Re.* 2000, *51,* 293.

[83] West, J.L.; Halas, N.J. *Applications of nanotechnology to biotechnology, Curr. Opin. Biotechnol.* 2000, *11,* 215.

[84] West, J.L.; Sershen, S.R.; Halas, N.J.; Oldenburg, S.J.; Averitt, R.D. *US Patent.* 2002, *642, 8811.*

[85] Rad,t B.; Smith, T.A.; Caruso, F. *Optically addressable nanostructured capsules, Adv. Mat.* 2004,*16 (23–24)*, 2184.

[86] Jang, B.; Park, J.Y.; Tung, Ch-H.; Kim, I.H.; Choi, Y. *ACSNano*. 2011, 5(2), 1086.

[87] Cheng, Y.; Meyers, J.D.; Broome, A-M.; Kenney, M.E.; Basilion, J.P.; Burda, C. *J. Am. Chem. Soc.* 2011, *133*, 2583.

[88] Cheng, Y.; Samia, A.C.; Meyers, J.D.; Panagopoulos, I.; Fei, B.; Burda, C. *J. Am. Chem. Soc,* 2008, *130,* 32.

[89] Kim, D.; Park, S.; Lee, J.H.; Jeong, Y.Y.; Jon, S. *J. Am. Chem. Soc.* 2007, *129,*.7661.
[90] Kim, D.; Jeong Y.Y.; Jon, S. *ACSNano*. 2010, *4,* 3689.
[91] Yigit, M.V.; Zhu, L, A. Ifediba, M.; Zhang, Y.; Carr, K.; Moore, A.; Medarova, Z. *ACSNano.* 2011,. *5* ,1056.
[92] Sun, I-Ch.; Eun, D-K.; Na, J.H.; Lee, S.; Kim, I-J.; Youn, I-Ch.; Ko, Ch-Y.; Kim, H-S.; Lim, D.; Choi, K.; Messersmith, P.B.; Park, T.G.; Kim S.Y.; Kwon, I.Ch.; Kim, K.; Ahn, Ch-H. *Chem. Eur. J.* 2009, *15,* 13341.
[93] Lee, J.; Yang, J.; Ko, H.; Jae Oh, S.; Kang, J.; Son, J-H.; Lee, K.; Lee, S-W.; Yoon, H-G.; Suh, J-S.; Huh, Y-M.; Haam, S. *Adv. Funct. Mater.* 2008, *18,* 258.

In: Hybrid Nanostructures in Cancer Therapy
Editor: Mohsen Adeli

ISBN: 978-1-62100-517-9
© 2012 Nova Science Publishers, Inc.

Chapter VIII

Application of TiO_2 Nanomaterials for Photocatalytic Destruction of Biological Species and Cancer Therapy

A. R. Khataee*[*] *and M. Fathinia

Department of Applied Chemistry, Faculty of Chemistry,
University of Tabriz, Tabriz, Iran

Abstract

Titanium dioxide (TiO_2), which is one of the most basic materials in our daily life, has emerged as an effective photocatalyst for environmental purification. In the past decade, research and development in the area of application of different nanostructured TiO_2 for photocatalytic destruction of biological species have become tremendous. This document briefly describes the applications of TiO_2 nanomaterials in photo-destruction of bacteria, fungi, and yeasts. Special emphasis is placed on the photocatalytic killing of cancer cells. Applications of TiO_2 nanomaterials in photocatalytic treating cancer through photodynamic and sonodynamic therapy (PDT) are discussed.

1. Introduction

There are many circumstances where it is necessary or desirable to remove or kill microorganisms found in environment. Disinfection of water is required for direct human consumption as well as in the production of products to be consumed by humans or animals. Disinfection of air is required in medical facilities and production processes where biological contamination must be prevented. Disinfection can require the removal or deactivation of pathogenic bacteria, viruses, protozoa, or fungi [1, 2]. As has been pointed out by Heller, all

[*] Email: a_khataee@tabrizu.ac.ir.

of the extensive knowledge that was gained during the development of semiconductor photoelectrochemistry during the 1970 and 1980s has greatly assisted the development of photocatalysis for disinfection of water and air [3]. In particular, it turned out that TiO_2 can be used for photocatalytic breaking down organic compounds [4-6]. For example, if one puts catalytically active TiO_2 powder into a shallow pool of polluted water and allows it to be illuminated with sunlight, the water will gradually become purified. Ever since 1977, when Frank and Bard first examined the possibilities of using TiO_2 to decompose cyanide in water [7], there has been increasing interest in environmental applications [8-11]. These authors quite correctly pointed out the implications of their result for the field of environmental purification. Their prediction has indeed been borne out, as evidenced by the extensive global efforts in this area [4, 12]. One of the most important aspects of environmental photocatalysis is the availability of a material such as titanium dioxide, which is close to being an ideal photocatalyst in several respects. For example, it is relatively inexpensive, chemically stable, and the photogenerated holes are highly oxidizing [13, 14]. In addition, photogenerated electrons are reducing enough to produce superoxide from oxygen. The status of methods to disinfect drinking water has been reviewed by several researchers [4, 8, 9, 15]. Disinfection of air can be accomplished by the use of germicidal lamps or size exclusion filters [16]. Photocatalytic methods are unique in having several modes of action that can be brought to bear on disinfection. The targets of disinfection processes are pathogenic organisms including viruses, bacteria, fungi, protozoa, and algae. Each presents a challenge in terms of the structure and defense mechanisms that must be overcome [17]. The current disinfection technologies rely on the chemical or photochemical induced damage or physical removal by filtration. Mechanisms for the killing of cells by conventional methods have been covered in earlier reviews [18-20]. As already mentioned, TiO_2 photocatalyst can be used to kill bacteria and, therefore, self-sterilizing surfaces can be prepared. Recently TiO_2 photocatalysis is used for cancer treatment which attracted global attention in this area. Although surgical, radiological, immunological, thermotherapeutic, and chemotherapeutic treatments have been developed and are contributing to patient treatment, cancer is among the leading causes of death worldwide and accounted for 7.6 million deaths (around 13% of all deaths) in 2008 [21]. As far back as the mid-1980s, when Fujishima et. al. reported using the strong oxidizing power of illuminated TiO_2 to kill tumor cells, photocatalytic cancer treatment became one of the most important topics [22]. They found that polarized, illuminated TiO_2 film electrode and an illuminated TiO_2 colloidal suspension could be effective in killing HeLa cells [23]. By following series of studies, they had examined various experimental conditions including the effect of superoxide dismutase, which enhanced the photocatalytic killing effect, due to the production of peroxide [24-26]. In addition, selective killing of a single cancer cell using a polarized, illuminated TiO_2 microelectrode was reported [23]. A detailed study by Fujishima et. al. on the implanted cancer cells under the skin of mice showed that a solution containing fine TiO_2 particles inhibited the tumor growth with irradiation-assistance [12]. However, their technique was not effective in stopping a cancer that had grown beyond a certain size. They then developed a device to allow the cancer to be exposed to light while TiO_2 powder was being added to the tumor. This device, built by modifying an endoscope, should make it possible to access various parts of the human body. There are still some problems to be solved before such a device can be put into practical use [12]. However, because the photocatalytic reactions only occur under illumination, it is possible to selectively destroy cancer cells, if there is a technique available for illumination of the tumor. Although this device requires further refinement, it appears likely that it can be used on many types of cancer. Tumors of organs (e.g. the digestive organs, such as the stomach and colon; respiratory organs, such as the pharynx and bronchus; urinary system organs, such as the bladder and ureter; reproductive organs, such as the uterus and cervix; and, of course, the skin) that are irradiated by the use of an endoscope can be treated in this way. Obviously, the excitation light should not cause mutations in normal cells. The results of animal experiments have shown that near-UV rays with wavelengths of 300–400 nm, which are used in photocatalytic reactions, were safe [12].

2. Photocatalytic Properties of TiO_2 Nanomaterials

Titanium dioxide has been used extensively as a white pigment and as a cosmetic ingredient. Photocatalytic chemistry of titanium dioxide has been extensively studied over the last 25 years for removal of organic and inorganic compounds from contaminated water and air [2, 27-29]. The literature for the photocatalytic oxidation or reduction of organic and inorganic compounds has been the subject of comprehensive bibliographies [30] and various reviews [31-34]. Also, engineering requirements for practical photocatalytic systems have been discussed by Delase et. al. [35]. A recent review includes some coverage of the photocatalytic disinfection processes [17].

TiO_2 is a wide-gap semiconductor material with photocatalytic ability. Crystals of titanium dioxide can exist in one of the three crystalline forms: rutile, anatase or brookite. In their structures, the basic building block consists of a titanium atom surrounded by six oxygen atoms in a more or less distorted octahedral configuration [4]. Anatase has a band gap of 3.2 eV and for rutile it is 3.02 eV. Anatase has been found to be the most active form. As it can be observed from Figure 1, when TiO_2 is illuminated with the light (λ < 390 nm), an electron excites out of its energy level and consequently leaves a hole in the valence band [4].

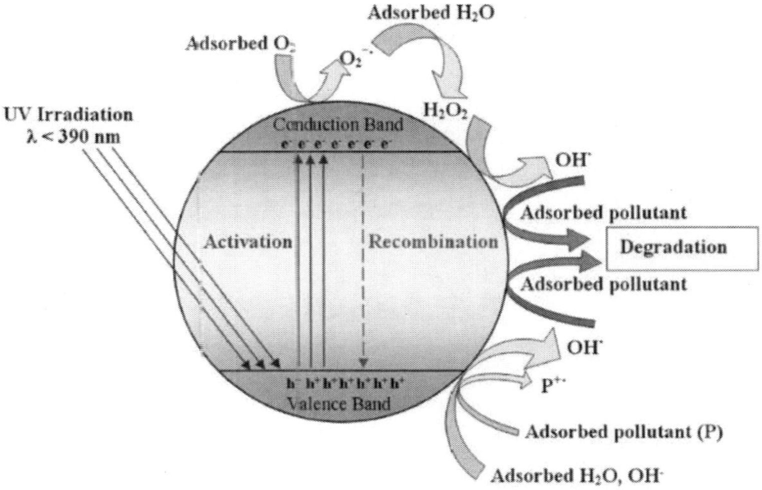

Figure 1. General mechanism of the photocatalysis on TiO2 nanomaterials [4]. (Adapted from Khataee et. al. [17] with permission from publisher, Elsevier. License Number: 2656881377519).

The photocatalytic process includes chemical steps that produce reactive species that in principal can impose fatal damage to microorganisms [17, 36-38]. The steps are summarized in Table 1 and include formation of the following species: hydroxyl radical, hydrogen peroxide, superoxide, conduction band electron, and valence band hole [39]. Formation of singlet oxygen on irradiated TiO_2 has also been reported but is not usually considered to be present under the usual conditions of disinfection reactions. The reactive oxygen species (ROS) can lead to oxidation of nearby biomolecules, may disrupt, damage various cell, viral functions and structures which can be useful for therapeutic purposes. The preponderance of evidence on photocatalytic chemistry in aqueous solution suggests that the hydroxyl radical formed by hole transfer does not diffuse from the surface of the TiO_2 into bulk aqueous phase [39]. For a cell or virus in contact with the titanium dioxide surface there may also be direct electron or hole transfer to the organism or one of its components.

Table 1. Elementary reaction equations used for oxidation of organic compounds. The subscript "ads" and S_{TiO2} refer to the adsorbed species and the surface of immobilized TiO_2 nanoparticles, respectively [39]

$TiO_2 + h\nu \xrightarrow{k_1} e^- + h^+$	(1)
$e^- + h^+ \xrightarrow{k_2} heat$	(2)
$H_2O + H^+ + OH^- + S_{TiO_2} \xrightarrow{k_3} H_2O_{ads} + OH^-_{ads} + H^+$	(3)
$h^+ + H_2O_{ads} \xrightarrow{k_4} {}^{\bullet}OH_{ads} + H^+$	(4)
$h^+ + OH^-_{ads} \xrightarrow{k_5} {}^{\bullet}OH_{ads} + H^+$	(5)
$C_nO_mH_{(2n-2m+2)} + S_{TiO_2} \xrightarrow{k_6} [C_nO_mH_{(2n-2m+2)}]_{ads}$	(6)
${}^{\bullet}OH_{ads} + [C_nO_mH_{(2n-2m+2)}]_{ads} + O_2 \xrightarrow{k_7} nCO_2 + (n-m+1)H_2O$ *Oxidation of Organic compounds*	(7)
${}^{\bullet}OH_{ads} \xrightarrow{k_8} OH^-_{ads} + h^+$	(8)
${}^{\bullet}OH_{ads} + e^- \xrightarrow{k_9} OH^-_{ads}$	(9)
$O_2 + e^- \xrightarrow{k_{10}} O_2^{\bullet-}$	(10)
$O_2^{\bullet-} + H^+ \xrightarrow{k_{11}} HO_2^{\bullet}$	(11)
$HO_2^{\bullet} + HO_2^{\bullet} \xrightarrow{k_{12}} H_2O_2 + O_2$	(12)
$HO_2^{\bullet} + O_2^{\bullet-} \xrightarrow{k_{13}} HO_2^- + O_2$	(13)
$HO_2^- + H^+ \xrightarrow{k_{14}} H_2O_2$	(14)
$H_2O_2 + e^- \xrightarrow{k_{15}} {}^{\bullet}OH_{ads} + OH^-$	(15)
$H_2O_2 + O_2^{\bullet} \xrightarrow{k_{16}} {}^{\bullet}OH_{ads} + OH^- + O_2$	(16)
$H_2O_2 + h\nu \xrightarrow{k_{17}} 2\,{}^{\bullet}OH_{ads}$	(17)

If titanium dioxide particles are of small size, they may penetrate into the cell and these processes can occur in the interior [40]. Since light is an essential component of the photocatalytic process, there can also be direct photochemistry from any UV source. There is also the possibility for enhanced or unique photochemistry resulting from the irradiation of the microbe while it is adsorbed on an oxide surface [35]. As can be seen in Table 1, hydroxyl radicals are highly reactive and therefore short-lived. Superoxide ions are more long lived; however, due to the negative charge they cannot penetrate the cell membrane. Upon the production of ROS on the TiO_2 surface, both hydroxyl radicals and superoxide would have to interact immediately with the outer surface of an organism unless the TiO_2 particle has penetrated into the cell.

Compared to hydroxyl radicals and superoxide ions, hydrogen peroxide is less detrimental. However, hydrogen peroxide can enter the cell and be activated by ferrous ion via the Fenton reaction (Eq. 1) [1].

$$Fe^{+2} + H_2O_2 \rightarrow OH^{\bullet} + OH^{-} + Fe^{+3} \quad (1)$$

The ability of bacteria, such as *Escherichia coli* (*E. coli*), to sequester iron is well documented [41]. Iron levels on the cell surface, in the periplasmic space or inside the cell, either as iron clusters or in iron storage proteins (such as ferritin) are significant and can serve as a source of ferrous ion. Therefore, while the TiO_2 is being illuminated to produce H_2O_2, the Fenton reaction may take place *in-vivo* and produce the more damaging hydroxyl radicals [42]. When the light is turned off, any residual hydrogen peroxide would continue to interact with the iron species and generate additional hydroxyl radicals through the Fenton reaction. When both H_2O_2 and superoxide ion are present, the iron-catalyzed Haber-Weiss reaction can provide a second pathway to form additional hydroxyl radicals (Eqs. 2 and 3) [43].

$$Fe^{+3} + O_2^{-} \rightarrow Fe^{+2} + O_2 \quad (2)$$

$$Fe^{+2} + H_2O_2 \rightarrow Fe^{+3} + OH^{-} + OH^{\bullet} \quad (3)$$

Since the initial actions of these reactive oxygen species target the outer surface of a cell, the rigidity and chemical arrangements of their surface structure will determine how effectively the TiO_2 photocatalytic disinfection process functions.

2.1. Photocatalytic Reactor Configurations

Photocatalytic reactors are designed to operate in either a liquid-solid system (e.g., water disinfection) or a gas-solid system (e.g., air disinfection). The two systems have implications with respect to reactor design. Another important distinction is whether the catalyst is immobilized on a support, or moveable. Therefore, photocatalytic reactors fall into four broad categories:

1) Liquid-solid, moveable bed reactors: These systems typically involve slurries of TiO_2 suspended in the liquid to be treated. The concentration of TiO_2 typically ranges between 0.05% and 1% by weight. Light penetration limitations prevent the use of high concentrations of TiO_2. The catalyst flows into and out of the reactor with the liquid being treated. Typically either natural or artificial irradiation sources are external to the system, and the photons are transmitted through UV-transparent ports. A subsequent separation step is necessary to remove the TiO_2 from the treated water [27, 44]
2) Liquid-solid, fixed bed reactors [6, 44]: Recent investigations on TiO_2 photocatalysis have been oriented towards the photocatalyst immobilization in the form of a thin film. This technique enables industrial application by eliminating the majority of the problems encountered. Liquid-solid fixed-bed reactor (LSFBR) is one of the most used solar photoreactor which has received an increasing interest as a suitable commercial application [6, 44-46]. Therefore, these reactors can employ both direct and diffuse portions of solar radiation as a light source and do not require the separation of the photocatalysts from the purified water, this problem presented a significant hurdle to commercial applications [47].
3) Gas-solid moveable bed reactors: Fluidized bed systems have been studied for destruction of chemicals in air. The catalyst particles are not entrained in the air stream. Rather, in a properly designed system, the catalyst is contained in the irradiated reactor vessel. An entrained bed system can also be envisioned since separating the catalyst particles from the air stream is easier than separation from water slurry. It has been postulated that a moveable bed reactor may benefit from the "light-dark" phenomena explored by Sczechowski and coworkers for the liquid solid system [48].
4) Gas-solid fixed bed reactors: Reactors of this type have been widely studied and fabricated in a variety of geometries. Annular reactors typically feature an inner annulus which is the light source or may have a UV-transparent sheath around the light source. The inside surface of the outer annulus is often coated with TiO_2 via a variety of methods, leading to even illumination of the coated surfaces. The annular region can also be filled with TiO_2 crystals or substrates coated with TiO_2. Other geometries include powder layer reactors in which the powder is supported on a frit, and the fluid to be treated flows normally through the powder and the frit. External illumination is provided through a UV-transparent window. UV-transparent tubes, filled with catalyst particles or coated with catalyst have also been externally illuminated with both natural and artificial light.

3. Photocatalytic Destruction of Biological Species Using TiO_2 Nanomaterials

3.1. Antibacterial Effect of TiO_2 Nanomaterials

Since most of the organic compounds are decomposed on photoexcited TiO_2, it is expected that microorganisms which also contain organic molecules should be destroyed on it. Therefore, photocatalysts are expected to play a major role in the destruction of bacteria and also in causing detoxification. This part briefly highlights some of the important studies in recent years on the bactericidal and detoxification effects of illuminated TiO_2 nanomaterials. As early as 1985, Matsunaga et. al. [49] reported that *Lactobacillus acidophilus*, *Saccharomyces cerevisiae* and *E.coli* were completely sterilized when incubated with platinum-loaded TiO_2 particles under metal halide lamp irradiation for 60–120 min. This has opened a new way for sterilization and motivated attempts to use this novel photocatalytic technology for disinfecting water and in the removal of bio-aerosols from indoor environments. A very comprehensive review of the application of TiO_2 photocatalysis for disinfection of water is given by Mccullagh et. al. [50] with many others available in the literature [1, 17, 51, 52].

Most of the reports on photocatalytic destruction of biological species are in aqueous phase, but there are some reports of bacteria removal from humid air [53]. Table 2 summarizes the photocatalytic degradation of bacterial species. Ireland et. al. [54] have confirmed the application of TiO_2 for inactivation of *E. coli*, under UV-A light irradiation in the wavelength range of 300–400 nm. A detailed study by Wei et. al. [55] on solar-assisted water disinfection system using TiO_2 photocatalyst corroborates the findings of Matsunaga et. al. [49] and Ireland et. al. [54] on the bactericidal activity, and established that irradiation of suspensions of *E. coli* and TiO_2 with UV-Visible light of wavelengths longer than 380 nm resulted in the complete killing of the bacteria. Studies with different compositions of the gas (O_2–N_2) flowing in the solutions exerted a considerable effect on the bactericidal activity of irradiated TiO_2 nanoparticles [55]. There was no bactericidal activity in the presence of 100% N_2, and the presence of O_2 was found to be a prerequisite for the bactericidal activity because of formation of reactive oxygen species. Kinetic studies revealed that the bacterial killing followed first order in *E. coli* concentration. The disinfection rate constant was proportional to the square root of the concentration of TiO_2 and proportional to the incident light intensity [56].

Caballero et. al. [57] have employed Degussa P25 TiO_2 as a suspension and a Hanau Sun-test lamp for the photocatalytic inactivation of *E. coli K12*. The researchers observed that the operational parameters such as light intensity, extent of continuous irradiation, catalyst concentration and temperature have a positive effect on disinfection. In order to mimic solar-UV power which varies with time, especially when cloud passes, intermittent illumination was employed and the results indicated that an increase in illumination time was required for *E. coli* inactivation. The interruption of illumination provides time for bacteria to recover by a self-defense mechanism against oxidation stress, resulting in the production of superoxide dismutase (SOD) enzymes and in some cases, catalyse. SOD enzyme accelerates the disproportionation of $O_2^{\bullet-}$ (precursors of $^{\bullet}OH$) into H_2O_2 and molecular oxygen (Eq. (4)) and catalyse eliminates the photogenerated H_2O_2 [38] (Eq. (5)).

$$2O_2^{\bullet-} + 2H^+ \xrightarrow{\text{SOD}} O_2 + H_2O_2 \qquad (4)$$

$$H_2O_2 + H_2O_2 \xrightarrow{\text{Catalyse}} O_2 + 2H_2O \qquad (5)$$

Table 2. Photocatalytic degradation of bacterial species using TiO_2 nanomaterials

Organism	Gram +/-	Light source	Kind of TiO_2	Irradiation time	Loss of bacteria (%)	Reference
Escherichia coli	-	UV-A: 2×15 W	Degussa P25	1h	91.6	[19, 57-60]
Pseudomonas aeruginosa	-	UV: 870 W/m^2	Degussa P25	8h	99.0	[61]
Pseudomonas putida	-	UV: 1.89 W/cm^2	Degussa P25	4 h (daily) for 4 days	99.8	[62]
Klebsiella pneumoniae	-	UV lamp	TiO_2 synthesized by sol-gel technique	20 min	99.0	[45]
Shigella flexnerii	-	Classictone incandescent lamp, 60W, 90 mw/cm^2	Mixed-phase TiO_2 nanocrystals	25 min	20.0	[46, 63]
S. dysenteriae	-	150 W Xenon arc lamp	Solar cells without TiO_2	1.5 h	70.0	[64]
Acinetobacter baumannii	-	Classictone incandescent lamp, 60W, 90 mW/cm^2	Mixed-phase TiO_2 nanocrystals	40 min	30.0	[63]
Salmonella typhimurium	-	UV-A	Degussa P25	40 min	100	[19]
S. choleraesuis	-	UV lamp, 20 W	Degussa P25	3 h	100	[47, 65]
Vibrio parahaemolyticus	-	UV lamp, 20 W	Degussa P25	3 h	100	[47, 66]
Enterobacter cloacae	-	UV-A: 5.5 W/cm^2	Degussa P25	40 min	100	[67]
Staphyloccus aureus	+	Classictone incandescent lamp, 90 mW/cm^2	TiO_2 synthesized by sol-gel technique	20 min	90.0	[63, 68, 69]
Streptococcus mutans	+	UV-A	Degussa P25	15 min	99.0	[70]
S. aureus	+	Sodium lamp, 400 W	Degussa P25	40 min	100	[36, 63, 71]
S. sobrinus	+	Fluorescent chemical lamp, 20 W	Degussa P25	60-120 min	100	[72]
Bacillus anthracis	+	Monochromati c UV: 7 mW/cm^2	Degussa P25	300 min	70.0	[51]
B. subtilis	+	Monochromati c UV: 7 mW/cm^2	Degussa P25	300 min	80.0	[73]
B. cereus	+	Monochromati c UV: 7 mW/cm^2	Degussa P25	300 min	80	[74]
Micrococcus luteus	+	UVA: 0.6 mW/cm^2	Degussa P25	24 h	15.0	[75]
Micrococcus lylae	+	UV: 2.6 W/m^2	Degussa P25	60 min	90.0	[76]

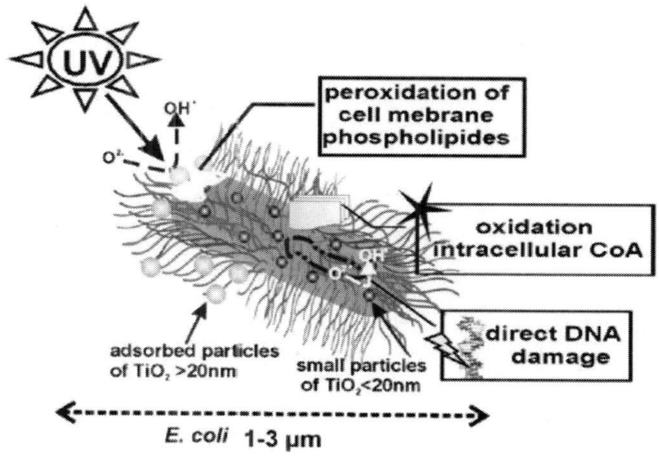

Figure 2. Photocatalytic degradation of *E. coli* cell. (Adapted from Markowska-Szczupak et. al. [78] with permission from publisher, Elsevier. License Number: 2670180565358).

Caballero et. al. [57] was also found that no bacterial growth was observed after illumination in suspended TiO_2 and then keeping in the dark for 3 h. This was in contrast to the complete recovery of bacteria on illumination in the absence of TiO_2 and after 3 h in the dark. These results confirm the previous findings about bactericidal activity of illuminated TiO_2 [38, 64]. Mannes et. al. [77] reported that disinfection was positively correlated with the TiO_2 dose used up to a concentration of 1 mg/mL. These authors presented evidence that the lipid peroxidation reaction is the underlying mechanism of *E. coli* K-12 cells death that was irradiated in the presence of TiO_2 nanoparticles. Figure 2, schematically illustrates the process of photocatalytic degradation of bacterial cells.

As can be seen in Figure 2, the killing mechanism assumes the oxidation/reduction of the intracellular Coenzyme A (CoA). This process causes the loss of bacterial respiratory activity and leads to cell death [49, 79, 80]. If the titanium dioxide particles are sufficiently small, they can penetrate in the cell giving rise to the photocatalytic process inside. This has been theorized to be another mechanism of bacterial death during photocatalytic processes [30, 79]. Free TiO_2 particles may also attack intracellular components directly. It is known that UV irradiation induces DNA and RNA physical and chemical damage. Pyrimidine and purine bases are converted to carbon dioxide and ammonia and nitrate ions [81-83]. Both ultrafine and nano size TiO_2 particles can cause bacterial plasmid DNA breakage [1, 84].

3.1.1. Photocatalytic Bactericidal Effect of TiO_2 Thin Films

Since supported photocatalyst is advantageous under continuous flow, as the recovery steps such as filtration and decantation can be avoided [5, 6, 44], so photocatalytic bactericidal effect of TiO_2 thin films will be discussed briefly in this part. However, the following factors that influence the photocatalytic activity of immobilized TiO_2 should also be taken into consideration:

(1) Diminution of specific surface catalyst accessible to light and bacteria; (II) Enhancing the recombination of photo-generated electron–hole pairs;
(2) Limitation of oxygen diffusion in the deeper layers of TiO_2;

(3) Mean distance between bacteria and immobilized TiO_2 increasing and causing a diminution of the probability of attack by $^{\bullet}OH$ compared to suspended TiO_2;
(4) Due to catalytic fixation, no penetration of the little TiO_2 beads (30–50 nm) into bacteria (~ 1 mm) possible to cause intercellular damage [85].

Matsunaga et. al. [64] successfully constructed a practical photochemical device in which TiO_2 powder was immobilized on an acetylcellulose membrane. Fujishima and co-workers [86] have extensively studied photocatalytic activity of TiO_2 thin films. TiO_2 thin films were prepared by a conventional dip-coating technique on silica-coated soda-lime glass plates. These films are transparent in the visible region and their high photocatalytic efficiency has been demonstrated. Fujishima and co-workers [86] observed that the survival ratio for *E. coli* in the liquid film on the illuminated (1 mW/cm^2) TiO_2 film decreased to a negligible level (i.e. essentially complete sterilization) within 1 h. In the absence of TiO_2, UV illumination caused only 50% sterilization in 4 h. Generally, antibacterial reagents inactivate cell viability, but pyrogenic and toxic ingredients such as endotoxins remain even after the bacteria are destroyed. Nearly 1800 people [38], including many children were hospitalized and twelve died in the summer of 1996 in Western Japan due to food poisoning by the toxin of *E. coli* [12]. The poisoning was caused by O-157 endotoxin and this inspired Fujishima's group to examine TiO_2 photocatalysis as a means of decomposing this deadly toxin [87]. On the other hand, on illuminated TiO_2 film the concentration of endotoxin in *E. coli* suspension decreased with concomitant decrease in the survival ratio of *E. coli*. The decomposition of endotoxin from *E. coli* cells certainly points out that the TiO_2 photocatalyst destroys the outer membrane of the *E. coli* cell. Therefore, the antibacterial effects of TiO_2-coated materials involve not only nullification of the viability of the bacteria, but also destruction of the bacterial cell. Another study by Sunada et. al. [85], indicated that the antibacterial effect of TiO_2-coated materials was not a simple bacteriostatic action. It was a bactericidal action that involved the decomposition of the cell wall. TiO_2 nanoparticles immobilized on Nafion membranes were used for deactivation of *E. coli* with efficiencies close to those observed for bacterial suspension containing the same concentration of suspended TiO_2. However, bactericidal effect for fixed TiO_2 on glass is diminished compared to that of with the suspended one [38].

3.2. Antivirus Effect of TiO_2 Nanomaterials

In comparison with bacteria, viruses are much smaller in size (from 0.01 to 0.3 μm) and can pass through filters that retard most of bacteria. Viruses infect all types of organisms, from bacteria and archean to animals and plants. TiO_2 nanomaterials possesses antivirus properties caused by photocatalytic reactions [88-90]. Table 3 summarizes the photocatalytic degradation of various viruses, yeasts and fungi species in the presence of TiO_2 nanomaterials. Most of the studies were performed under UV light irradiation [91, 92] But, TiO_2 nanomaterials under visible light irradiation also deactivated some viruses. Sjogren and Sierka [93] reported inactivation of Phage MS2 by Iron-Aided TiO_2. Their results showed that inactivation of phage MS2 increased from 90% to 99.9% after 2 μM ferrous sulfate was added after 30 min.

In some studies, viral deactivation rates were found to be even higher than those for bacteria [89]. Li et. al. [94] demonstrated that the use of visible-light photocatalysis with

TiON/PdO fibers allowed reaching the final virus MS2 phage removal efficiency of 99.75–99.94% in 1 h of contact time. Subsequently, Mazurkowa et. al. [95] proved that the TiO_2 nanoparticles destroyed the influenza virus after 30 min of incubation with removal efficiency of 100%. However, the mechanism of virus destruction by photocatalysis is poorly understood. It has been demonstrated that viruses respond differently from bacteria, when come in to contact with TiO_2. It was well documented that the MS2 phage was inactivated by free surface-bound hydroxyl radicals as a major path and by ROS as a minor path [93]. Kashige et. al. [96] suggested that the mechanism of *Lactobacillus casei* phage deactivation by TiO_2 under UV-A irradiation was primarily caused by the damage to the capsid protein by ROS such as $^{\bullet}O_2^-$ and $^{\bullet}OH$. In the next stage of the virus destruction, the genome DNA or RNA inside the viral particles was considerably fragmented as observed electrophoretically [92, 95, 96]. It is believed that among biological species, viruses are the most photocatalysis-sensitive species [78]. Several studies revealed the deactivation of viruses by TiO_2 depending on different factors such as the concentration of TiO_2 nanoparticles, incubation period, solution composition, light source, etc. Sang et. al. [97] reported that the addition of bovine serum albumin could protect the FCV virus against deactivation by TiO_2 in a dose-dependent manner. In the presence of UV-A light, TiO_2 oxidizes and destroys organic substances, including infectious agents such as prions (proteinaceous infectious particle). They reported that completed degradation of proteins PrP^{Sc} have been achieved after treatment with 4g/L TiO_2 (P25) and 4 g H_2O_2 diluted in distilled water and irradiated with UV-A lights for 12 h [98].

Table 3. Photocatalytic degradation of viruses, yeasts and fungi species using TiO_2 nanomaterials

Organism	Light source	Kind of TiO_2	Irradiation time	Degradation efficiency (%)	Reference
Phage Qβ	Near UV black light, 3.6 mW/cm^2	Degussa P25	1h	70	[98, 99]
Phage MS-2	Near-UV	Degussa P25	30 - 210 min	99.9%	[92, 93]
Poliovirus 1	Fluorescent or sun light	Degussa P25	30 min	60	[89]
Lactobacillus phage PL-1	UV-A	Mixture of TiO_2, Al_2O_3, SiO_2	10 days	100	[17, 100]
Saccharomyces cerevisiae	Sodium lamp, 400 W	Degussa P25	120 min	100	[36]
Candida albicans	UV-A	TiO_2 synthesized by sol-gel technique	30 min	100	[101]
Penicillium expansum	Solar light	Degussa P25	1 week	100	[102]
Daporthe actinidiae	UV lamp, 6 W	Synthesized TiO_2	5 min	95	[74]
Aspergillus niger	UV lamp	Rutileand anatase	72 h	100	[66, 67]
Fusarium solani	Solar light	Degussa P25	3 h	100	[103, 104]
F. anthophilum	Solar light	Degussa P25	4 h	100	[103]
F. equiseti	Solar light	Degussa P25	6 h	100	[104]
F. oxysporum	Solar light	Degussa P25	2 h	100	[104]
F. verticillioides	Solar light	Degussa P25	1 h	100	[104]
Penicillium chrysogenum	UV lamp	Rutileand anatase	72 h	100	[67]

3.3. Antifungal Effect of TiO_2 Nanomaterials

Fungi (i.e. filamentous forms and yeasts) are very diverse in their morphology. There are almost 200,000 fungal species described all over the world [78]. About 500 species are presently known to be pathogenic or potentially pathogenic to animals, including humans, and plants [78]. Fungi have been identified as a primary contributor to the problem of indoor air quality. In fact, the term "sick building syndrome" is used to describe buildings, in which various physical, chemical and biological factors, including fungi (their spores and mycotoxins), considerably decrease the indoor air quality. It consequently, leads to discomfort or illness of the occupants [78]. Allergies, asthma, infections, and the long-term repercussions of mycotoxins are just a few of the many real health effects associated with fungal contamination of indoor environments. Outdoor environments can also be negatively affected by these organisms. Fungi can destroy wood, fibbers and other materials; causing severe damage to buildings and technical materials. Most antifungal chemicals are non-specific to the organism affected and can be detrimental to the environment, including toxicity to plants and animals [71]. Photocatalysis using TiO_2 has been suggested as effective method for removal of fungal cells from the environment (see Table 3) [66, 67, 74, 103]. However, the available literature contains little data on the deactivation of fungi and/or fungal spores by TiO_2-mediated photocatalysis.

The first research on the photocatalytic destruction of fungi, specifically the yeast *Saccharomyces cerevisiae*, was carried out by Matsunga et. al. in 1985 [49]. They found that Degussa P25 enhanced the killing of the yeast from 80% to 100% over 120 min of the reaction time. The antifungal activity of TiO_2 nanomaterials has been examined intensively on other fungal species which have been reported in Table 3. Chen et. al. [105] found that the photocatalytic sensitivity of fungi to be considerably weaker than that of bacteria. TiO_2 irradiated with UV and visible light rarely induced photoreaction for fungal inhibition [61, 104, 106]. This probably resulted from different chemical composition, structure and thickness of cell walls in these organisms. One major difference is that fungal cells have cell walls that contain chitin, unlike the cell walls of bacteria, which contain peptidoglycan. Furthermore, due to the structural differences between fungal groups (e.g. filamentous and yeast species) and also between fungal spores (conidia) and filaments (hyphae), these organisms display different reactions to the photocatalysis. Seven et. al. [36] demonstrated that the photocatalytic process could not completely inactivate the *Aspergillus niger* spores, while this process killed the *Candida albicans* cells. Akiba et. al. [107] proved that the photocatalytic antifungal effect resulted from the denaturation of the *Candida* cell. The antifungal and protein degradation effects increased with increasing the concentration of TiO_2 (10 nm), and radiation time. After 90 min radiation the viability of *C. albicans* was reduced to 16.2% [107.]. Sichel et. al. [75], demonstrated that from 1 to 6 h were necessary to inactivate *Fusarium sp.* spores in water solution by solar photocatalysis. Subsequently, Chen et. al. [105] reported that *A. niger* mycelium, which grown on the wood surface, was completely inhibited with TiO_2 coated film under UV-A irradiation after 20 days. However, after that time the spores of *A. niger* were still viable and the fungal re-growth was observed. Similar findings were reported by Wolfrum et. al. [51] and Mitorajetal [73]. The photocatalysis was found to be ineffective in controlling latent infections of *Daporthe actinidiae* in kiwifruit [74]. Maneerat and Hayata [102] reported that TiO_2 alone did not affect the growth of *Penicillium expansum*. This finding is consistent with previous data, which showed that TiO_2

itself did not act as germicide or fungicide in the dark. When UV-A was combined with TiO_2, the viable number of this fungus apparently decreased [108].

3.4. Photocatalytic Destruction of Cancer Cells Using TiO_2 Nanomaterials

Cancer treatment is one of the most important topics associated with photocatalysis [12, 22, 109, 110]. The cancer cells are eukaryotic cell (containing the nucleus) and their structure is complex. Based on this knowledge it is thought that killing cancer cells might be more difficult than killing microorganisms (bacteria and viruses) by the photocatalytic reaction with TiO_2 nanoparticles. In all probability, in the presence of UV light titanium dioxide induces the apoptosis of cancer cells. Cancer cells die, if their membranes are damaged or if the oxidation/reduction compounds needed for adenosine triphosphate (ATP) production in the cell are depleted or exhausted. The cancer cells which had been destroyed by TiO_2 photocatalysis were reported in Table 4. Human U937 monocytic leukaemia cells were treated with 1 mg/mL of colloidal TiO_2 for 2 h at 37 °C followed by irradiation with UV light (300–400 nm). About 80% of the cells were killed after 10 min of illumination and complete destruction of leukaemia cells were obtained after 30 min [111]. Titanium dioxide nanomaterials showed the evidence of the membrane damage and DNA fragmentation, especially the formation of DNA ladder. All these effects are characteristics for apoptosis. It has been suggested that reactive oxygen species are responsible for this process [81]. Zhang and Sun [112] found that photoexcited TiO_2 induced series of oxidized chain reactions, which damaged cancer cells. The human carcinoma cell damages occurred in two stages. The initial oxidative damage took place on the cell membranes, where the TiO_2 nanoparticles (21.2 nm) had its first contact with intact cells. At this stage, the cells did not lose their viability but the membranes became somewhat permeable.

Table 4. Photocatalytic destruction of cancer cells using TiO_2 nanomaterials

Cancer cell	Light source	Kind of TiO_2	Irradiation time	Treatment efficiency (%)	Reference
HeLa	100 W long-wave UV lamp	Degussa P25	30 min	63	[119]
T24	500 W high pressure mercury lamp	Degussa P25	5 min	70	[120]
Ls-174-t	UV-A	Degussa P25	30 min	88	[112]
MCF-7 and MDA-MB-468 breast cancer epithelial cells	UV-A	TiO_2 synthesized by sol-gel technique	20 min	50	[114]
Human LoVo cancer	UV-A	Degussa P25	90 min	100	[121]
Hamster CHL/IU cells	UV/visible	Degussa P25	1 h	80	[122]
Alveolar macrophage Chinese	UV lamp	Degussa P25	24 h	70	[123]
Bel 7402 human hepatoma	15 W fluorescent lamp	Cerium doped TiO_2	24 h	100	[124]
U937 monocytic leukaemia cells	UV-A	Degussa P25	10 min	80	[111]

Subsequently, TiO_2 nanoparticles diffused into the damaged cells and directly attacked intracellular components. These findings are in agreement with those of Fujishima et. al. [113] and other authors [114-116]. Specifically, Lagopati et. al. [114] reported that TiO_2 nanoparticles (above 10 nm) exerted cell-dependent effects on cellular functions such as proliferation and viability. The limitation of cancer treatment by photocatalysis generally consists of the weak penetration of UV and visible light through the skin. The cerium doped TiO_2 nanoparticles (13 nm) induced the apoptosis of Bel 7402 human hepatoma cells in the presence of visible light [117]. Xu et. al. [118] showed that the deposition of gold on TiO_2 nanoparticles greatly increased the photocatalytic deactivation effect of TiO_2 on tumor cells. The optimum Au content in the Au/TiO_2 nano-composites was about 2 wt. %.

3.5. Photocatalytic Destruction of Microcystins

Microcystins are toxins produced in freshwater systems as secondary metabolites by various cyanobacteria (blue-green algae) belonging to the genera Microcystis, *Anabaena*, *Nostoc* and *Oscillatoria*. The increasing eutrophication of natural water has led to an increase in the incidence of algae blooms and the consequent increased risk of microcystin contamination of water. It has been reported that the presence of microcystins in water bodies has caused illness and death of wild and domestic animals [125] and recently their presence in dialysis water resulted in human fatalities [126]. Microcystins are cyclic heptapeptides and generally contain five invariant amino acids (or derivatives of them) and two variable L-amino acids, whose one-letter nomenclature abbreviations are used to name the various analogues. Thus, microcystin-LR contains leucine and arginine, microcystin-YR, tyrosine and arginine and microcystin-YA, tyrosine and alanine. They are hepatotoxic due to their inhibition of protein phosphates 1 and 2A and are potent promoters of liver cancer. Microcystins are chemically very stable over a wide range of pH and temperature due to their cyclic structure. Conventional water treatment with chlorine and ozone has limited degree of success for the destruction of microcystins in drinking water. The microcystins which had been destroyed by TiO_2 photocatalysis were reported in Table 5. The photolysis of microcystin using sunlight resulted in relatively slow decomposition in pure solution. The use of powdered and granulated activated carbon has only limited efficacy. In 1999, WHO suggested a guideline value of 1 μg/L for microcystin-LR [127]. It is essential to establish a reliable treatment strategy that can remove microcystin from water. The most commonly occurring cyanobacterial toxin, microcystin-LR, was effectively destroyed under the irradiation in the presence of TiO_2 [38]. Though the concentrations employed (μM) in the photocatalytic destruction of this toxin exceeded those occurring naturally (nM–pM), it has been shown that the much lower concentrations which can be present in drinking water will be rapidly removed by this technique. The samples that were illuminated without TiO_2 displayed no degradation. Shephard et. al. [128] reported the decomposition of microcystins-LR,-YR and -YA from contaminated water using a photocatalytic 'falling film' reactor in which an oxygen purge, UV radiation and TiO_2 were used to oxidatively decompose the microcystin pollutants. The decomposition followed first order kinetics with half-life of less than 5 min, with the reactor operating in a closed-loop mode. It was also observed that the reaction rates were strongly dependent on the amount of TiO_2 catalyst (1–5 g/L), but only marginally influenced by a change in gas purge from oxygen to compressed air.

It is generally believed that the hydroxyl radicals generated at the semiconductor surface may be responsible for the photo-destruction process.

Table 5. Photocatalytic destruction of microcystins using TiO_2 nanomaterials

Organism	Light source	Kind of TiO_2	Irradiation time	Treatment efficiency (%)	Reference
Microcystin-LR	Xenon UV lamp	Degussa P25	30 min	100	[38, 129]
Microcystin -RR	Xenon UV lamp	Degussa P25	30 min	83	[125, 129]
Microcystin-LW	Xenon UV lamp	Degussa P25	30 min	100	[38, 129]
Microcystin-LF	Xenon UV lamp	Degussa P25	30 min	100	[38, 129]
Microcystins-YR and -YA	UV-light	Degussa P25	Less than 5 min	100	[128]

From the above-mentioned explanations, it can be concluded that TiO_2 nanomaterials can effectively be used for destruction of different biological species (e.g. bacteria, viruses, fungi, yeasts and microcystins) and cancer cells. In the next sections, we will discuss about biomolecules-conjugated TiO_2 nanomaterials and their applications in treatment and therapy of cancer.

4. Photodynamic Therapy Using TiO_2 Nanoparticles

Photodynamic therapy (PDT) has been shown to be an effective therapeutic approach for the treatment of various cancers, cardiovascular, dermatological, and ophthalmic diseases [130]. PDT induces cancer cell death through a combination of light, photosensitizes, and oxygen. The disadvantage of this therapeutic method is the challenge of targeting local tumor tissue without damaging adjacent healthy tissues. Photodynamic therapy is a promising noninvasive treatment for cancer. It has been studied in a variety of nononcologic applications. The process is a two step method, in which a combination of a photosensitizer (PS) agent and UV-Visible light are used in the presence of molecular oxygen to obtain a therapeutic effect [131]. The PDT effect occurs when the PS absorbs photons and the ground singlet state becomes excited. A fraction of the excited single-state molecules is transformed via intersystem crossing into excited triplet state, forming free radicals or ions. Then, the hydrogen atom is removed and an electron is transferred to biological substrates such as membrane lipids, solvent, or molecular oxygen [130]. These radicals interact with molecular oxygen in two steps: (I) A free electron or hydrogen atom is transferred to membrane and/or (II) the excited triplet state transfers its energy to molecular oxygen in singlet state ($^1O_2$) to form a highly reactive nonradical in triplet state ($^3O_2$). Both processes can be occurring simultaneously, and the ratio between them depends on the nature of the PS as well as substrate properties. A great majority of photosensitizers tested for their photodynamic activities are more or less complex organic or organometallic compounds (mainly tetrapyrrols, phthalocyanines, naphthalocyanines, texapyrines, and others) [131]. Although their long-lived triplet excited states enable efficient energy or electron transfer processes leading to formation of reactive oxygen species (ROS; $^{\bullet}OH$, $O_2^{\bullet-}$, H_2O_2, $^1O_2$, etc.), there are still serious limitations for the use of this type of compounds in therapy. For instance, limited stability and photostability, insufficient light absorption, or low yields of ROS generation hinder applications of these classes of compounds as drugs [131]. Development of a new class of photosensitizers based on inorganic micro- or nano-assemblies that are stable and nontoxic in the dark can be a good approach to overcome such problems. Titanium dioxide, known for its photocatalytic activity, can be a good candidate. Excited TiO_2 with its unique redox properties is already used for numerous practical applications [132, 133]. The main disadvantage of neat crystalline TiO_2 is the fact that its photoactivity is limited to only ultraviolet light. However, a spectral photosensitization of TiO_2 to visible light may be achieved by proper modification [131]. Titanium dioxide shows a very weak or no toxicity *in-vitro* and *in-vivo* but TiO_2 particles irradiated with UV light exhibit a significant cytotoxicity, attracting studies on TiO_2 applications in PDT. The majority of *in-vitro* studies on phototherapeutical applications concern unmodified TiO_2 excited with UV light which were reported in Table 4. In comparison with homogeneous sensitizers irradiated TiO_2 favors formation of at least the same broad variety of ROS. The mechanism of the cellular death induced by TiO_2 is that the photodynamic effect can be strengthened by incorporation of titanium dioxide particles into cells [132]. Janczyk et. al. [134] tested the visible light-induced phototoxicity of TiO_2 (sample TH-0 (Kerr-McGee)) modified with platinum(IV) chloride complexes, [$TiO_2/PtCl_4$]. Their results have demonstrated phototoxicity of the [$TiO_2/PtCl_4$] material with the mouse melanoma cells (S-91). Detection of efficiently generated various reactive oxygen species ($^{\bullet}OH$, $O_2^{\bullet-}$, H_2O_2, $^1O_2$) and also reactive chlorine species had proven the photodynamic activity of the tested material, induced by visible light. They reported the cellular death (recognized as a necrosis) was a result of the cell membrane peroxidation. Recently, sensitization of wide–band gap semiconductors with organic and inorganic dyes have been demonstrated [132]. In this system, a PS adsorbed at the support surface is excited by visible light, and an intercomponent electron transfer is realized in the couple molecular semiconductor–semiconductor oxide, extending the useful wavelength of TiO_2 from the UV to the visible region. Lopez et. al. [132] investigated the possible synergy of zinc-phthalocyanines (ZnPc) supported on nanostructured TiO_2 to increase the photochemical performance in killing cancer cells and pathogen microorganisms. They probed *in-vitro* photoactivity of modified TiO_2 under visible light on killing of cancer cells and Leishmania parasites [132]. By characterization of supported ZnPc they found that phthalocyanine was linked by the N-pyrrole to the support and could be used in PDT. The preferential localization in target organelles such as mitochondria or lysosomes determined the cell death mechanism after PDT. Their results suggested that nanoparticulated TiO_2 sensitized with ZnPc was an excellent candidate as sensitizer in PDT against cancer and infectious diseases.

In another study it was reported that TiO_2 phototoxicity depends not only on the photocatalyst concentration and light dose but as well on its crystalline form [130]. Furthermore, it was shown that TiO_2 particles can be incorporated into cells. Hydroxyl radical was proposed to be the main species responsible for cellular death due to lipid peroxidation. However, it was also reported that the photokilling mechanism of TiO_2 involved different photogenerated reactive oxygen species such as $^{\bullet}OH$, $O_2^{\bullet-}$ and $HO_2^{\bullet-}$ [135].

5. Conjugation of Biomolecules to the Surface of TiO_2 Nanoparticles

The most common cancer treatments are limited to chemotherapy, radiation, and surgery. Frequent challenges encountered by current cancer therapies include nonspecific systemic distribution of antitumor agents, inadequate drug concentrations reaching the tumor, and the limited ability to monitor therapeutic responses. Poor drug delivery to target special site of cancer cells leads to significant complications, such as multidrug resistance. Greater targeting selectivity and better delivery efficiency are the two major goals in the development of therapeutic agents and imaging contrast formulations. Ideally, a therapeutic drug would be selectively enriched in the tumor lesions with minimal damage to normal tissues. Several ligand-targeted therapeutic strategies, including immunotoxins, radioimmunotherapeutics, and drug immunoconjugates are being developed [136]. Ligand-targeted therapeutic strategies have demonstrated promising efficiency compared with conventional chemotherapy drugs in preclinical and clinical trials. For example, *in-vivo* studies have shown that only one to 10 parts per 100,000 of intravenously administered monoclonal antibodies (or mAbs), therapeutic and imaging agents can reach their parenchymal targets [136]. At present, noninvasive imaging approaches, including X-ray-based computer-assisted tomography (CT), positron emission tomography (PET), single-photon emission tomography and magnetic resonance imaging (MRI) are used as important tools for detection of human cancer. Recent developments in nanotechnology have provided researchers with new tools for cancer imaging and treatment. This technology has enabled the development of nanoscaled devices that can be conjugated with several functional molecules simultaneously, including tumor-specific ligands, antibodies, anticancer drugs, and imaging probes. Since these nanodevices are 100 to 1000-fold smaller than cancer cells, they can be easily transferred through leaky blood vessels and interact with targeted tumor-specific proteins both on the surface of and inside cancer cells. Therefore, their application as cancer cell-specific delivery vehicles are a significant addition to the currently available armory for cancer therapeutics and imaging [136]. The development of tumor-targeted contrast agents based on a nanoparticle formulation may offer enhanced sensitivity and specificity for *in-vivo* tumor imaging using currently available clinical imaging modalities. By applying a vast and diverse array of nanoparticles, whose design derives from the engineering, chemistry, and medicine fields, to molecular imaging and targeted therapy, cancer nanotechnology promises solutions to several of the current obstacles facing cancer therapies. Nanoparticles have a mesoscopic size range of 1 to 100 nm, allowing their imaging. Because of their material composition, nanoparticles are capable of self-assembly and maintaining stability and specificity, which are crucial to drug encapsulation and biocompatibility. Hereafter, the aim is to introduce the TiO_2 nanomaterials as drug delivery systems and, how TiO_2 nanomaterials can be used as therapeutic systems and imaging devices to destroy the cancerous cells or imaging contrast agents. We will also explain how TiO_2 nanoparticles can be further developed to improve their functionality in cancer treatment and imaging. Over the past 20 years, the field of nanoparticle-based drug delivery focused on two chemically distinct colloidal particles, liposomes and biodegradable polymers. Both delivery systems encapsulate/entrap the active drug within their structures and release the active agent as the particle lyses, in the case of liposomes, or disintegrate as described for biodegradable polymers. A recent newcomer to this field is the metallic nanoparticles and semiconductor nanoparticles such as gold, iron oxide, TiO_2 and ZnO nanoparticles [136]. The schematic multifunction of TiO_2 nanoparticles had been depicted in Figure 3. The scheme illustrates the fabricated multifunctional TiO_2 nanoparticles with different receptor targeting, multimodality imaging, and multiple therapeutic entities. All of the functional moieties are not necessary and only suitably selected components are needed for each individual application.

Particular attention is given to a different type and size of TiO_2, which is easily functionalized by both optically fluorescent agents and molecules for subcellular targeting and treatment. The surface characteristics of TiO_2 nanomaterials allow efficient conjugation to nucleic acids (PNA, DNA) proteins, sugars, fluorescent agents and monoclonal antibodies, which enables their retention in specific subcellular compartments. Uunderstanding of the interactions between nanoparticles and cells is the first step toward mechanistic understanding of the relationship between organisms and nanomaterials. Therefore, cellular studies provide a preliminary step for nanoparticles used *in-vivo* therapeutic or imaging purposes. Although cytotoxicity and the effects of cell loading by TiO_2 nanoparticles are of little consequence in fixed cells, nanoparticle biocompatibility and cellular uptake mechanisms are particularly relevant to live cell studies. Surface modification of TiO_2 nanoparticles serve to (I) increase cellular uptake of TiO_2-nanoconjugates, (II) increase the specificity of cellular uptake, and (III) increase the efficiency of intracellular targeting or retention of TiO_2-nanoconjugates.

In this part of the document, several methods for conjugation of antibody to the surface of TiO_2 nanoparticles are discussed. Bioconjugation can take place by means of adsorption (at the isoelectrical point of the antibody via electrostatic interaction or physisorption), by direct covalent linkage between the surface of the nanoparticle and the antibody, or by using adapter molecules. The use of adapter molecules generally involves dopamine, streptavidin and biotin for the formation of the complex. Biotinylated antibodies are commercially provided [137].

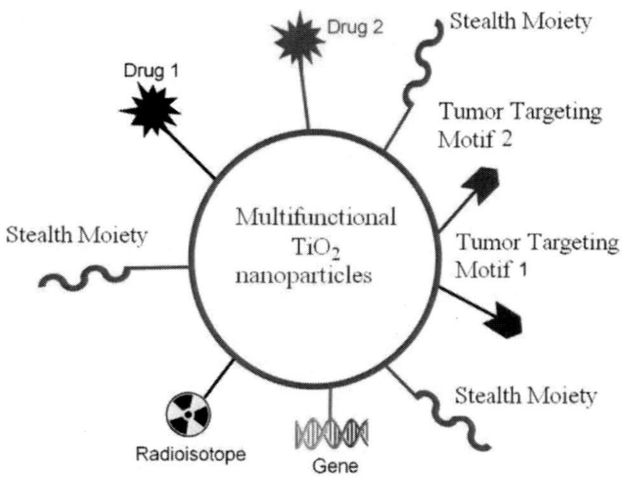

Figure 3. Schematic of a multifunctional TiO2 nanoparticle.

One of the advantages of using covalent bound compared to physical adsorption is that the linkage prevents the competitive displacement of the adsorbed antibodies by blood components, which occurs for adsorbed antibodies. In addition, the use of a spacer for surface modification of TiO_2 nanoparticles is highly recommended to enhance the probabilities of the antibody finding its corresponding antigen. Hence, oriented covalent binding can increase antibody stability and control the available protein binding sites.

It is possible to prepare antibody-conjugated nanoparticles, where the antibodies are randomly attached to the surface of the nanoparticle, by using numerous approaches. However, the following points should be considered:

I. Formation of a Schiff's base between the primary amine of the antibody and the free aldehyde groups of the glutaraldehyde (bifunctional cross-linker) present on the surface of the amino-functionalized nanoparticle.
II. Formation of an amide bond between the carboxylated nanoparticles and the amino groups of the antibodies, using EDAC (1-Ethyl-3-(3-dimethylaminopropyl) carbodiimide hydrochloride) as cross-linking agents [138].

Oriented conjugation of the antibody on the surface of TiO_2 nanomaterials is another strategy. This strategy includes the surface functionalization of TiO_2 nanoparticles to render aldehydes, epoxides, thiols, etc. It is possible to achieve an oriented conjugation with those functional groups using the following bonds: aldehydes to the lysine-rich region of the antibody; epoxides to the histidine-rich region of the antibody and thiols to the centre thiol groups of the antibody obtained by reduction [138]. The surface chemistry of TiO_2 nanoparticles smaller than 20 nm relies on formation of ''corner defects'' on the surface of TiO_2 nanoparticles which are very reactive with bidentate ligands; for example dopamine can be easily attached to the surface of TiO_2 nanoparticles [136]. This approach was used for attachment of DNA oligonucleotides enabling subcellularly specific retention of TiO_2-DNA oligonucleotide nano-conjugates, to target nanoparticles to specific cell types, in order to increase uptake efficiency and bypass intracellular obstacles [136]. Polyacrylic acid-coated TiO_2 nanoparticles were covalently coupled to anti-estradiol mouse antibodies with an amide bond, and used not only in the recognition of the estradiol, but also in its destruction by using the previously mentioned photocatalytic properties of TiO_2. There are clear applications for these carriers in medical [76]. Lai and Lee [119] reported coupleing of folic acid (FA) onto TiO_2 nanoparticles (28 nm) to provide a specificity of cell targeting. Modification was confirmed by infrared absorption spectra and zeta potential that suggested a formation of linkage between carboxylic acid of FA and TiO_2. Their results showed that the FA-modified TiO_2 nanoparticles could be internalized by cells at a much faster rate than the unmodified TiO_2, due to the mediation of folate receptor on the cancer cells. The UV irradiation caused death of HeLa cells pretreated with FA-modified TiO_2 more effectively than that of HeLa cells treated with unmodified TiO_2. The results suggested that to modify TiO_2 with folic acid using appropriately the FA-to-TiO_2 mass ratio of 0.2 could yield nanoparticles having higher cytotoxicity under photoexcitation. Results from flow cytometry-based analysis indicated that the mechanism of cell death was a combination of necrosis and apoptosis.

Recently, Rozhkova et. al. [115] reported the development of the first nanoparticles that seek out and destroy brain cancer cells without damaging nearby healthy cells. The authors utilized the TiO_2 nanoparticles (5 nm) covalently conjugated with antihuman- IL13α2R via dihydroxybenzene bivalent linker. The linker application enables absorption of a visible part of the solar spectrum by the nanobiohybrid TiO_2. The phototoxicity is mediated by reactive oxygen species that initiate programmed death of the cancer cell without damaging nearby healthy cells. The researchers found that after a 5-min exposure to polychromatic visible light, titanium dioxide initiated the production of reactive oxygen species, which damaged the cancer cells and induced their programmed death [115]. Moreover, even after 48 h light exposure, the TiO_2 toxicity to cancer cells was still high.

Xu et. al. [121] attached anti-carcinoembryogenic antibodies of human LoVo cancer cells to TiO_2 nanoparticles (25 nm), which improved the photokilling selectivity and efficiency of photoexcited TiO_2 on cancer cells in the photodynamic therapy. The antibodies were also labeled with Fluorescein isothiocyanate (FITC) for improving optical detection by using confocal laser microscopy. Their results approved that conjugation of the TiO_2 nanoparticles with monoclonal antibodies increased the photokilling selectivity of TiO_2 nanoparticles to cancer cells. Electroporation (use of electric stimulation to deliver moieties through the micropores on the cell membrane) was used to accelerate the internalization of the conjugated nanoparticles into cancer cells. It was observed that by combination of electroporation method, 100% human LoVo cancer cells were photokilled within 90 min, while only 39% of the normal cells were killed under the irradiation of the UV light (365 nm). Furthermore, the combination method may be used to photokill of various kinds of cancer cells only if the antibody conjugated on the TiO_2 nanoparticles is changed [121].

Huang et. al. [139] showed that biotin could be directly bound to the TiO_2 surface by coupling the biotin COOH to the titanol groups in phosphate-buffered saline. The results showed that the surface of the thin titania coating was fully covered by a biotin monolayer. Dimitrijevic et. al. [140] and Rajh et. al. [141] have modified TiO_2 with enediol ligands, typically dopamine, to give terminal amines that can react with N-droxy-succinimidemodified biotin. In these cases, dopamine acts as a ligand for the free surface sites of TiO_2 and forms chemical bonds between the ligand and TiO_2. Ye et. al. [137] reported that improved control in the creation of TiO_2/biological composites could be provided by the use of silane coupling agents as linkers. Silane coupling agents are widely used to modify the surface of mineral oxides including silica, alumina and titania. A variety of organic functional groups can be introduced to the surface using mild conditions. Thus, the traditional silane-coupling agent provides a route to bind biotin molecules to TiO_2 surface. Typically, the inorganic surface is first modified with a silane coupling agent to introduce appropriate functional groups, and then a biotin reagent is tethered to the functional surface. Finally, the biotin-modified inorganic material is exposed to streptavidin/avidin. It can be challenging to control the molecular densities of silane agents applied to titania surface. The choice of silane coupling agent, humidity, temperature, and reaction time all affect the efficiency of the surface modification in subtle ways [136].

In addition to targeted cancer therapy, imaging of cancerous cells with modified TiO_2 nanoparticles is possible. Paunesku et. al. [142] synthesized nanoconjugates composed of TiO_2 nanoparticles (6 nm). They used DNA oligonucleotides and a gadolinium (Gd) contrast agent for magnetic resonance imaging. Paunesku stated "Transfection of cultured cancer cells with these nanoconjugates showed them to be superior to the free contrast agent of the same formulation with regard to intracellular accumulation, retention, and sub cellular localization". Their results have shown that 48 h after treatment, the concentration of Gd in nanoconjugate-treated cells was 1000-fold higher than in cells treated with contrast agent alone [142]. Endres et. al. [143] have prepared a Gd(III)-modified DNA-TiO_2 semiconducting nanoparticle (3-5 nm), that functioned in a targeted and therapeutic capacity and also was detectable in cells by MR imaging. They described that targeting was accomplished via oligonucleotide hybridization to an intracellular organelle's matching DNA sequence, and therapeutic activity was elicited by light-induced scission of the nanoparticle-bound DNA. To assess the biocompatibility and MR image contrast of the modified nanoparticles in vitro, PC3M cells were imaged after incubation with the nanoconjugates in their experiments. Comparison of the images with and without nanoconjugates, revealed that the cells incubated with the modified nanoparticles displayed a greater contrast enhancement over control cells.

Wang et. al. [144] studied the interaction of a model cell with TiO_2-nanotubes (TiO_2-NTs). TiO_2-NTs (less than 10 nm) firstly have been conjugated with a fluorescent label, fluorescein isothiocyanate (FITC). FITC-conjugated TiO_2-nanotubes (FITC-TiO_2-NTs) have been internalized in mouse neural stem cells which can be directly imaged by confocal microscopy. The confocal imaging showed that FITC-TiO_2-NTs readily have been entered into the cells. The results approved that FITC-TiO_2-NTs localized around the cell nucleus without crossing the karyotheca after co-incubation with cells for 24 h. The researchers also reported that TiO_2 nanotubes passed through the karyotheca entering the cell nucleus after co-incubation for 48 h. The atomic force microscopy (AFM) and transmission electron microscopy (TEM) images approved existence of the TiO_2 nanotubes in the cell [144].

Photocatalyzed TiO_2 nanoparticles have been shown to eradicate cancer cells. However the required *in-situ* introduction of UV light limits the use of such a therapy in patients. Thevenot et. al. [145], examined the non-photocatalyic anti-cancer effect of surface functionalized TiO_2 nanoparticles (21 nm) bearing -OH, $-NH_2$, or -COOH surface groups, and they tested their effect on *in-vitro* survival of several cancer and control cell lines.

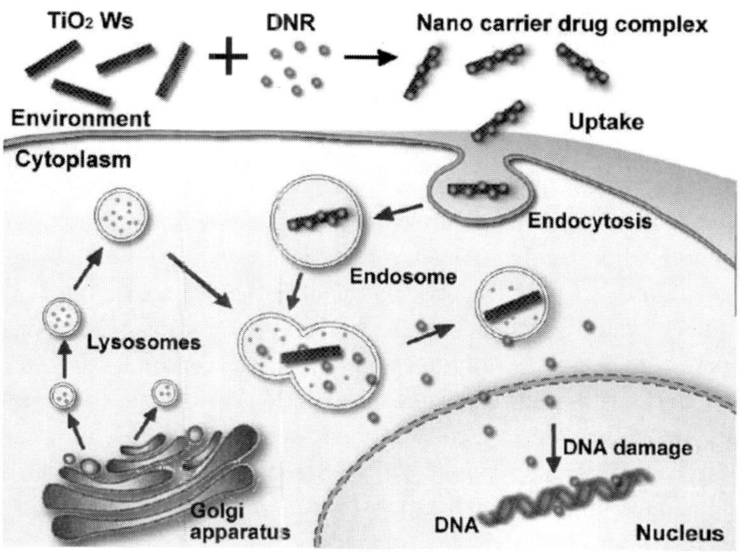

Figure 4. Illustration of the possible mechanism accounted for the enhancing uptake of DNR into cells via TiO_2 whiskers drug delivery. (Adapted from Li et. al. [146] with permission from publisher, Elsevier. License Number: 2655890596046).

The cells tested included B16F10 melanoma, Lewis lung carcinoma (LLC), JHU prostate cancer cells, and 3T3 fibroblasts. Cell viability was observed to depend on particle concentrations, cell types, and surface chemistry. They reported $-NH_2$ and -OH groups exhibited significantly higher toxicity than -COOH. Microscopic and spectrophotometric studies revealed that nanoparticle-mediated cells membrane disruption leaded to 50-75% of the mentioned cells death after 24h of incubation. Their results suggested that functionalized TiO_2 can be used for targeted cancer therapy [145].

In addition to targeted cancer therapy and imaging of cancerous cells with modified TiO_2 nanoparticles, chemotherapeutic drugs like doxorubicin can also be attached to TiO_2 nanoparticles surface. For example, Li et. al. [146] reported fabrication of the one-dimensional TiO_2 whiskers (about 80 nm and length range from 200 to 5000 nm) for drug delivery application and anti-tumor function combined with daunorubicin (DNR). Their results showed that TiO_2 whiskers can obviously increased the intracellular concentration of DNR and enhanced its potential anti-tumor efficiency. They reported that indicating TiO_2 whiskers could produce an efficient drug delivery carrier for importing DNR into target cells. Furthermore, the photocatalytic activity of TiO_2 whiskers had led to the enhanced mortality of cancer cells under UV irradiation. Figure 4 illustrates the possible mechanism accounted for the enhancing uptake of DNR into cells via TiO_2 whiskers drug delivery.

In conclusion, the above-mentioned explanations reveal that surface modification of TiO_2 nanomaterials with different biomolecules lead to produce multifunctional TiO_2 nanomaterials for use *in-vivo* targeted cancer therapy and imaging of cancerous cells.

6. Sonodynamic Therapy for Cancer Treatment Using TiO_2 Nanoparticles

Recently, the sonocatalytic technology using TiO_2 nanomaterials combined with ultrasonic radiation has been received much attention to introduce another way for cancer treatment. Sonodynamic therapy (SDT) for cancer is based on the activation of sono-sensitizers by ultrasound. This is a new approach for cancer therapy derived from photodynamic therapy [135].

In the treatment of malignant gliomas, there have been several preliminary studies of PDT using 5-aminolevulinic acid (5-ALA), a porphyrin derivative [147, 148]. However, the limited tissue penetrability of light has been a crucial problem because the malignant gliomas often develop in deep brain tissue, such as the basal ganglia or the brainstem. In this regard, ultrasound can penetrate deeply into tissues and, moreover, can be focused to the tumor site [149]. Therefore, SDT with sonosensitizers is expected to become a novel and effective therapeutic arm. Recently, the effects of sonocatalytic reagents in combination with ultrasound on glioma cells were reported [150]. Some photo-sensitizers such as porphyrin derivatives demonstrate ultrasound-induced cytotoxic reactions [135]. TiO_2 is one of the photo-sensitizer that can produce oxidative radicals under irradiation of UV light [19]. In the previous sections, the photocatalytic application of TiO_2 nanomaterials in cancer treatment was explained.

Ultrasound radiation is an alternative energy source for activation of TiO_2 nanomaterials [124, 151, 152]. Therefore, sonocatalytic process using TiO_2 nanomaterials supposes a promising method for various cancers treatment. Wang et. al. [153] detected and analyzed reactive oxygen species generated by nano-sized TiO_2 powder under ultrasonic radiation by the method of Oxidation–Extraction Photometry (OEP). They also studied the effect of operation parameters such as ultrasonic radiation time and amount of TiO_2 on the generation of ROS. The results indicated that the quantities of generated ROS increased with increasing of ultrasonic radiation time and amount of TiO_2.

Yamaguchi et. al. [135] have developed a novel water-dispersed TiO_2 nanoparticles (40 nm) modified by polyethylene glycole (PEG). A comparison was made between the photodynamic and sonodynamic damages on U251 human glioblastoma cell lines using modified TiO_2 nanoparticles. Their results showed that ultrasound-treated cells lost their viability immediately after irradiation, and cell membranes were especially damaged in comparison with ultraviolet-treated cells. Their findings showed a potential application of TiO_2/PEG to sonodynamic therapy as a new treatment of malignant gliomas and suggested that the mechanism of TiO_2/PEG mediated sonodynamic cytotoxicity differs from that of photodynamic cytotoxicity.

Harada et. al. [154] determined the therapeutic effect of ultrasound combined with TiO_2 nanoparticles (6 nm) on melanoma C32 cells under *in-vitro* and *in-vivo* conditions. Melanoma cells (C32) were irradiated with ultrasound in the presence and/or absence of TiO_2. Cell viability was measured immediately after ultrasound irradiation (1 MHz, 0.5 and 1.0 W/cm^2 for 10 s). The effect of the combination of TiO_2 and ultrasound exposure (1 MHz, 1.0 W/cm^2, 2 min duration) on subcutaneously implanted C32 solid tumors in mice have been investigated by measuring tumor volume regression. The results show that the cell viability is significantly decreased only after ultrasound radiation in the presence of TiO_2. Their *in-vivo* results show significant inhibition of tumor growth in groups treated with TiO_2 and ultrasound. This technique may offer a new and non-invasive therapy for malignant melanoma in the near future.

Acknowledgments

We are grateful to the University of Tabriz, Iran for the all supports.

References

[1] D.M. Blake, P.-C. Maness, Z. Huang, E.J. Wolfrum, J. Huang, Application of the photocatalytic chemistry of titanuim dioxid to disinfection and killing of cancer cells, *Separation and Purification Methods*, 28 (1999) 1-50.

[2] A.R. Khataee, M.B. Kasiri, *Artificial neural network modeling of water and waste water treatment processes*, Nova Science Publishers, Inc. New York, (2010).

[3] A. Heller, Conversion of sunlight into electrical power and photoassisted electrolysis of water in photoelectrochemical cells, *Accounts of Chemical Research*, 14 (1981) 154-162.

[4] A.R. Khataee, M.B. Kasiri, Photocatalytic degradation of organic dyes in the presence of nanostructured titanium dioxide: Influence of the chemical structure of dyes, *Journal of Molecular Catalysis A: Chemical*, 328 (2010) 8-26.

[5] A.R. Khataee, M. Zarei, M. Fathinia, M.K. Jafari, Photocatalytic degradation of an anthraquinone dye on immobilized TiO_2 nanoparticles in a rectangular reactor: Destruction pathway and response surface approach, *Desalination*, 268 (2011) 126-133.

[6] A.R. Khataee, M. Fathinia, S. Aber, M. Zarei, Optimization of photocatalytic treatment of dye solution on supported TiO_2 nanoparticles by central composite design: Intermediates identification, *Journal of Hazardous Materials*, 181 (2010) 886-897.

[7] S.N. Frank, A.J. Bard, Heterogeneous photocatalytic oxidation of cyanide ion in aqueous solutions at titanium dioxide powder, *Journal of American Chemical Society,* 99 (1977) 303-304.

[8] S. Ahmed, M.G. Rasul, R. Brown, M.A. Hashib, Influence of parameters on the heterogeneous photocatalytic degradation of pesticides and phenolic contaminants in wastewater: A short review, *Journal of Environmental Management*, 92 (2011) 311-330.

[9] S. Ahmed, M.G. Rasul, W.N. Martens, R. Brown, M.A. Hashib, Heterogeneous photocatalytic degradation of phenols in wastewater: A review on current status and developments, *Desalination,* 261 (2010) 3-18.

[10] U.G. Akpan, B.H. Hameed, Parameters affecting the photocatalytic degradation of dyes using TiO_2-based photocatalysts: A review, *Journal of Hazardous Materials*, 170 (2009) 520-529.

[11] I.K. Konstantinou, T.A. Albanis, TiO_2-assisted photocatalytic degradation of azo dyes in aqueous solution: kinetic and mechanistic investigations: *A review, Applied Catalysis B: Environmental,* 49 (2004) 1-14.

[12] A. Fujishima, T.N. Rao, D.A. Tryk, Titanium dioxide photocatalysis, Journal of Photochemistry and Photobiology C: *Photochemistry Reviews*, 1 (2000) 1-21.

[13] M. Fathinia, A.R. Khataee, M. Zarei, S. Aber, Comparative photocatalytic degradation of two dyes on immobilized TiO_2 nanoparticles: Effect of dye molecular structure and response surface approach, *Journal of Molecular Catalysis A: Chemical*, 333 (2010) 73-84.

[14] A.R. Khataee, M.B. Kasiri, Artificial neural networks modeling of contaminated water treatment processes by homogeneous and heterogeneous nanocatalysis, *Journal of Molecular Catalysis A: Chemical*, 331 (2010) 86-100.

[15] O. Legrini, E. Oliveros, A.M. Braun, Photochemical processes for water treatment, *Chemical Reviews*, 93 (1993) 671-698.

[16] R.C. Brown, D. Wake, Air filtration by interception theory and experiment, *Journal of Aerosol Science*, 22 (1991) 181-186.

[17] J. Gamage, Z. Zhang, Applications of photocatalytic disinfection, Review article, *International Journal of Photoenergy*, 2010 (2010) 1-11.

[18] R.A. Larson, M.R. Berenbaum, Environmental phototoxicity, *Environmental Science and Technology,* 22 (1988) 354-360.

[19] S.B. Farr, T. Kogoma, Oxidative stress responses in *Escherichia coli* and *Salmonella typhimurium*, *Microbiological Reviews*, 55 (1991) 561-585.

[20] A.R. Khataee, H.R. Khataee, Mechanical and Dynamical Principles of Protein Nanomotors: *The Key to Nano-Engineering Applications*, Nova Science Publishers, Inc. New York, (2010).

[21] Globocan (IARC) *Section of Cancer Information*, (2008).

[22] A. Fujishima, J. Ohtsuki, T. Yamashita, S. Hayakawa, Behavior of tumor cells on photoexcited semiconductor surface, *Photomedicine and Photobiology*, 8 (1986) 45-46.

[23] H. Sakai, R. Baba, K. Hashimoto, Y. Kubota, A. Fujishima, Selective killing of a single cancerous T24 cell with TiO_2 semiconducting microelectrode under irradiation, *Chemistry Letters*, (1995) 185-186.

[24] R. Cai, K. Hashimoto, K. Ito, Y. Kubota, A. Fujishima, Photokilling of malignant cells with ultra-fine TiO_2 powder, *Bulletin of the Chemical Society of Japan*, 64 (1991) 1268-1273.

[25] R. Cai, K. Hashimoto, Y. Kubota, A. Fujishima, . Increment of photocatalytic killing of cancer cells using TiO_2 with the aid of superoxide dismutase, *Chemistry Letters,* 3 (1992) 427-430.

[26] R. Cai, H. Sakai, K. Hashimoto, Y. Kubota, A. Fujishima, Phagocytosis of titanium dioxide particles chemically modified by hematoporphyrin, *Journal of the Electrochemical Society of Japan*, 60 (1992) 314-321.

[27] R. Pourata, A.R. Khataee, S. Aber, N. Daneshvar, Removal of the herbicide Bentazon from contaminated water in the presence of synthesized nanocrystalline TiO2 powders under irradiation of UV-C light, *Desalination*, 249 (2009) 301-307.

[28] A.R. Khataee, M. Zarei, Photocatalysis of a dye solution using immobilized ZnO nanoparticles combined with photoelectrochemical process, *Desalination*, 273 (2011) 453-460.

[29] K.-P. Yu, G.W.-M. Lee, S.-Y. Lin, C.P. Huang, Removal of bioaerosols by the combination of a photocatalytic filter and negative air ions, *Journal of Aerosol Science*, 39 (2008) 377-392.

[30] D.M. Blake, Bibliography of work on the photocatalytic removal of hazardous compounds from water and air, *National Renewable Energy Laboratory*, (2001) 1-58.

[31] A.L. Linsebigler, G. Lu, J. John T. Yates, Photocatalysis on TiO2 surfaces: principles, mechanisms, and selected results, *Chemical Reviews*, 95 (1995) 735-758.

[32] X. Chen, S.S. Mao Titanium dioxide nanomaterials: synthesis, properties, modifications, and applications, *Chemical Reviews*, 107 (2007) 2891-2959.

[33] T.L. Thompson, J.T. Yates, Surface science studies of the photoactivation of TiO2 new photochemical processes, *Chemical Reviews*, 106 (2006) 4428-4453.

[34] M.R. Hoffmann, S.T. Martin, W. Choi, D.W. Bahnemann, Environmental applications of semiconductor photocatalysis, *Chemical Reviews*, 95 (1995) 69-96.

[35] H. Delase, B. Serrano, M. Salaices, *Photocatalytic reaction engineering*, springer, (2005).

[36] O. Seven, B. Dindar, S. Aydemir, D. Metin, M. A. Ozinel, S. Icli, Solar photocalytic disinfection of a group of bacteria and fungi aqueous suspensions with TiO2, ZnO and sahara desert dust, *Journal of Photochemistry and Photobiology: A-Chemistry*, 165 (2004) 103-107.

[37] L.K. Adams, D.Y. Lyon, P.J.J. Alvarez, Comparative Ecotoxicity of Nanoscale TiO2, SiO2, and ZnO Water Suspensions, *Water Research*, 40 (2006) 3527-3532.

[38] C. Srinivasan, N. Somasundaram, Bactericidal and detoxification effects of irradiated semiconductor catalyst, TiO2, *Current Science*, 85 (2003) 1431-1438.

[39] A.R. Khataee, M. Fathinia, S. Aber, Kinetic modeling of liquid phase photocatalysis on supported TiO2 nanoparticles in a rectangular flat-plate photoreactor, *Industrial and Engineering Chemistry Research*, 49 (2010) 12358-12364.

[40] P.V. Kamat, Photochemistry on nonreactive and reactive (semiconductor) surfaces, *Chemical Reviews*, 93 (1993) 267-300.

[41] S.D. Aust, A sources of iron for lipid peroxidation in biological systems, Federation of American Societies for Experimental Biology, *Bathesda*, (1987) 27-33.
[42] J.B. Neiland, Microbial envelope proteins related to iron, *Annual Review of Microbiology,* 36 (1982) 285-309.
[43] R.J. Youngman, Oxygen activation: Is the hydroxyl radical always biologically relevant, *Trends in Biochemical Sciences*, 9 (1984) 280-283.
[44] A.R. Khataee, M.N. Pons, O. Zahraa, Photocatalytic degradation of three azo dyes using immobilized TiO2 nanoparticles on glass plates activated by UV light irradiation: Influence of dye molecular structure, *Journal of Hazardous Materials*, 168 (2009) 451-457.
[45] M. Bekbolet, M. Lindner, D. Weichgrebe, D.W. Bahnemann, Photocatalytic detoxification with the thin-film fixed-bed reactor (TFFBR): Clean-up of highly polluted landfill effluents using a novel TiO2 photocatalyst, *Solar Energy*, 56 (1996) 455-469.
[46] A.J. Feitz, B.H. Boyden, T.D. Waite, Evaluation of two solar pilot scale fixed bed photocatalytic reactors, *Water Research*, 34 (2000) 3927.
[47] G. Zayania, L. Bousselmia, F. Mhennib, A. Ghrabia, Solar photocatalytic degradation of commercial textile azo dyes: Performance of pilot plant scale thin film fixed-bed reactor, *Desalination,* 248 (2009) 23-31.
[48] J.G. Sczechowski, C.A. Koval, R.D. Noble, A taylor vortex reactor for heterogeneous photocatalysis, *Chemical Engineering Science*, 50 (1995) 3163-3173.
[49] T. Matsunaga, R. Tomoda, T. Nakajima, H. Wake, Photoelectrochemical sterilization of microbial cells by semiconductor powders, *FEMS Microbiology Letters*, 29 (1985) 211-214.
[50] C. Mccullagh, J. M. C. Robertson, D. W. Bahnemann, P. K. J. Robertson, The application of TiO2 photocatalysis for disinfection of water contaminated with pathogenic micro-organisms: A review, *Research on Chemical Intermediates*, 33 (2007) 359-375.
[51] E.J. Wolfrum, J. Huang, D.M. Blake, P.C. Maness, Z. Huang, J. Fiest, W.A. Jacoby, Photocatalytic oxidation of bacteria, bacterial and fungal spores, and model biofilm components to carbon dioxide on titanium dioxide-coated surfaces, *Environmental Science Technology*, 36 (2002) 3412-3419.
[52] S. Malato, J. Blanco, D. C. Alarcon, M. I. Maldonado, P. Fernandez-Ibanez, W. Gernjak, Photocatalytic decontamination and disinfection of water with solar collectors, *Catalysis Today,* 122 (2007) 137-149.
[53] C. Guillard, T.-H. Bui, C. Felix, V. Moules, B. Lina, P. Lejeune, Microbiological disinfection of water and air by photocatalysis, *Comptes Rendus Chimie*, 11 (2008) 107-113.
[54] J.C. Ireland, P. Klosterman, E.W. Rice, R.M. Clark, Inactivation of Escherichia coli by titanium dioxide photocatalytic oxidation, *Applied and Environmental Microbiology,* 59 (1993) 1668-1670.
[55] C. Wei, W.Y. Lin, Z. Zainal, N.E. Williams, K. Zhu, A.P. Kruzic, R.L. Smith, K. Rajeshwar, Bactericidal activity of TiO2 photocatalyst in aqueous media: Toward a solar-assisted water disinfection system, *Environmental Science and Technology*, 28 (1994) 934-938.

[56] A. Rincon, C. Pulgarin, Bactericidal action of illuminated TiO2 on pure Escherichia coli and natural bacterial consortia: Post-irradiation events in the dark and assessment of the effective disinfection time, *Applied Catalysis B-Environmental*, 49 (2004) 99-112.

[57] L. Caballero, K.A. Whitehead, N.S. Allen, J. Verran, Inactivation of Escherichia coli on immobilized TiO2 using fluorescent light, *Journal of Photochemistry and Photobiology A-Chemistry*, 202 (2009) 92-98.

[58] A.-G. Rincon, C. Pulgarin, Use of coaxial photocatalytic reactor (CAPHORE) in the TiO2 photo-assisted treatment of mixed E. coli and Bacillus sp. and bacterial community present in wastewater, *Catalysis Today*, 101 (2005) 331-344.

[59] T. Yuranova, A.G. Rincon, C. Pulgarin, D. Laub, N. Xantopoulos, H.-J. Mathieu, Bactericide cotton textiles active in E. coli abatement prepared under mild preparation conditions, *Journal of Photochemistry and Photobiology A-Chemistry*, 181 (2006) 363-369.

[60] A.K. Benabbou, Z. Derriche, C. Felix, P. Lejeune, C. Guillard, Photocatalytic inactivation of Escherischia coli. Effect of concentration of TiO2 and microorganism, nature, and intensity of UV irradiation, *Applied Catalysis B-Environmental*, 76 (2007) 257-263.

[61] J. Lonnen, L.J. Kilvington, S.C. Kehoe, F. Al-Touatj, K.G. Mcguigan, Solar and photocatalytic disinfection of protozoan, fungal and bacterial microbes in drinking water, *Water Research*, 39 (2005) 877-883.

[62] J.M.C. Robertson, P.K.J. Robertson, L.A. Lawton, A comparison of the effectiveness of TiO2 photocatalysis and UVA photolysis for the destruction of three pathogenic micro-organisms, *Journal of Photochemistry and Photobiology: A-Chemistry*, 175 (2005) 51-56.

[63] C.L. Cheng, D.S. Sun, W.C. Chu, Y.H. Tseng, H.C. Ho, J.B. Wang, P.H. Chung, J.H. Chen, P.J. Tsai, N.T. Lin, M.S. Yu, H.H. Chang, The effects of the bacterial interaction with visible-light responsive titania photocatalyst on the bactericidal performance, *Journal of Biomedical Science*, 16 (2009) 7.

[64] T. Matsunaga, R. Tomoda, T. Nakajima, N. Nakamura, T. Komine, Continuous sterilization system that uses photosemiconductor powders, *Applied and Environmental Microbiology*, 54 (1988) 1330-1333.

[65] B. Kim, D. Kim, D. Cho, S. Cho, Bactericidal effect of TiO2 photocatalyst on selected food-borne pathogenic bacteria, *Chemosphere*, 52 (2003) 277-281.

[66] M-S. Wong, W-C. Chu, D-S. Sun, H-S. Huang, J-H. Chen, P-J. Tsai, N-T. Lin, M-S. Yu, S-F. Hsu, S-L. Wang, H.-H. Chang, Visible-Light-Induced Bactericidal Activity of a Nitrogen-Doped Titanium Photocatalyst against Human Pathogens, *Applied and Environmental Microbiology,* 72 (2006) 6111-6116.

[67] L. Hochmannova, J. Vytrasova, Photocatalytic and antimicrobial effects of interior paints, Review article, *Progress in Organic Coating*, 67 (2010) 1-5.

[68] K. Shiraishi, H. Koseki, T. Tsurumoto, Antibacterial metal implant with a TiO2-conferred photocatalytic bactericidal effect against Staphylococcus aureus, *Surface and Interface Analysis*, 41 (2009) 17-22.

[69] S.S. Block, D.Y. Goswami, Chemical enhanced sunlight for killing bacteria, *Journal of Solar Energy Engineering,* 1 (1995) 431-437.

[70] T. Morioka, T. Saito, Y. Nara, K. Onoda, Antibacterial action of powdered semiconductor on a serotype Streptococcus mutans, *Caries Research*, 22 (1988) 230-231.

[71] K. Ulfig, Keratinolytic and keratinophilic fungi in sewage sludge: factors influencing their occurrence in fungi from different environments, *Science Publishers*, U.S., (2009) 4-45.

[72] T. Saito, T. Iwase, J. Horie, T. Morioka, Mode of photocatalytic bactericidal action of powdered semiconductor TiO2 on mutans streptococci, *Journal of Photochemistry and Photobiology B: Biology*, 14 (1992) 369-379.

[73] D. Mitoraj, A. Janczyk, M. Strus, H. Kirsch, G. Stochel, P.B. Heczko, W. Macyk, Visible light inactivation of bacteria and fungi by modified titanium dioxide, *Photochemical and Photobiological Sciences*, 6 (2007) 642-648.

[74] J.-S. Hur, S.-O. Oh, K.-M. Lim, J.S. Jung, J.-W. Kim, Y.J. Koh, Novel effects of TiO2 photocatalytic ozonation on control of postharvest fungal spoilage of kiwifruit, *Postharvest Biology and Technology*, 35 (2005) 109-113.

[75] C. Sichel, J. Tello, M. DeCara, P. Fernandez-Ibanez, Effect of UV solar intensity and dose on the photocatalytic disinfection of bacteria and fungi, *Catalysis Today*, 129 (2007) 152-160.

[76] C. Ogino, K. Kanehira, R. Sasai, S. Sonezaki, N. Shimizu, Recognition and effective degradation of 17β-estradiol by anti-estradiol-antibody-immobilized TiO2 nanoparticles, *Journal of Bioscience and Bioengineering*, 104 (2007) 339-342.

[77] P.-C. Mannes, S. Smolinski, D.M. Blake, Z. Huang, E.J. Wolfrum, W.A. Jacoby, Bactericidal activity of photocatalytic TiO2 reaction: Toward an understanding mechanisms, *Applied Environmental and Microbiology*, 65 (1999) 4094-4098.

[78] A. Markowska-Szczupak, K. Ulfig, A.W. Morawski, The application of titanium dioxide for deactivation of bioparticulates: *An overview, Catalysis Today*, Article in press (2010).

[79] Z. Huang, P.-C. Maness, D.M. Blake, E.J. Wolfrum, S.L. Smolinski, W.A. Jacoby, Bactericidal mode of titanium dioxide photocatalysis, *Journal of Photochemistry and Photobiology A: Chemistry,* 130 (2000) 163-170.

[80] J. Blanco-Galvez, P. Fernandez-Ibanez, S. Malato-Rodriguez, Solar photocatalytic detoxification and disinfection of water: Recent overview, *Journal of Solar Energy Engineering,* 129 (2007) 4-15.

[81] H. Hidaka, S. Horikoshi, N. Serpone, J. Knowland, In vitro photochemical damage to DNA, RNA and their bases by an inorganic sunscreen agent on exposure to UVA and UVB radiation, *Journal of Photochemistry and Photobiology A: Chemistry*, 111 (1997) 205-213.

[82] G. Gogniat, S. Dukan, TiO2 photocatalysis causes DNA damage via fenton reaction-generated hydroxyl radicals during the recovery period, *Applied and Environmental Microbiology,* 73 (2007) 7740-7743.

[83] K. Hirakawa, M. Mori, M. Yoshida, S. Oikawa, S. Kawanishi, Photo-irradiated titanium dioxide catalyzes site specific DNA damage via generation of hydrogen peroxide, *Free Radical Research*, 38 (2004) 439-447.

[84] T. Ashikaga, M. Wada, H. Kobayashi, M. Mori, Y. Katsumura, H. Fukui, S. Kato, M. Yamaguchi, T. Takamatsu, Effect of the photocatalytic activity of TiO2 on plasmid

DNA, *Mutation Research/Genetic Toxicology and Environmental Mutagenesis*, 466 (2000) 1-7.

[85] K. Sunada, T. Watanabe, K. Hashimoto, Studies on photokilling of bacteria on TiO2 thin film, *Journal of Photochemistry and Photobiology* A, 156 (2003) 227-233.

[86] Y. Kikuchi, K. Sunada, T. Iyoda, K. Hashimoto, A. Fujishima, Photocatalytic bactericidal effect of TiO2 thin films: dynamic view of the active oxygen species responsible for the effect, *Journal of Photochemistry and Photobiology A: Chemistry*, 106 (1997) 51-56.

[87] K. Sunada, Y. Kikuchi, K. Hashimoto, A. Fujishima, Bactericidal and detoxification effects of TiO2 thin film photocatalysts, *Environmental Science and Technology*, 32 (1998) 726-728.

[88] D. Gerrity, H. Ryu, J. Crittenden, M. Abbaszadegan, Photocatalytic inactivation of viruses using titanium dioxide nanoparticles and low-pressure UV light, Journal of Environmental Science and Health, Part A: *Toxic/Hazardous Substances and Environmental Engineering*, 43 (2008) 1261-1270.

[89] R.J. Watts, S. Kong, M.P. Orr, G.C. Miller, B.E. Henry, Photocatalytic inactivation of coliform bacteria and viruses in secondary wastewater effluent, *Water Research*, 29 (1995) 95-100.

[90] W. Heaselgrave, N. Patel, S Kilvington, S.C. Kehoe, K.G. Mcguigan, Solar disinfection of poliovirus and Acanthamoeba polyphaga cysts in water a laboratory study using simulated sunlight, *Letters in Applied Microbiology*, 43 (2006) 125-130.

[91] I.B. Ditta, A. Steele, C Liptrot, Photocatalytic antimicrobial activity of thin surface films of TiO2, CuO and TiO2 /CuO dual layers on Escherichia coli and bacteriophage T4, *Applied Microbiology and Biotechnology*, 79 (2008) 127-133.

[92] M. Cho, H. Chung, W. Choi, J. Yoon, Different inactivation behaviors of MS-2 phage and Escherichia coli in TiO2 photocatalytic disinfection, *Applied Environmental and Microbiology*, 71 (2005) 270-275.

[93] J.C. Sjorgren, R. Sierka, Inactivation of phage MS2 by iron-aided titanium dioxide photocatalysis, *Applied Environmental and Microbiology,* 60 (1994) 344-347.

[94] Q. Li, M.A. Page, B.J. Marinas, J.K. Shang, Treatment of Coliphage MS2 with palladium-modified nitrogen-doped titanium oxide photocatalyst illuminated by visible light, *Environmental Science and Technology*, 42 (2008) 6148-6153.

[95] N.A. Mazurkowa, Y.E. Spitsyna, N.V. Shikina, Z.R. Ismagilov, S.N. Zagrebelnyi, E.I. Ryabchikova, Interaction of titanuim dioxid nanoparticles with influenza virus, *Nanotechnologies in Russia*, 5 (2010) 417-420.

[96] N. Kashige, Y. Kakita, Y. Nakashima, F. Miake, K. Watanabe, The mechanism of the inactivation of Lactobacillus casei phage PL-1 suspended in a phosphate buffer by by black-light, *Current Microbiology*, 42 (2001) 184-189.

[97] X. Sang, T.G. Phan, S. Sugihara, F. Yagyu, S. Okitsu, N. Maneekarn, Photocatalytic inactivation of diarrheal viruses by visible-light-catalytic titanium dioxide, *Clinical Laboratory*, 53 (2007) 413-421.

[98] I. Paspaltsis, K. Kotta, R. Lagoudaki, N. Grigoriadis, I. Poulios, T. Sklaviadis, Titanuim dioxid photocatalytic inactivation of prions, *Journal of General Virology*, 87 (2006) 3125-3130.

[99] S. Lee, K. Nishida, M. Otaki, S. Ohgaki, Photocatalytic inactivation of phage QB by immobilized titanium dioxide mediated photocatalyst, *Water Science and Technology,* 35 (1997) 101-106.

[100] Y. Kakita, N. Kashige, F. Miake, K. Watanabe, Photocatalysis-dependent inactivation by a ceramics preparation, *Bioscience, Biotechnology, and Biochemistry*, 61 (1997) 1947-1948.

[101] J.Y. Yang, H.J. Kim, C.H. Chung, Photocatalytic antifungal activity against Candida Albicans by TiO2 coated acrylic resin denature base, *The Journal of Korean Academy of Prosthodontics*, 44 (2006) 284-294.

[102] C. Maneerat, Y. Hayata, Antifungal activity of TiO2 photocatalysis against Penicillium expansum in vitro and in fruit tests, *International Journal of Food Microbiology*, 107 (2006) 99-103.

[103] C. Sichel, M. DeCara, J. Tello, J. Blanco, P. Fernandez-Ibanez, Solar photocatalytic disinfection of agricultural pathogenic fungi: Fusarium species, *Applied Catalysis: B-Environmental,* 74 (2007) 152-160.

[104] P. Fernandez-Ibanez, C. Sichel, M.I. Polo-Lopez, M. De Cara-Garcia, J.C. Tello, Photocatalytic disinfection of natural well water contaminated by Fusarium solani using TiO2 slurry in solar CPC photo-reactors, *Catalysis Today*, 144 (2009) 62-68.

[105] F. Chen, X. Yang, Q. Wu, Antifungal capability of TiO2 coated film on moist wood, *Building and Environment*, 44 (2009) 1088-1093.

[106] C. Hu, J. Guo, J. Qu, X. Hu, Photocatalytic degradation of pathogenic bacteria with AgI/TiO2 under visible light irradiation, *Langmuir*, 23 (2007) 4982-4987.

[107] N. Akiba, I. Hayakawa, E.S. Keh, A. Watanabe, Antifungal effects of a tissue conditioner coating agent with TiO2 photocatalyst, *Journal of Medical and Dental Sciences,* 52 (2005) 223-227.

[108] A.G. Rincon, C. Pulgarin, Photocatalytical inactivation of E. coli: Effect of (continuous-intermittent) light intensity and of (suspended-fixed) TiO2 concentration *Applied Catalysis B: Environmental*, 44 (2003) 263-284.

[109] O. Carp, C.L. Huisman, A. Reller, Photoinduced reactivity of titanium dioxide, *Progress in Solid State Chemistry*, 32 (2004) 33-177.

[110] T.Y. Lai, W.C. Lee, Killing of cancer cell line by photoexcitation of folic acid-modified titanium dioxide nanoparticles, *Journal of Photochemistry and Photobiology A: Chemistry* 204 (2009) 148-153.

[111] C. Guillard, J. Disdier, J.M. Herrmann, C. Lehaut, T. Chopin, S. Malato, J. Blanco, Comparison of various titania samples of industrial origin in the solar photocatalytic detoxification of water containing 4-chlorophenol, Catalysis Today, 54 (1999) 217-228.

[112] A.P. Zhang, Y.P. Sun, Photocatalytic killing effect of TiO2 nanoparticles on Ls-174-t human colon carcinoma cells, *World Journal of Gastroenterology*, 10 (2004) 3191-3193.

[113] A. Fujishima, R.X. Cai, J. Otsuki, K. Hashimoto, K. Itoh, T. Yamashita, Y. Kubota, Biochemical application of photoelectrochemistry: photokilling of malignant cells with TiO2 powder, *Electrochimica Acta*, 38 (1993) 153-157.

[114] N. Lagopati, P.V. Kitsiou, A.I. Kontos, P. Venieratos, E. Kotsopoulou, A.G. Kontos, D.D. Dionysiou, S. Pispas, E.C. Tsilibary, P. Falaras, Photo-induced treatment of breast epithelial cancer cells using nanostructured titanium dioxide solution, *Journal of Photochemistry and Photobiology A: Chemistry*, 214 (2010) 215-223.

[115] E.A. Rozhkova, I. Ulasov, B. Lai, N.M. Dimitrijevic, M.S. Lesniak, T. Rajh, A high-performance nanobio photocatalyst for targeted brain cancer therapy, *Nano Letters*, 9 (2009) 3337-3342.

[116] Y. Chihara, K. Fujimoto, H. Kondo, Y. Moriwaka, T. Sasahira, Y. Hirao, H. Kuniyasu, Anti-tumor effects of liposome-encapsulated titanium dioxide in nude mice, *Pathobiology,* 74 (2007) 353-358.

[117] L. Wang, J. Mao, G.H. Zhang, M.J. Tu, Nano-cerium-element-doped titanium dioxide induces apoptosis of Bel 7402 human hepatoma cells in the presence of visible light, *World Journal of Gastroenterology*, 13 (2007) 4011-4414.

[118] J. Xu, Y. Sun, Y. Zhao, J. Huang, C. Chen, Z. Jiang, Photocatalytic inactivation effect of gold-doped TiO2 (Au/TiO2) nanocomposites on human colon carcinoma lovo cells, *International Journal of Photoenergy*, 2007 (2007) 1-7.

[119] T.Y. Lai, W.C. Lee, Killing of cancer cell line by photoexcitation of folic acid-modified titanium dioxide nanoparticles, *Journal of Photochemistry and Photobiology A: Chemistry,* 204 (2009) 148-153.

[120] Y. Kubota, T. Shuin, C. Kawasaki, M. Hosakal, H. Kitamura, R. Cail, H. Sakai, K. Hashimoto, A. Fujishima, Photokilling of T-24 human bladder cancer cells with titanium dioxide, *British Journal of Cancer*, 70 (I 994) 1107-1111.

[121] J. Xu, Y. Sun, C.C. Junjie Huang, G. Liu, Y. Jiang, Y. Zhao, Z. Jiang, Photokilling cancer cells using highly cell-specific antibody–TiO2 bioconjugates and electroporation, *Bioelectrochemistry,* 71 (2007) 217-222.

[122] Y. Nakagawa, S. Wakuri, K. Sakamoto, N. Tanaka, The photogenotoxicity of titanium dioxide particles, *Mutation Research*, 394 (1997) 125-132.

[123] O.V. Salata, Application of nanoparticles in biology and medicine, *Journal of Nanobiotechnology*, 2 (2004) 3-6.

[124] J. Wang, J. Wu, Z. Zhang, X. Zhang, Z. Pan, L. Wang, L. Xu, Sonocatalytic damage of bovine serum albumin (BSA) in the presence of nanometer anatase titanium dioxide (TiO2), *Ultrasound in Medicine and Biology*, 32 (2006) 147-152.

[125] K. Sivonen, G. Jones, *In toxic cyanobacteria in water E and FN Spon*, London, (1991) 41.

[126] E.M. jochimsen, W.W. Carmichael, J. An, Liver failure and death after exposure to microcystins at a hemodialysis center in brazil, *The New England Journal of Medicine,* 338 (1998) 873-878.

[127] World Health Organization, *Guidelines for drinking-water quality, health criteria and other supporting information,* Geneva, 2nd edition (1998).

[128] G.S. Shephard, S. Stockenstrm, D. De Villiers, W.J. Engelbrecht, E.W. Sydenham, G.F.S. Wessels, Photocatalytic degradation of cyanobacterial microcystin toxins in water, *Toxicon*, 36 (1998) 1895-1901.

[129] L.A. Lawton, P.K.J. Robertson, B.J.P.A. Cornish, I.L. Marr, M. Jaspars, Processes influencing surface interaction and photocatalytic destruction of microcystins on titanium dioxide photocatalysts, *Journal of Catalysis*, 213 (2003) 109-113.

[130] L. Chen, M.X. Liao, J.W. Xiong, Experiment research of the vivo destruction of HL60 cells by use of TiO2 and iron-doped TiO2-based photodynamic therapy, Guangdianzi Jiguang/*Journal of Optoelectronics Laser*, 19 (2008) 278-281.

[131] A. Janczyk, A. Wolnickaglubisz, K. Urbanska, H. Kisch, G. Stochel, W. Macyk, Photodynamic activity of platinum(IV) chloride surface-modified TiO2 irradiated with visible light, *Free Radical Biology and Medicine*, 44 (2008) 1120-1130.

[132] T. Lopez, E. Ortiz, M. Alvarez, J. Navarrete, J.A. Odriozola, F. Martinez-Ortega, E.A. Paez-Mozo, P. Escobar, K.A. Espinoza, I.A. Rivero, Study of the stabilization of zinc phthalocyanine in sol-gel TiO2 for photodynamic therapy applications, *Nanomedicine: Nanotechnology, Biology and Medicine*, 6 (2010) 777-785.

[133] O.L. Kaliya, E.A. Lukyanets, G.N. Vorozhtsov, Catalysis and photocatalysis by phthalocyanines for technology, ecology and medicine, *Journal of Porphyrins and Phthalocyanines*, 3 (1999) 592-610.

[134] A. Janczyk, A. Wolnickaglubisz, K. Urbanska, G. Stochel, W. Macyk, Photocytotoxicity of platinum (IV)-chloride surface modified TiO2 irradiated with visible light against murine macrophages, *Journal of Photochemistry and Photobiology B: Biology*, 92 (2008) 54-58.

[135] S. Yamaguchi, H. Kobayashi, T. Narita, K. Kanehira, S. Sonezaki, N. Kudo, Y. Kubota, S. Terasaka, K. Houkin, Sonodynamic therapy using water-dispersed TiO2-polyethylene glycol compound on glioma cells: Comparison of cytotoxic mechanism with photodynamic therapy, *Ultrasonics Sonochemistry*, Article in Press (2010).

[136] K.T. Thurn, E.M.B. Brown, A. Wu, S. Vogt, B. Lai, J. Maser, T. Paunesku, G.E. Woloschak, Nanoparticles for applications in cellular imaging, *Nanoscale Research Letters,* 2 (2007) 430-441.

[137] L. Ye, R. Pelton, M. A. Brook, Biotinylation of TiO2 nanoparticles and their conjugation with streptavidin, *Langmuir,* 23 (2007) 5630-5637.

[138] M. Arruebo, M. Valladaresb, A.G. Fernandez, Antibody-conjugated nanoparticles for biomedical applications, *Journal of nanomaterials*, 1 (2009) 1-74.

[139] J. G. Huang, I. Ichinose, T. Kunitake, *Biomolecular modification of hierarchical cellulose fibers through titania nanocoating*, Angewandte Chemie International Edition, 45 (2006) 1-5.

[140] N. M. Dimitrijevic, Z. V. Saponjic, B. M. Rabatic, T. J. Rajh, Assembly and charge transfer in hybrid TiO2 architectures using biotin–avidin as a connector, *American Chemical Society*, 127 (2005) 1344-1345.

[141] T. Rajh, L. D. I. Garza, Z. V. Saponjic, N. M. Dimitrijevic, M. C. Thurnauer, Surface states of titanium dioxide nanoparticles modified with enediol ligands, *Journal of Physical Chemistry: B*, 110 (2006) 680-686.

[142] Tatjana Paunesku, Tianyi Ke, Rohan Dharmakumar, Nicole Mascheri, Aiguo Wu, Barry Lai, Stefan Vogt, Jörg Maser, Kenneth Thurn, Barbara Szolc-Kowalska, A. Larson, Raymond C Bergan, Reed Omary, Debiao Li, Zheng-Rong Lu, Gayle E. Woloschak, Gadolinium conjugated TiO2-DNA oligonucleotide nanoconjugates show prolonged intracellular retention period and T1-weighted contrast enhancement in magnetic resonance images, *Nanomedicine,* 4 (2008) 201-207.

[143] P.J. Endres, T. Paunesku, S. Vogt, T.J. Meade, G.E. Woloschak, DNA-TiO2 Nanoconjugates labeled with magnetic resonance contrast agents, *Journal of American Society,* 129 (2007) 15760-15761.

[144] Y. Wang, J. Wang, X. Deng, J. Wang, H. Wang, M. Wu, Z. Jiao, Y. Liu, Direct imaging of titania nanotubes located in mouse neural stem cell nuclei, *Nano Research*, 2 (2010) 543-552.

[145] P. Thevenot, J. Cho, D. Wavhal, R. Timmons, L. Tang, Surface chemistry influences cancer killing effect of TiO2 nanoparticles, *Nanomedicine: Nanotechnology, Biology and Medicine*, 4 (2008) 226-236.

[146] Q. Li, X. Wang, X. Lu, H. Tian, H. Jiang, G. Lv, D. Guo, C. Wu, B. Chen, The incorporation of daunorubicin in cancer cells through the use of titanium dioxide whiskers, *Biomaterials,* 30 (2009) 4708-4715.

[147] H. Inoue, Y. Kajimoto, M.A. Shibata, N. Miyoshi, N. Ogawa, Y.O. S. Miyatake, T. Kuroiwa, Massive apoptotic cell death of human glioma cells via a mitochondrial pathway following 5-aminolevulinic acid-mediated photodynamic therapy, *Journal of Neuro-Oncology*, 83 (2007) 223-231.

[148] S.J. Madsen, C.H. Sun, B.J. Tromberg, V.P. Wallace, H. Hirschberg, Photodynamic therapy of human glioma spheroids using 5-aminolevulinic acid, *Photochemistry and Photobiology*, 72 (2000) 128-134.

[149] Z.R. Cohen, J. Zaubermann, S. Harnof, Y. Mardor, D. Nass, A.H. E. Zadicario, D. Castel, M. Faibel, Z. Ram, Magnetic resonance imaging-guided focused ultrasound for thermal ablation in the brain: a feasibility study in a swine model, *Neurosurgery,* 60 (2007) 593-600.

[150] S. Dai, S. Hu, C. Wu, Apoptotic effect of sonodynamic therapy mediated by hematoporphyrin monomethyl ether on C6 glioma cells in vitro, *Acta Neurochirurgica,* 151 (2009) 1655-1661.

[151] M.F. Dadjour, C. Ogino, S. Matsumura, S. Nakamura, N. Shimizu, Disinfection of Legionella pneumophila by ultrasonic treatment with TiO2, *Water Research,* 40 (2006) 1137-1142.

[152] M. Kubo, R. Onodera, N. Shibasaki-Kitakawa, K. Tsumoto, T. Yonemoto, Kinetics of ultrasonic disinfection of Escherichia coli in the presence of titanium dioxide particles, *Biotechnology Progress*, 21 (2005) 897-901.

[153] J. Wang, Y. Guo, B. Liu, X. Jin, L. Liu, R. Xu, Y. Kong, B. Wang, Detection and analysis of reactive oxygen species (ROS) generated by nano-sized TiO2 powder under ultrasonic irradiation and application in sonocatalytic degradation of organic dyes, *Ultrasonics Sonochemistry*, 18 (2011) 177-183.

[154] Y. Harada, K. Ogawa, Y. Irie, H. Endo, L.B. Feril Jr, T. Uemura, K. Tachibana, Ultrasound activation of TiO2 in melanoma tumors, *Journal of Controlled Release*, 149 (2011) 190-195.

Index

A

D

E

F

G

H

I

J

K

L

M

N

O

P

Q

R

T

U

V

W

X

Y

Z